THE
AGED
ILL

Coping with Problems
in Geriatric Care

ABOUT THE AUTHORS

DOROTHEA JAEGER *is a graduate of Barnard College where she majored in sociology. She has an M.A. degree in Nursing Education from Teachers College, Columbia University, and did post-master's work in research and the social sciences at Columbia. Born in Germany, she received her early schooling in that country.*

Her professional activities have included hospital and public health nursing, both on the staff and the administrative level. She has taught public health nursing, and has been involved in research on the university level. Her most recent position, from 1964 to 1967, was that of Research Associate at Yale University.

LEO W. SIMMONS *received his Ph.D. in Sociology and Anthropology from Yale University and served there on the faculty, 1937 to 1959 and 1964 to 1967. He was, on leave of absence, Visiting Professor of Anthropology at Cornell Medical College from 1950 to 1952. In 1959 he joined the faculty at Teachers College, Columbia University where he served as Director of the Institute of Nursing Research until 1963. In the summer of 1967 he held the appointment of Sloan Visiting Professor at the Menninger Foundation. Presently, he is Professor Emeritus at Columbia University and Visiting Professor at Case Western Reserve University.*

His publications include: Nursing Research: A Survey and Assessment *(with Virginia Henderson)*; Social Science in Medicine *(with Harold G. Wolff, M.D.)*; Sun Chief: Autobiography of a Hopi Indian; *and* The Role of the Aged in Primitive Society.

THE
AGED
ILL

Coping with Problems
in Geriatric Care

DOROTHEA JAEGER

LEO W. SIMMONS

APPLETON-CENTURY-CROFTS
EDUCATIONAL DIVISION/MEREDITH CORPORATION
New York

Preface

This book is designed to shed some light on better things to come in the care of the aged ill. Our aim has been four-fold: to identify certain of the crucial problems of coping with illness, infirmity, and dying in old age; to learn how select nursing personnel in geriatric institutions of recognized repute deal with these problems; then to compare certain aspects of their practice with what should be done, as recommended by degree-holding registered nurses who occupy positions of leadership in the profession; and finally, to examine certain psychosociological concepts as these relate to present-day geriatric care.

While major consideration in this discourse is given to the challenge of geriatrics to the nursing profession, hopefully, this book will commend itself to a readership beyond the field of nursing: health professionals involved in geriatrics and gerontology; individuals who may be considering institutionalization for themselves or for an aged kinsman; or persons still in the vigor of life who contemplate what life may have in store for them if and when they reach a venerable age and can no longer "go it alone."

By virtue of the lengthening span of life, greater proportions of the population can count on facing illness and infirmity, prior to death in their old age. Nevertheless, the achievement of a "good" life up to the very end remains a praiseworthy goal — "the last of life for which the first was made." (Robert Browning)

With the increasing perplexities, pressures, and hazards of modern life, however, this goal becomes neither a certain, nor an easy accomplishment. Indeed, for many aged individuals, the odds seem to be against attainment of a good ending, *unless* organized society and skilled personnel provide the help oldsters need when their resources waste away and the going gets really tough—for then the fulfillment of a good life unto its closure generally becomes dependent upon and beholden to caregiving institutions and talented attendants who are able and committed to providing the comprehensive and personalized care that is required.

Although the studies out of which the book evolved were directed largely to the care of the aged within the context of nursing homes and

v

similar geriatric facilities, there was no intent to disparage the recent rapid development of such institutions as a potential expedient of merit in coping with illness, infirmity, and death in old age. Such organized care of the aged ill may prove, in time and on the whole, to be among the more satisfactory solutions to many of the problems involved; but it certainly is not, as yet, without its particular problems and pitfalls, especially in the area of personality impacts, interpersonal relationships, and the peace of mind of either patients or their families. This being so, and institutionalization of the aged ill being the trend, attention has been directed especially to the psychosocial aspects of senescent patient care— but with no intention of negating the importance of physical care.

Certain features of the exposition deserve an early comment. The first two chapters (Part I) lay the foundation for what follows. They elucidate the broader aspects of aging into decrepitude, including society's accommodation to the plight of the aged ill, and make possible a fuller understanding of and wider perspective on the central theme. In subsequent chapters (Part II, Chapters 4 to 14), two, and on occasion three, major positions on the practice and thinking of the four ranks of nursing personnel are discussed in detail. In general, the discussion proceeds from what appears to be the least effective to the most desirable nursing care, as revealed by the accumulated data. In Chapters 15 and 16, some consideration is given to certain needs and compensations of the geriatric nurse practitioner. In the final two chapters (Part III), attention returns to the broader perspective of gerontology, geriatrics, and death within societal and cultural contexts.

The authors are indebted to many people. They are deeply grateful to the administrators and nursing directors in the selected geriatric institutions who provided untold hours and even days of on-duty time for individual staff members to be interviewed; to their staffs—nurse aides, licensed practical nurses, and registered nurses—who shared so freely their experiences and ideas; and to the degree registered nurses who responded to the questionnaire, and whose often lengthy and detailed responses contributed immeasurably to the project. Because major contributions come from the nurses themselves, this is, in a very real sense, their book.

Since the participating geriatric institutions and their staffs were assured of anonymity, they are not further identified. It should be noted, however, that much of the case material presented (except where otherwise indicated) was contributed by the nurse practitioners. The participating degree registered nurses, with very few exceptions, granted permission to be quoted, and credit is given whenever possible.

Very special gratitude must go to two nurse specialists in geriatrics,

Lois N. Knowles and Doris Schwartz, who, in addition to contributing to the original data, reviewed large sections of the manuscript and proposed some valuable revisions which were made.

Commendations should go, also, to the physicians, clergymen, social workers, researchers, and nurses (other than those referred to above), comprising too large a number to be cited by name, who shared so freely their interests and ideas on geriatrics and gerontology.

Charles F. Bollinger, Editor-in-Chief, Nursing Education Department of Appleton-Century-Crofts, saw the book through from the beginning to the end and left something of his influence on almost every page.

Yale University, through its School of Nursing, under the deanship of Florence S. Wald, sponsored the project. The study was made possible by a grant from the Elida B. Langley Charitable Trust, with additional funding provided through university auspices.

Dorothea Jaeger and Leo W. Simmons

Contents

CONTENTS

APPENDICES

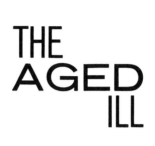

THE
AGED
ILL

Coping with Problems
in Geriatric Care

part I
THE ISSUE

1 Society and the Aged

Growing old is like walking over a bridge that becomes ever narrower so that there is progressively less range. . . . The bridge slowly tapers to a log, then a tightrope, and finally a thread. But we must go on till it breaks or we lose our balance. Some keep a level head and go farther than others, but all go down sooner or later.

G. STANLEY HALL

One of the most striking aspects of modern society, in contrast to earlier and more primitive cultures, is the increased proportion of a population that can reasonably be assured of reaching a venerable age. In the United States, the percentage of older citizens has more than doubled during the past half century and at present is approaching a ratio of 1 to 10. In 1900 the average span of life was 43 years, today it is 73 years. It is estimated that every 20 seconds someone in this country reaches the age of 65, whereas every 30 seconds an older citizen dies. By the end of this century the number of Americans 65 or over is expected to reach 32 million.

Modern science has succeeded in helping many more people reach an extended age; but as a society we have been remiss in giving meaning and fullness to the extra years. In spite of all that is being done in the area of geriatrics and gerontology, our aged countrymen stand a good chance of becoming *forgotten* men and women, subjected to a life of idleness, loneliness, and near poverty within this affluent society. Very likely, the older American will end his days in an institution. If he is fortunate, he will receive adequate physical care and even, perhaps, good psychosocial care; but chances are that he will not. Then, uprooted, depressed, or subdued, and feeling unwanted, he may withdraw into himself and become progressively enfeebled and desolate in mind and body. With such prospects, it may be pertinent and useful to compare the issue of aging in an anthropologic perspective broader than contemporary American society.

Aging as an Achievement

Whenever and wherever an individual "makes it" into a venerable age, it is never entirely his own doing; rather, it is a joint accomplishment. While realizing certain of his potentials for longevity by his own strivings, he is significantly helped along by his group through its organizational structure and its culture, and the gamble can be lost by remissness on the part of either. Indeed, it is more than probable that the remote past of all peoples included a period when attainment of great chronological age was not possible for any member of the group because adverse circumstances did not permit it.

A good and rounded off old age implies that the individual live *long and well* and *die timely and well.* These two achievements, also, are never arrived at by individual endeavor alone. Whether the added years bring further fulfillments to the ager* or are barren and empty, and whether senescent death be timely and appropriate or marred and defeative, depend upon the combined efforts of the individual *and* his society.

Another relationship of teamlike enterprise is a requisite for aging well. The human cycle begins with dependency of the young upon those who are older; and it ends, especially in the extremities of aging, with dependency of the old upon those who are younger. Both dependencies are deeply rooted in close human ties and stable culture patterns. This should be clearly kept in mind by anyone who would aspire to a long and worthwhile life without the benefit of intergenerational bonds and family obligations within his society. When society provides mutually supportive relationships between its youth and its elders, old age rests upon firm foundations. In contrast, when the old have found themselves without strong and binding ties with the young and able-bodied to rely upon, they have encountered the severest hazards.

There is considerable evidence that long before societies anywhere could assure many of their people a chance to reach any substantial age, human groups actually solved the problem of survival into senescence for a few of their members, with certain safeguards for living and for dying well according to their particular standards. Elders in some rather primitive societies have had assurances of remarkable security, exercising privileges that reached even past their old age into "dead-hand" prerogatives. Societal forms and functions, however, shift with time and place, and frequently these changes work dire consequences on the elders with

---

* Ager in our usage is meant to signify any person 65 or older.

respect to the length and value of their lives and in the manner of their deaths. It is sobering to contemplate that there are no perfect or permanent solutions to the problem of aging, short of death, partly because no cultural system is entirely stable or static. Change is the great disrupter of individual adaptation, including adaptation to aging into senescence.

Every conceivable coping pattern and attitude toward the vicissitudes of old age appear to have been tried out or expressed sometime, somewhere, in human endeavors to enrich and conclude a venerable age. In any comparative review, either of many different peoples and cultures or a long historical survey of a particular people and their changing cultural patterns, the attitudes held toward old age and its final termination can be plotted along a continuum between two extremes of viewing these experiences of life as a curse on the one hand or good fortune on the other; and the image a people hold of old age considerably effects the treatment afforded the elders by their younger associates.

On the basis of attitudinal appraisals, old age is variously defined as beginning fairly early or quite late in life and lasting a very short or an overly long period of time. The onset of old age may be welcome and treasured or resented and resisted—even camouflaged or denied to absurd degrees. When it is recognized and duly accepted, old age may be considered a fruitful period; when it is not, an idle and well-nigh intolerable one. In one society, people may anticipate a full and productive old age; in another, only empty days for killing time until time kills them. Some elders may welcome death or be induced or coerced to die in a commendable way, while others may prefer or be impelled, even compelled, to cling to life deep into its dregs.

Constructive answers to the problem of aging into senescence are nearly always relative, but they are especially relevant to the particular society and culture in which they apply. A specific coping pattern, even in the nursing care of a dying elder, may be adequate and right at one time and place in a culture and prove entirely inadequate and inappropriate for a similar problem in another culture or even at another time and place in the same culture. No society is without culturally determined attitudes and stances which sway between two poles of viewing the circumstances of aging, especially of extreme and enfeebled aging, as a living curse or a vital challenge—and what happens in the way of dying is not unrelated.

Threats to Good Living

On the curse side of the conventionalized, and often stereotyped, evaluation of old age and its corresponding coping patterns are encountered certain common pitfalls or major threats to human welfare that are potentially ever-present within the life cycle, but which loom with more ominous import as one approaches senescence. Almost universally they constitute threats to good living. Four of them can be identified as:

> loss in position and useful occupation or activity
> loss of family and kinship ties
> loss of vigor and health
> loss of incentive or purpose in life.

While these losses can be traumatic at any stage of life, the impact of any one of them can be far greater when striking during one's later years. Moreover, an uncanny relationship exists between these four threats: any three of them coming close together tend to bring on the fourth; any two may lead into a third, and then the fourth; and any one of them often paves the way for a second.

Loss of position or occupational status relates mainly to the disappearance of meaningful interests associated with retirement from habitual roles of participation that are, in turn, associated with feelings of worth. In our modern society there appear to be two types of retirement: technological or occupational retirement, linked significantly to chronological age, and psychological retirement, which involves a form of personal resignation and perhaps withdrawal from productive participation and which is more highly individualized. Should technological and psychological retirement come close together in time, both close personal ties and zest for living may suffer serious jeopardy. But should technologic retirement precede psychological resignation by a substantial margin, the chance exists for something like a silver lining with yet precious time for achieving further goals, some of which may be within reach of individuals despite increasing handicaps and dwindling resources.

Essentials for Further Achievements

Concerning advanced aging with accompanying disease and disabilities, certain dominant themes can be identified which relate to further achievements, especially for those who strive for a life that is "good to the last."

First, there are equilibriums to be maintained where the balance becomes ever more delicate or even precarious. There are equilibriums between passivity and self-assertion: when to ease up and when to keep on trying; when to yield and retreat and when to stand up and be bold; when to save and reserve one's energy and when to extend and spend oneself? Forfeiting too early the zest for what one considers worthwhile in life can become as detrimental as asserting oneself overly late.

Then there is the critical equilibrium between making one's own decision and relying upon the decision of others. The problem of independence versus dependence in interpersonal relationships, especially for those who are ailing, is not easily resolved. Even when a person is very old and enfeebled, self-decision-making often remains a treasured prerogative, though the risks involved may be considerable. When exercised overly long, however, the dangers inherent in such self-reliance become magnified.

Other equilibriums to be contended with by older persons relate to the balance of detriments with increments such as canes or walkers for weak legs and hearing aids for ears that are impaired. For the chairbound and the bedfast, there are even more finely balanced maneuvers, such as bargaining at the bedside with many *quid pro quos*. Indeed, some of the finest victories achieved by enfeebled agers have come to them through the exercise of their wits more than by their works. Even within an institutional setting some exciting and poignant dramas take place, as when a spirited old man or woman gives of whatever is left in order to get whatever is still wanted.

Another theme in the data on aging concerns a timeliness in senescence that may be golden and that, per chance, may be lost. There is a timeliness in the rites of passage when one faces, accepts, and assumes the role of an ager; there is a timeliness for the peak of aging when opportunities for that period in life are optimal; and, finally, there appears to be a timeliness for dying; for aging is rarely, if ever, very good when it lasts overly long. As the timeliness of these phases in aging fades away and is lost, one's position in senescence may shift away from the challenge and toward the curse side of existence.

INSTRUMENTAL AND FUNDAMENTAL NEEDS

The longer one lives, the more individual, different, or unique one may become—even to the extent of being somewhat of a "character" and possibly possessing certain outlandish traits and propensities for atypical wish-fulfillments. Consequently, uniform programs and procedures in health care and social welfare routines organized to serve the elderly can turn into serious disservice simply by stereotyping all old people as alike.

Aged persons should be spared such a fate, by either concept or practice, and thought should be given to regard every aged man and woman as a unique individual with deeply imprinted continuities in his or her style of life. When attempts are made to do this, however, the task of classifying and cataloging the needs of large numbers of aged and enfeebled individuals, especially within different social settings, becomes a difficult and discouraging commitment.

One way to solve this problem is the recognition of two types of needs of aged and infirm persons: *instrumental* and *fundamental.* These needs are more or less related, but they do afford useful differentiation.

Although somewhat arbitrarily defined, the *instrumental needs* are perceived to be the wants that constitute the more variable, immediate or short-term, and provisional goals of the aging person, which serve mainly as *means* for obtaining the more constant, far-reaching or continuing strivings that characterize older people. Instrumental needs are relevant to, and constantly modified by, the society and culture of which the elder person is a part. Their pertinence to the particular person's way of life is, substantially, an outgrowth of the norms and patterns of that culture. In some cultures, for instance, the acquisition of money is a dominant and extremely apt need; but this is not true for all cultures. The degree to which it is true in different cultures also varies. In cultures that are characterized by the exchange of goods and services almost solely by barter and where the concept of money barely exists, any strivings for the "money stuff" may be inept and all but meaningless; it therefore constitutes no important instrumental need. But within the same society where money is meaningless, the ownership and use of certain materials or implements and the existence of certain safeguards to socially established claims and prerogatives, such as family support and sustaining care in advancing age, may constitute major need instrumentalities. Indeed, for the individual ager such needs may be the major means or "lifeline" in his strivings during senescence. The noteworthy point of emphasis here is that instrumental needs are culturally derived. They differ from culture to culture and often, within the same culture, adapt in different ways to social change that occurs over spans of time. They *can,* however, be identified and classified, with focus and relevance for a given culture within a particular epoch.

To illustrate a sampling of instrumental needs within contemporary American culture: in the 1959 Report to the President, *Program and Resources for Older People,* prepared by the Federal Council on Aging, instructive data are provided. After calling attention to the fact that about one twelfth of the population is 65 or older, the statement is made that, while the concept of "average" is inaptly applied to older Americans and no uniform list of their needs can be compiled, nevertheless, certain problems are found to occur among them more often or with greater intensity than among those who are younger.

Among the problems cited—and identified for our purpose as instrumental needs—are these: suitable employment; adequate income maintenance; effective health and medical care; suitable housing; and adult education adapted for the elderly. These problems, or instrumental needs, relate characteristically to our American society and its culture. They might not be applicable in cultures unlike ours, particularly those of a very primitive type. However, it would not be too difficult to identify and classify such useful instrumental needs for particular societies and their cultures.

Instrumental needs, being adaptations of particular groups of people to their way of life, are as variable as are different cultures; however, there is a common base. Herein lies the key for determining so-called *fundamental needs*—the underlying, universal needs and wants that are characteristic of the strivings of all aging individuals in all cultures and that are reflected in the different cultures as a common denominator of late-age motivations. They are the mainsprings that impel and sustain old people, regardless of cultural setting or of time and place, to press on toward the limits of longevity.

There are many facets to motivation, but the parts overlap for individuals as well as for groups, especially when attempts are made to identify the common components across cultural lines. However, this has been attempted, albeit in an approximate manner, from masses of data gathered and assembled over many years (Human Area Files, Yale University). The objective has been to identify common underlying incentives or fundamental needs for which satisfactions were apparently sought in the adaptive behavior of old people. The project included a worldwide sample of seventy-odd societies—primitive and contemporary, agricultural and industrial. (Leo W. Simmons, 1945)

For the purpose at hand, the findings indicate at least five fundamental needs or motivational drives:

1. To live as long as possible, or at least until life's satisfactions no longer compensate for its privations or the advantages of death seem to override the burdens of life. Barring the burdens, life generally remains highly prized up to or beyond the point where the group recognizes the individual's potential for achievements or contributions.

2. To preserve and conserve one's energies and potentials, physical and otherwise, against depletion. This basic idea and age-old necessity connotes rest, relaxation, recuperation, renewal of health.

3. To safeguard and strengthen, wherever possible, prerogatives acquired earlier in life, such as knowledges and skills, possessions,

rights, and authority or prestige. The aged, far and wide, need to hold onto and jealously guard any seniority assets.

4. To continue some pertinent participation in group affairs either in an operational or supervisory role. Almost any sharing of interests and activities is preferred for its own sake, regardless of secondary gain therefrom, over sheer idleness on the part of the aged or indifference on the part of associates significant to them.

5. Finally, to find a closure to one's life, when necessity calls for it, that is as creditable and satisfying as circumstances permit and that has maximum prospects for an attractive and rewarding hereafter. Everywhere, there appears a valued difference between dying in victory or at least with dignity and dying in defeat or with degradation.

These five underlying incentives or components of basic motivations in old age, labelled here as fundamental needs (care for life, conservation of energy and resources, safeguards for capabilities and prerogatives, participation to some degree in current affairs, and a closure to life that is creditable and timed appropriately to circumstances) can be summed up more concisely in just three words: security, achievement, fulfillment. This uniformity in the fundamental or basic needs appears to cut across all cultural demarcations.

Significantly, a counterpart to the fundamental needs in aging is that in all human groups and their cultures there exist, to a greater or lesser degree, social capabilities and sanctioned practices for providing support for these needs. And, in apparent contrast, no other grouping of living species, except man, is found to be very supportive of their aged members. It appears that all lower forms of life leave their aged forebears to shift for themselves in their age extremities.

It should be remembered that any substantial aging in the history of mankind has come about, in all probability, as a reciprocal individual-group accomplishment, at times perhaps as a by-product of human strivings for group survival. However, it should not be overlooked that some societies or groups, in certain times and places, have ignored, neglected, even exploited their enfeebled forebears. It may be that human offspring can be, or become, more abusive and actually cruel to their elders—especially in the subtle refinements of cruelty—than can be the offspring of any other creature known. Lastly, it should not be forgotten that in the destiny of human societies and their cultures, the securities, achievements, and fulfillments that are won by, and vouchsafed to, the aged may be lost again within the shifts and changes of the norms of particular cultures.

LONGEVITY: PROBLEM AND CHALLENGE

Sooner or later for everyone, and relatively soon for ailing elderly individuals, the time comes for coping with the closure of one's life. Death can hardly be a stranger to really old people. Any long life has had some close calls; and part of the price for long life is to witness the passing of loved ones, be they relatives, friends, or associates.

In a society that prizes youth above age, that venerates knowledge more than wisdom, that accords status to work over leisure, and that, above all, abhors and rejects death, the aged find themselves at a culturally imposed disadvantage that is not equally shared in all human societies. It is true, nevertheless, that among all people with ample records, primitive or civilized, a state is reached in aging when further worthwhileness of living is difficult to discern, at least from the vantage point of one's associates. Then the encumbent is likely to become regarded as a surviving liability, perhaps to himself and certainly to most around him; and at some point the prospects for further meaningful activities appear uniformly dismal, no matter what the society or culture.

It is difficult, cross-culturally, to find conventionalized exceptions to this social decision on the dire extremities of aging; but great differences are encountered from culture to culture with respect to the point in longevity when the label of superannuation is applied and, also, with respect to what may be done by way of coping with the critical situation.

A significant fact is that until fairly recent times the "overaged" or "useless" phase in life was of no major importance because relatively few persons reached such a stage and almost none lasted very long into it. When such situations did arise, societies usually did something about it; but if they did not, a harsh natural environment resolved the matter. Even among groups of people where nature brooked few delays, some primitive societies seemed to face the issue of death with greater realism and philosophical composure than do some contemporary societies. We tend more to withdraw from or to deny, at least symbolically, the reality of the issue, in spite of the fact that the helpless and hopeless period in life is taking on vastly greater importance.

One notable outgrowth of our present-day values and norms has been the geriatric care-giving institution, a "need instrumentality" devised by society for the care of its aged and infirm members. The significance of this development is that relatively fewer and fewer elderly Americans are privileged to live out their lives at home amid family and friends. Conversely, current trends toward institutional care for persons in the extremities of aging seem destined to accelerate under the influence of today's health and welfare programs. As the aged in growing numbers find themselves spending their declining period of life in an institutional setting, they are faced with a real problem of achieving a worthwhile life during the time left to them and, also, an appropriate death—in a manner compatible with their style of life.

As was noted earlier in this chapter, attainment of great age requires joint endeavor; that of the individual *and* his society. By the same token, an aged person's attainment of further meaningful life experiences and a fulfilling and timely death within the institutional milieu requires reciprocal strivings; that of the aged resident or patient on the one hand and of the geriatric facility in which he is being cared for on the other. And the responsibility of the care-giving institution is, to say the least, considerable.

Some Problems in Institutionalized Geriatrics

Man does not live by bread alone.
THE BIBLE

An ever increasing number of people are living past the Biblical age of three score years and ten, and growing numbers of them are spending their last days and dying in a hospital, nursing home, or similar institution, instead of in their home among family or friends. To be sure, not all nursing home residents are very aged or terminally ill, unless the concepts of "aged" and "terminally ill" are stretched beyond meaningful limits. Some elderly persons are admitted to extended care-giving institutions for curative reasons—following major surgery, cerebrovascular accident, hip fracture, or the like. Others are institutionalized because of personal or social factors. But no matter what the immediate reason for admission, for a great many individuals the institution becomes their last place of residence—their final coping place.

THE GERIATRIC INSTITUTION

When an elderly person is in need of skilled nursing care, his family often finds itself unable to provide such care at home amid accustomed surroundings. A nursing home becomes more and more the practical solution, even when it is viewed as a compromise by the family or the patient. Often a proprietary nursing home is the only facility which will admit an aged ill or infirm person on a long-term basis, except when one is forced by circumstances to seek shelter and care in a tax-supported institution such as a city hospital or a county home. Relatively few voluntary institutions in this country are organized to provide long-term care for an elderly person who is ill or infirm and in need of skilled nursing care.

13

Voluntary, nonprofit homes for the elderly have a long history. Many of them were established—some more than a hundred years ago—by churches or religious orders; others were organized by fraternal societies such as the Masons, by groups sharing a common-nationality background, or by those having a common interest, such as benevolent associations or unions organized by professional or vocational groups. Their major purpose was to provide a "home" for elderly persons who were well but who could no longer maintain a home of their own or who, bereft of family or other close ties, sought companionship as well as shelter. Today, most of these institutions provide nursing care units for their residents in case of illness, but, with very few exceptions, they do not *admit* a person in need of skilled nursing care.

In recent years, some of the nonprofit institutions have made changes in their admission policies and have enlarged existing, or built new, nursing care units to accommodate the growing number of aged persons in need of nursing care. However, they have not been able to keep up with the changing and growing needs.

To meet the demands, the establishment of proprietary nursing homes, operated for profit, has become a dominant trend. They constitute a fairly modern innovation in American society due to rapid social changes and growth of interest in, as well as financial gains from, such services. The trend has been intensified also by the fact that many of the existing voluntary institutions for the aged continue to require that those seeking admission be well enough not to need much nursing service; and relatively few nonprofit facilities for the aged ill have been established.

The immensity of the problem of providing adequate facilities and services for the aged ill and infirm is reflected in the phenomenal rise in the number of nursing homes over the past 10 years. According to a recent publication of the U.S. Department of Health, Education and Welfare,* the number of nursing homes in this country increased during the period 1954 to 1965 from 6,539 to 11,981. Since the new institutions tend to be larger, the increase in available beds is even more striking— an increase from 171,816 in 1954 to 330,981 in 1961 and a second increase to 512,052 in 1965 show respective gains of 92 percent and 55 percent.†

---

* *Nursing Home Utilization and Costs in Selected States.* Health Series No. 8, February 1968. Washington, U.S. Government Printing Office.

Data for this report were drawn mainly from 2,616 nursing homes from the following states: California, Colorado, Massachusetts, Missouri, and North Carolina. Added to this were summary statements drawn from relevant information reports in other states from 1960 to 1965.

† This rise has continued unabated, and today there are reported to be some 860,000 nursing home beds. This figure does not include the thousands of beds occupied by aged patients in mental institutions. These are people who, because of brain damage rooted in physical illness or severe emotional pressures or both, have become severely

This large expansion is attributed in the report to: the rapid extension of the human life span; the increased prevention or control of chronic disease; and the shifts of the elderly from familial surroundings, stimulated in part by housing inadequate for sharing with older family members. More recently, too, the Medicare program has added new stimulus to the expansion of nursing homes.

As of 1963, 87 percent of these nursing homes were proprietary in ownership, operation, and private profit gains, and they provided 70 percent of all nursing home beds. Voluntary, nonprofit homes amounted to about 8 percent and provided approximately 15 percent of the beds, while institutions owned and operated by public agencies (local, state, and federal government) provided the remaining 15 percent of the beds. The average size of nursing homes varied somewhat with the type of ownership: proprietary institutions averaged 32 beds; voluntary nonprofit homes averaged 78 beds, and public institutions averaged 125 beds.

It is recognized in the report that the standards and quality of nursing care vary widely from home to home, and, in general, from state to state, and that nursing homes in the United States have "for a long time been outside the mainstream of health care" (page 3).

It seems pertinent at this point to summarize briefly from the report some of the characteristics of the nursing home population. About 9 out of 10 patients were 65 years or older, and 1 out of 3 was 85 or over. About 2 out of 5 came from hospitals, a similar proportion was admitted directly from their own homes, and the remainder came from other nursing homes. There were nearly three times as many women as men. Often only about one half were ambulatory, nearly as many were unable to dress themselves, and about 1 in 7 was unable to feed himself. Of every 4, 1 or more was mentally confused at least part of the time, and 1 out of 4 (often more) was incontinent. Length of stay ranged from 3 days to 32 years, with a median stay of 18 months. Nearly one third were discharged to their own homes; another third died while patients in a nursing home; and the remaining third were transferred either to another nursing home or to a hospital.

---

confused. Most nursing homes reject such patients, and if a nursing-home-resident's mental condition worsens to the point where staff considers him difficult to handle, more often than not, he is transferred to a mental hospital. "There they join longtime bonafide psychotics—schizophrenics and others—who have grown old in the hospital and together these two groups dominate the patient population." (*The New York Times*, December 1, 1968.)

THE AGED PATIENT

Removing enfeebled elders from their accustomed home surroundings and placing them together in strange institutional settings, where they are to live out the rest of their days, is nearly always accompanied by disruptive stress for those who are personally involved, be they the ailing patients or their responsible relatives.

In a group-living situation such as a nursing home, a person's individuality is apt to become submerged, and it is also difficult to preserve one's personal privacy. A nursing home is *not* a family, although the staff sometimes refer to it as such. In a family situation one lives with one's own kith and kin, while in a nursing home one is called upon to live with large numbers of unrelated persons. This is an entirely different kind of living situation from family life, and one which makes enormous adjustment demands upon the individual patient. It can be an especially traumatic experience for an older person, whose long life-span has left imprints and habits that have become ever more ingrained upon his personality as the years passed.

The perils arise, in large measure, because of the divergencies and conflicts that exist between two contrasting sets of values and behavioral patterns; those of the institution on the one hand and the home and family setting on the other. Some of the contradictions and incompatibilities can be sharp and quite disturbing to the aged person who suspects or realizes that this is a permanent move, and that the new and strange setting is to become his final "coping place" for achieving, to whatever extent he can, a suitable closure for his life. The dissimilarities in the situations and their impact upon the patient are all the more striking when one realizes that most other crises the elderly person has faced and survived have been within the home and family context. It is no wonder, then, that the prospect of confronting one's final crisis in life within an unfamilial setting can constitute a "cultural shock" for the person who is already disabled and without prospects of much improvement.

Under such circumstances, an aged patient may feel impelled to fear, resent, or even subjectively "withdraw" from his new surroundings. The situation can easily appear to him ill-fitted and ill-fated as a satisfactory or even tolerable completion to his life. Indeed, it may well be that this upsetting transitional phase in the life of the patient will bring for him subjective stresses more severe than those he will face during his final days, when he faces death.

The following illustrations each tell a story of adjustment of an aged ill person to an institutional setting—a story that may well be repeated in any nursing home anywhere in this country. They are important if we are to appreciate and understand the significance of illness and infirmity in old age and their implications:

> Mrs. F., an attractive, gregarious widow in her seventies, was admitted to the nursing home from a nearby hospital with a diagnosis of hip fracture. Full of hope that before long she would be able to return to her own home, she conscientiously followed her rehabilitative regimen. She seemingly accepted the idea that she would be less independent than she had been before she sustained the fracture. A niece, who lived nearby and visited her regularly, offered to assist with shopping and household chores which Mrs. F. would no longer be able to do. Mrs. F. seemed very happy when she was discharged, and looked forward with eagerness to being back in her own home.
>
> In less than three weeks Mrs. F. was readmitted to the nursing home. She refused to talk about the time she had been home and kept repeating that she had come back here "to die." Her former gaiety had given way to a moroseness which she seemed unable to dispel. Whereas formerly she had sought out others, she now refused to mingle with the other residents and insisted upon being left in her room, alone. She ate poorly and claimed that she was too weak to follow the exercises that had been prescribed. Her niece rarely visited. Mrs. F. resisted all attempts by doctors and nurses to help her regain her former joy of living. She steadily grew weaker, and died about 10 weeks after her readmission to the nursing home.
>
> Mr. C., a seventy-two-year-old was admitted to the institution after he had fallen while taking a walk near his home. He was not hurt, but his daughter and her husband, with whom he had been making his home, felt that he would be better off in a nursing home, where he would be in a more protective environment and have the companionship of people his own age.
>
> Mr. C.'s wife had died some 5 years before, at which time he had sold his home; his daughter and her husband also sold theirs; together they had purchased one that would accommodate grandfather, parents, and their three children. This living arrangement apparently had worked out well.
>
> Mr. C., who had been a quiet and unassuming person, became markedly more so after being admitted to the nursing home. He was considered a model resident by the staff and not at all "troublesome" as were some of his fellow residents. He seldom went out of doors, spoke very little, and sat in a chair for hours at a time quietly watching the activities about him. His memory had been failing during the last year he had been living with his daughter and family. This condition worsened considerably after he entered the nursing home. In addition he became subject to periods of confusion, when he did not know where he was or why he was there; but he was not "difficult" and always did what the staff asked of him. He remained in the nursing home until he died—a little less than 2 years after he entered it.

Following major surgery, Mrs. P. had been transferred from a nearby general hospital to the nursing home. From the moment she entered the institution, Mrs. P. had "felt at home." A woman of European birth, and a widow, she had worked hard all of her life. Until her recent surgery, she had kept house for her only daughter and her daughter's husband, both of whom worked.

Now she enjoyed and actively participated in the various activities organized for the residents. She repeatedly told the staff and her fellow residents how lucky she considered herself to be in such a fine institution.

Mrs. P. had been in the nursing home for some weeks, when one day she discovered that public funds were used to pay for her stay in the institution. Deeply hurt, she confronted her daughter with this and asked to return to her daughter's home. When the daughter explained that she would not be able to have her mother live with them again, and, furthermore, that she did not have the means to pay for her mother's upkeep in the institution, Mrs. P. became a "changed person." She refused to go out. During her daughter's visits, Mrs. P. remained silent. She lost all interest in her surroundings, and despite encouragement from the staff, she ate less and less. As the weeks and months went by, Mrs. P. grew steadily weaker. Despite psychiatric consultation, infusions, and other life-sustaining measures, Mrs. P. died because, as one nurse put it, "she willed to die."

White-haired and walking as erect as always, 87-year-old Mrs. N. was a lady of independent spirit who had remained quite active in the various civic organizations she had joined during her younger days. She made hand-sewn articles for charitable bazaars and continued to sew for the hospital auxiliary. She no longer went out, but family and friends visited her in her home. After the death of her husband, she had continued to live in the attractive white house which had been her home since her husband had brought her there as a bride some 60 years before. For several years they had had a housekeeper on an 8-hour, 5-day-a-week basis. A son and his wife who lived next door visited when they came home from work and on weekends.

Several months after Mr. N.'s death, the housekeeper left quite suddenly, and the family decided that Mrs. N. would be better cared for in a nursing home. She did not want to go, and went only when her children assured her that it was to be for a limited time—until they found another housekeeper for her.

About a week after Mrs. N. entered the nursing home, several members of the hospital auxiliary to which she belonged visited her. They found Mrs. N. sitting in a corner of her room, which she shared with a seriously ill woman who was expected soon to die. She seemed overjoyed to see her friends. During the visit she constantly spoke of going back to her own home, and she seemed confident that this would be very shortly. She brushed aside her friends' suggestions that her son bring her television set from home or that she join the other residents in watching television, a pastime she had always enjoyed. On subsequent visits Mrs. N. became ever more quiet and apathetic: she spoke less and less about going home; her previously always busy hands remained idle; and she appeared to take little interest in her surroundings. Despite various medicines her physician prescribed to improve her appetite, she ate poorly. She began having periods of disorientation, and it would take a while before she would recognize friends when they visited. Then she would just sit quietly in a wheelchair, her face set in an expression of blankness. When someone said "hello," she would look up and her face would soften to a faint smile. Her family visited regularly. They were assured by the physician and the staff that "everything" was being done for her. Mrs. N. died quietly, in her sleep, about 9 months after she had been taken to the nursing home.

It is common practice in nursing homes to have patients up and about whenever possible, and there is considerable evidence that keeping them out of bed and active prevents physical complications. A search of the literature, however, reveals little that suggests that such practices are always appreciated by patients who are aged and often "weary to death." It may well be, however, that institutional rules and regulations, if very rigidly enforced, have adverse effects and add to the strain and stress of a person who is already overwrought because of the move from home to institution.

There was, for instance, Mrs. Z., who at the age of 84 had fallen and sustained a hip fracture. For many years she had lived alone in the rambling white house, spending much of her leisure time reading while reclining on the living room couch. By choice she did not venture out of doors very often, but enjoyed seeing her children and grandchildren, who visited frequently. She remained keenly interested in community and world affairs.

When Mrs. Z. reached the age of 84, her daughter, who with her husband lived in a neighboring village, prevailed upon her mother to live with them. In her daughter's home, Mrs. Z. continued her way of living until she was hospitalized following the accident, which caused her hip fracture.

Mrs. Z. remained in the hospital for about a month, and then was transferred to a nursing home. Her family physician found the trip to the nursing home too far to travel and the nursing home administrator recommended another doctor to take over her medical regimen.

According to Mrs. Z.'s daughter, no one in the institution showed any interest in her mother's previous pattern of living; no one inquired about her habits, likes, and dislikes. The staff gave her excellent physical care, for Mrs. Z. was neat and clean whenever the daughter visited, but they seemed uninterested in her emotional well-being. The family had no contact with the physician who now attended Mrs. Z. until the daughter made a specific request to see him.

Mrs. Z. continually complained of feeling tired, and she found the geriatric chair, in which she spent most of her days, very uncomfortable. She could not understand why the staff refused to let her spend at least some of the time reclining on her bed, as had been her custom for many years. She ate poorly and, at times, needed to be fed. She voiced her resentment when she was wheeled into the dining room for her meals, for she had been accustomed to eating alone, and found the dining room noisy and the company, which included several senile patients, unattractive. She would not look at a book, though previously she had been an avid reader. She refused to mingle with the other residents. She was constantly begging to be left alone. She said that she had lived a full and long life and was ready to die. Her lament to her family was, "If only they would leave me alone." Then she began to be quite apathetic and even drowsy. She spent much of her time napping, while sitting in her chair. Upon being aroused, her first words were apt to be: "If only I would die."

The family then had Mrs. Z. transferred to another nursing home and the services of another physician were procured. In the second home a more congenial atmosphere seemed to prevail than in the previous institution. The daughter was made to feel much more welcome to visit, and the staff encouraged her to assist with arranging social and recreational endeavors the home was planning for the residents. Within a short time Mrs. Z.'s complaints became fewer, and after several weeks, she began to join in group activities. She ate much better and her drowsiness, which had been pronounced in the previous institution, became noticeably less. She continued to spend the better part of her day in the wheelchair. Mrs. Z. has not resumed her former reading habit, nor does she show any interest in what goes on outside of the institution. Her former zest for living seems to have gone, but she does appear to have come to terms with herself and with the situation in which she finds herself.

A very different experience in accommodation to institutional living was that of Miss L., who died at the age of 99, having been a resident in a church-affiliated home for the aged for more than 30 years.

Miss L. had entered the institution following her retirement from teaching in the hope that she would find companionship, opportunity for social activities, relief from housekeeping chores, and economic security in her old age, for she would be unable to maintain a home for herself on her meager retirement income. She had no close relatives. Within a relatively short time, the institution had become "home" to Miss L.

For many years Miss L. was an active participant in the various activities of the home. The residents had freedom to come and go, much as Miss L. had had when she had lived in a residential hotel. She enjoyed excellent health, and had remained remarkably active until her mid-nineties, when within a short time she became quite frail and was transferred to the nursing care unit of the home. Here she took to spending most of her time in a rocking chair which she had brought with her when she entered the home. As Miss L. grew older, she ate less and less, and, for almost a year prior to her death, her sole nourishment consisted of ice cream mixed with milk, which she enjoyed. On the morning of her death her usual routine had been followed, and the aide had assisted her to her rocking chair and then busied herself with giving care to the other patients in the room. Soon the aide became conscious of the fact that Miss L.'s rocking chair had come to a halt. She went over to Miss L., who kept her eyes closed and did not respond when spoken to. Miss L. had died quietly while rocking in her favorite chair.

Finally, there were Mr. and Mrs. A., both in their late seventies, who realized that the burdens of homemaking had come to outweigh the joy and pleasure of independent living. They had no children and no close relatives. Many of their friends had moved away or had died. Mrs. A. had arthritis and found it increasingly difficult to attend to her household chores. Their decision to enter a home for the aged had not been a hasty one, but they were able to face the future realistically and saw the necessity of living in a place where they would be cared for in the event of illness or infirmity. They discussed their plans with their pastor, their family physician, and with their lawyer. They also visited a variety of places established for the elderly and selected a church-related institution which had a large infirmary and a physician in attendance on schedule.

Their adjustment to group living was easier than they had thought possible. They found among the residents congenial friends with whom to play games, attend church services, and go shopping. Before long Mrs. A. was helping with caring for the many plants which were in the halls and living rooms.

Mr. and Mrs. A. had been residents in the home for about a year when Mr. A died following a brief illness. Death came to him in the home infirmary where he had been taken and where his wife could be with him much of the time.

Mrs. A. continued to live in the home among friends and people she knew, secure in the knowledge that she would receive warm and supportive care when she needed it.

No one single illustration or any group of illustrations can convey what it means to an aged ill or infirm person to be admitted to a nursing home or other extended care facility. Factors such as whether the move is a temporary or permanent one, and whether he has been allowed to participate in the decision-making or the decision has been made for him, play a large part in how he feels about the move. What the elderly person's adjustment to an institutional setting will be, however, is determined in large measure by the patient himself—the kind of person he is, the way he envisions whatever life remains to him, and all of his past experiences and how he has reacted to them. But it also depends to a very considerable degree upon the institution and the kind of environment it provides, not only in the physical arrangements, but also—and this is much more important—in the sociopsychological atmosphere; for in addition to such tangible requirements as proper housing and adequate medical care the aged person has need for affection, understanding, dignity, status, and the like.

Three leading ideas that are applicable to such institutional contexts have been analyzed perceptively by the late psychiatrist Ewen Cameron. These concepts are: *needs, demands,* and *setting.*

Cameron reports that two ever-present needs of human beings are affection and understanding. Both phenomena defy precise definition and it has been difficult to explore them on an experimental basis; however, certain definable defects regularly result if these needs are not met. Affection can be observed in the giving and receiving in terms of touching, handling, and holding of a young child by its mother; in adulthood a fair amount of it becomes symbolized in the form of words and of actions that do not necessarily involve touch. The second need, understanding, defies even such cursory description. Cameron suggests that both phenomena require further study for fuller comprehension of what is involved.

The second concept, demand, would seem to have more tangibility than the two needs discussed above. The implication of this concept on the revolutionary changes in patient care that have taken place during the past two decades is significant and noteworthy. Cameron writes: "Previously we had gone very far and, as circumstances have demonstrated, much too far in the direction of taking all demands off the patient. He was kept in bed and waited on hand and foot. We have gradually come to realize that if you make no demands on the individual's musculature, i.e., if you keep him in bed day after day and sometimes month after month, not only does his musculature atrophy, but his cardiovascular control also becomes impaired. Perhaps it has not been quite so apparent that to make no demands means to lose skills. The simplest example, of course, is the skill of walking, but any other skill also disappears if we make no demands."*

Following Kurt Lewin's idea of group anticipated response, Cameron then extends this concept into the ideological realm: "If the group anticipates that the individual will maintain a reasonable level of behavior, and if the individual accepts this, his behavior will remain at a much higher standard than otherwise. . ."*

As for the third concept, setting, considerable strides have been made in the knowledge of the importance of the setting in which action takes place. In a care-giving institution, the action may consist of therapeutic procedures, rehabilitative measures, or the ordinary physical and psychological processes of daily living. *But whatever the action, the setting in which it occurs greatly affects the outcome.* Accordingly, the major needs the aged carry with them into the institutional milieu and the demands, exemplified by what "others" expect of them become more or less modified and grounded by the institutional setting. Hence, a

* Cameron, E. Personal communication.

patient's accommodation to this final coping place must be viewed in terms of these three concepts, e.g., the patient's major needs, the demands imposed upon him by the staff, and the setting—the institutional context.

The decisive move of an older person from home to institution may prove stress laden for other family members as well. This is especially likely to happen when the separation of patient from family is clearly touched with a sense of finality and engenders feelings of guilt in the relatives and of abandonment in the patient. And when the relatives enter the institution in their new roles as visitors, subject to institutional rules and regulations, the contrast can become further imprinted upon them. In their adaptation to their new relationship with the patient, the relatives frequently tend to feel out of place, sense their inadequacies for being of any assistance in the new situation, and see themselves more as a hindrance than as a help either to the patient or to the busy staff. Feelings of detachment, even alienation, may arise if they come to sense something of mere toleration of their presence in a setting that is characterized for them by its sterile and disciplined atmosphere, its formidable apparatus, its complex and somewhat mysterious technical practices, and its tightly scheduled and more or less ritualized procedures and routines. For the visitor kinsman the effect of all this, with apparent violation of folkways and values to which the family is accustomed, may be dismay, even discord. Even the attitude toward, and approaching prospect of, the death of the patient may appear quite foreign to the relatives and strike them as unorthodox, strange, or somewhat inhuman.

Furthermore, medical diagnoses are now more expertly determined than ever before, and the tentative prolongation of life can be more significantly controlled by expert therapy and ingenious devices that are increasingly at the command of the physician. Medical attempts to prolong life are not limited to persons still in the fullness of their lives, nor exclusively to those with good prospect for recovery or cure. Persons of advanced age, some of them with little promise for further meaningful or satisfying existence, are known to have been kept alive by means of mechanical and electronic devices that can artificially prolong respiration and circulation almost indefinitely. So it appeared with certain patients in a long-term care facility which one of the authors had occasion to visit. The scene was a 40-bed floor, where 14 of the 40 patients either had had nasogastric feeding tubes inserted or were being given intravenous infusions. The youngest of these patients was 71; the oldest, 85 years of age. Three of them responded with lucidity when spoken to; the others remained more or less unresponsive. Several seemed to be in a deep coma. A 73-year-old patient with a history of senility and advanced cancer had managed to pull the tube from her nose. She seemed unresponsive, and the blank expression on her face never changed when the nurse asked her whether she found the tube in her nose uncomfortable. The 85-year-old patient had been in a coma since her admission some 2 weeks before, following a cerebrovascular accident. Being very restless, the nurses feared she might pull out the catheter which had been inserted because of incontinency, or disturb the nasogastric tube through which she was being fed at two-hour intervals. For this reason the patient had been placed in a restraining sheet. A number of these patients were on antibiotics, given intramuscularly, to prevent infection. One of the nurses commented:

> In this place there is no dignity in death; the doctors here just cannot bear to lose a patient to death and so insist on keeping the patients' bodies warm—to keep the heart beating, though the soul has already departed. Most of these doctors will not admit that a patient is terminally ill, and with the advent of Medicare some of them seem to be trying even harder to keep a patient's heart beating, showing little regard for the person in that body. If the doctors would only permit nursing to continue *ordinary* lifesaving measures such as nourishing, protecting, and supporting the aged ill person with maximum skill and consideration—as the founder of modern nursing, Florence Nightingale, admonished, "to put the patient in the best condition for nature to act upon."

In terminal illness, the issue often arises whether priority of staff attention should go to the patient expected soon to die or to those with greater potential for recovery. Concurrently, another decision-making dilemma is likely to ensue: whether attempts should be made to prolong the life of the patient into its utter extremity and by all possible means, or to permit and support a "natural" and possibly earlier death with emphasis upon personal comfort, propriety, and emotional support to the expiring patient and his immediate survivors.

Still another conflict may arise in situations of terminal illness which may be discerned by the patient, if he is alert and conscious, and by any relatives who continue to visit. This is if major concerns of the staff appear to shift from goals of recovery and possible cure to those of comfort during the process of dying; or, what is worse for the relatives and the patient, a shift is made toward withdrawal from, and possibly isolation and "forgetting" of the patient as death draws near.

It is of manifest importance that health professionals in positions of responsibility and trust recognize, understand, and anticipate such upsetting and damaging reactions to both the patient and his relatives. Recognition of the need for sustained care of the aged patient, and sometimes of his close of kin, on a supportive and interpersonal basis is becoming more and more widespread, and justified emphasis is being placed upon such concepts as "individualized," "personalized," and "comprehensive" care.

Geriatric Nursing

In a great many geriatric institutions the organization and the staffing differ from what is usually found in hospitals. Nurses in supervisory positions in nursing homes, for example, have a greater responsibility than their hospital counterparts where, more often than not, a medical resident or intern is available to verify untoward signs and symptoms that a nurse has observed in a patient and to make the major decisions. In a nursing home, evaluations and judgments in emergency situations and in referring matters to the attending physician are dependent more upon the nurse. The realization of these factors makes one aware of the need for well-prepared professionals in the nursing role.

This is not the place to comment in detail upon the social organization of nursing homes—an area in need of systematic exploration if the aged ill in our country are to receive the optimum care that government and society profess to be the right of all citizens. Suffice it to state that the expressed philosophy and policy of a specific institution do not always permeate the entire system; nor are they always observed within particular nursing units. Inadequate communication within the nursing service as well as between nurses and attending physicians is also encountered in many of these institutions. Better social organization, improved communication, and well-prepared professionals in the nursing role would no doubt go a long way to prevent situations such as the following—one of many encountered during the course of the project, in which the patient was an innocent sufferer. Two registered nurses were interviewed: one was in charge of a patient unit during the A.M.; the other, in charge of the same unit during the P.M. tour of duty. Each related a problem which concerned a patient for whom a pain-relieving medication on a p.r.n. basis had been prescribed by his physician. The one nurse believed that the patient, who was aged and considered terminally ill, should be kept free of pain as much as possible, and administered the drug as often as permitted under the prescription. The other nurse feared that the patient might become addicted to the drug and withheld the medication for long periods of time—until the patient would cry with pain. Each thought the other "wrong," and thus a feud was carried on with the patient caught in the middle. Neither felt that it was her responsibility to contact the physician, and the director of the nursing service, who worked the A.M. tour of duty, believed that the decision as to whether to give or to withhold the drug should be made by whoever was in charge of the floor at the time the drug might be given.

The care provided for the elderly in nursing homes, or in nursing units of homes for the aged, may or may not be under the direct supervision of a registered nurse. Particularly during the afternoon or night tour of duty, a licensed practical nurse may be in charge. Furthermore, actual care is, in most instances, in the hands of nursing assistants with little or no formal training. The proportion of licensed practical nurses and other ancillary personnel to the number of registered nurses has been mounting in hospitals as well as in long-term care institutions such as nursing homes. In a recent survey, which included about 100 proprietary nursing homes, it was found that twice as many practical nurses and seven times as many nurse aides worked in these homes as did registered nurses. To be sure, no one seems to know as yet the required ratio of nurse aides, licensed practical nurses, and registered nurses to the number of patients which provides optimum or adequate nursing care.

Moreover, most nursing personnel of all ranks are relatively ill prepared to cope constructively with either the patient or the relative in the event of pending death and family bereavement. It could be assumed that the nurse aide and licensed practical nurse are far less prepared than is the registered nurse for ministering to patients in such crises; but no one knows for sure how much help they do or could provide with proper preparation. Indeed, the possibility is recognized, that some NA's and LPN's do as well or even better than do some of the RN's in these dire and delicate situations. But when this occurs, it would appear to be, by all odds, more a matter of personal concern and human warmth than of training in nursing skills.

However this may be, it is now well known that there are many aspects in which the preparation of nurses of all ranks for the care of fatally ill patients can be greatly improved through planned educational programs. This is a timely and crucial issue, especially since the aged ill and the ancillary nursing personnel are being brought together in increasing numbers by the force of current circumstances and trends in medical and nursing care. And in spite of their limitations, for the foreseeable future at least, the nursing home is likely to remain a major facility for coping with the problem of terminal care in senescence.

Because of this and related issues and trends in the provision of long-term geriatric care, it would seem that major prospects for early improvement in the quality and quantity of care for aged patients will rest largely with the nursing profession and its ancillary personnel. The probability is strong that anything resembling comprehensive and supportive care for these patients will be left primarily to the responsibility of the professional nurse, be she at the bedside or in a position of leadership within the hierarchy of the nursing service.

part **II**

GERIATRIC NURSING: TODAY AND TOMORROW

③ Project Plans and Problems Raised

The study which forms the basis for this section of the book was designed to survey and appraise particular aspects of geriatric nursing. Since increasing numbers of elderly Americans are spending their last days in institutions such as hospitals and nursing homes instead of in their own homes among family and friends, and since current trends toward institutional care for persons in the extremities of aging and infirmity seem destined to accelerate under today's health- and medical-care programs, attention was directed primarily to the care of aged, terminally ill patients within the institutional context.

In the beginning, the purpose had been to limit the project largely to nursing-care problems of aged patients during the terminal phase of their fatal illness; but it soon became obvious that in order to consider carefully the problem of terminality, it was necessary to broaden the inquiry.

The major reasons for shifting our approach to encompass, also, some of the wider aspects of geriatric care were the following:

First, we found the use of the word "terminal" as applied to aged patients by nurses to be much more generalized than when applied to younger patients. Elderly patients may be regarded as terminal in the sense that they may not be expected to recover from a chronic ailment, or even to improve very much; but they are not viewed or treated as critically ill or placed on any "danger list." Even when a patient was medically diagnosed as terminal, many of the nursing respondents preferred not to be made aware of this fact. Moreover, with inquiry pointed directly to the problem of terminality, their responses often continued to relate to the broader context of geriatric care.

Second, a prominent, though by no means uniform, point of view reflected by the nursing personnel is that of dying being a part of living until death actually occurs, while death is a physical state that calls for new criteria. This way of looking at the conclusion of life, sometimes labelled as part of the developmental process, places the whole of dying within the framework of living, and makes the fact of death a sharply defined point in time just outside this framework. Such implied divorcement of dying and death, whether valid or not, appears over and over in the nursing comments and seems to affect definitions, attitudes, and usage of the concept of "terminal."

Third, as implied above, most of the nursing responses to the scheduled inquiries tended to reflect strongly our American cultural de-emphasis on death, with something of a denial or refusal to take note of what are called the negative aspects of dying. Instead, there were stressed the positive aspects of living and of making something good come of life to its very end.

It thus became clear that the wiser course was to enlarge upon the scope of the exposition, so that a broader range of involvements than the strictly defined terminal phase in geriatric nursing care would be encompassed.

Our aim was *not* to gather and evaluate a representative cross-section of typical nursing practices existing in contemporary institutions caring for the aged ill. It was to assemble firsthand information and report on current geriatric patient care that may be regarded as "good," or perhaps the "best," that is presently practiced by selected nursing personnel within a circumscribed group of institutions chosen because of their high repute. Interest was directed primarily to a limited number of identified issues that appear to be challenging and somewhat controversial within the nursing profession.

The interview material that was gathered from the nursing staff within the chosen geriatric facilities was to be matched, for comparative purposes, with information assembled on the basis of a mailed questionnaire to a selective group of degree-holding registered nurses throughout the country.* They were requested to express their views on what would constitute for them good or superior geriatric nursing care concerning the same problems dealt with in the interviews.

For obtaining the pertinent information, four important steps were taken:

First, relevant data from three major sources, including ideas, were gathered and reviewed: geriatric literature in the fields of medicine, nursing, and the behavioral sciences; conferences with leaders in health and welfare programs for the aged, including some clergymen, physicians, nurses, social workers, and researchers in geriatrics and gerontology; and repeated visits to geriatric institutions for observation, consultation, and trial interviews. At two of these facilities, a detailed examination was made of records of aged patients who had closed out their lives within their walls. These patient records numbered slightly more than 100 in one institution and about 20 in the other.

On the basis of this background information, 31 long-term care

* For statistical profile of the study participants, see Appendix C, Tables 2 to 12.

facilities for the elderly—homes for the aged having large nursing-care units, nursing homes, and geriatric hospitals—were selected on the basis of their high repute and, with one exception, of their location within a radius of 150 miles of New York City. Specified numbers of nursing personnel (nurse aides, licensed practical nurses, and registered nurses), depending upon the size of staff, were then chosen by the heads of the nursing department within these institutions for interviews.* Interviews were scheduled at the convenience of the particular institution and of the individual staff member. Approximately one hour was allowed for each interview, but the sessions often lasted longer. All interview sessions were conducted by the research staff on an individual basis and in the privacy of a room provided by the institution. In order to eliminate a possible barrier to free expression, the institutions and the interviewees were promised anonymity.

Next, a roster was made up of 300 academic-degree-holding registered nurses, occupying positions of leadership in the profession or, in a few instances, preparing for such positions. The roster was obtained through information from professional organizations and academic institutions.

Fourth, the key and perhaps most crucial step was the construction of a schedule of inquiry to serve as a standard guide for interviewing practitioners in the selected institutions and also as a questionnaire, similar to the interview guide in structure and content, to be mailed to the potential degree registered nurse respondents. The major difference between the two schedules was that the nurse practitioners were asked, in effect, "what do you do" about specific nursing problems, and the nursing leadership was asked, "what would you do" or "what may one say that should be done" about the same problem.†

DEFINITIONS

It seems pertinent at this point to clarify our meaning and use of the following terms: 1) terminal illness; 2) best geriatric nursing practice; 3) nurse and nursing personnel; and 4) registered and degree registered nurses.

A considerable diversity of opinion concerning the diagnostic concept of *terminal illness* as associated with a poor prognosis for elderly patients, already commented upon in a foregoing paragraph, mandated that for the purpose of this study a more precise interpretation be formulated.

---

* For selection formula, see Appendix C, Table 1.
† For copies of interview guide and questionnaire, see Appendix E.

Consequently, commitment is made to an operational definition of terminal illness: namely, that "terminal," as defined by medical diagnosis, is perceived to encompass that phase in the life of the patient which may be relatively indefinite in time, but which connotes a professional judgment of irreversibility of the illness, disability, or infirmity and carries a sense of immediacy (imminence) to impending death. The validity of the prognosis is viewed as resting upon less than total, but significant, degrees of dependability that justify taking the situation seriously. Medical prognoses will vary with the nature of the illness and the skill and experience of the physician, of course, but in the extremes of aging and decrepitude these prognoses probably reach higher degrees of dependability, generally, than in the lives of younger patients.

Our operational definition of the *best geriatric nursing care existing today* is: the reported practices on specific problems by the selected nurse practitioners engaged in geriatric nursing in long-term-care institutions which were, in turn, selected for their high repute in the quality of care provided. The reported "best" practices were then analyzed and compared with the "best" or "ideal" nursing care for the same particular problems as they are conceived of by selected prominent and interested degree registered nurses.

Apropos of the issues raised in this study, certain other terms need to be defined. Except where specifically defined, the words *nurses* and *nursing personnel* are used throughout in a very loose sense as a person or persons engaged in nursing activities, irrespective of vocational or professional preparation of the person. The reason for this has been to avoid the cumbrousness of spelling out each of the different categories of nursing personnel whenever reference is made to them. It also becomes important to remember that these terms, as used in this book, refer to the participants in the present study.

One further explanation is in order. While a few of the registered nurse practitioners have earned academic degrees, they are not singled out but are included in the registered nurse group engaged in geriatric nursing in the selected institutions. To distinguish between those employed in the participating geriatric facilities and the RN's who were selected specifically because of their academic or professional degrees and their leadership positions, only this latter group is designated as the degree registered nurse group.

ISSUES EXPLORED

The chief geriatric-care problems raised in this study and explored through the experience of the nurse practitioners (NA's, LPN's, and

RN's) and the expert opinions of qualified degree registered nurses (DRN's) were the following, in the order in which they are dealt with in the chapters of this section.

1. Under what conditions, if any, do or should aged patients be treated like children? How controversial is this issue among nursing personnel? What qualifying circumstances justify such treatment or discredit it? Where differences in practice and opinion do exist, do they correspond to the different ranks of nursing personnel? (Chapter 4.)

2. Do or should nurses resort to the use of good-natured banter and humor when caring for geriatric patients? Under what conditions, if any, may a nurse justifiably "kid" or "josh" with such patients? Is there any reason to expect greater or less agreement on this issue than that of treating aged patients like children? (Chapter 5.)

3. Three especially difficult problems in geriatric nursing were selected with the purpose of exploring in greater detail the concrete proposals made by nurses for coping with them. They were: What do you do or what may one say that should be done when an elderly patient a) shows mistrust or aggression toward those caring for him; b) undergoes a breakdown in conventional proprieties; c) hallucinates (has visions or other delusory experiences)? Which of these types of patient behavior produces the most critical coping problem for nursing personnel, and why? (Chapters 6, 7, 8.)

4. How may one say that nursing care "differs" or "does not differ" for an aged, critically-ill person who is conscious and mentally alert in contrast to one who is semi- or unconscious or under heavy sedation? Why can a majority of nurse practitioners say there is no difference and an even larger majority of degree registered nurses claim there are differences? (Chapter 9.)

5. Is geriatric nursing related to the nurse's knowledge of the medical prognosis? What are the possible differences, if any, in caring for an elderly person expected soon to die and one who is expected to recover? (Chapter 10.)

6. Do or should nurses take a stand on the use of artificial (unnatural, extraordinary, heroic) as opposed to natural lifesaving measures to prolong the life of an aged patient? If so, how far into the terminal phase of life is it important to support or urge the use of

such measures? Should there be any limits from the point of view of nursing? What kind of issues arise from this question, and under what circumstances? If in conflict, what should the geriatric nurse do? (Chapter 11.)

7. Should an aged patient be told, or have the right to know, when he is diagnosed as having a poor prognosis and considered to be terminally ill? Under what conditions should a nurse discuss, or not discuss, with her aged patient his prospects of dying in the near future? Would she welcome such opportunities? Does she perceive any need for this on the part of aged patients? If she is permitted or encouraged to do so, how may she prepare herself for this function? (Chapter 12.)

8. How concerned or affected are elderly patients in institutional settings when death takes one of them? What are the effects of staff attempts to hide or disguise the event, as opposed to their dealing openly with it? Under what conditions can knowledge about, and reaction to a fellow-patient's death become a constructive experience? What skills and opportunities are available to the nurse for coping constructively with this situation? (Chapter 13.)

9. How do geriatric nurses view the presence, attitudes, and reactions of relatives when death takes an aged family member? How much responsibility do nurses assume in providing comfort and support for relatives when an aged kinsman dies? What skills and guidelines are suggested for coping with these problems? (Chapter 14.)

The search for constructive solutions to these nursing problems, to which Chapters 4 to 14 are committed, provides no single answer to any of the above issues. Individual respondents within each of the four nursing ranks, as well as the separate nursing ranks per se, differ significantly on preferable nursing practices. These differences, when classified and analyzed, tend to cluster around two, sometimes three, distinct positions, and make it imperative that each of the major stances receive serious consideration. In the next eleven chapters, what may appear to be the least desirable position taken in nursing practice is generally reviewed first, followed by consideration of a "middle" stance, if any, and that is followed by a more thorough consideration of a final and usually more strongly supported position (by the DRN's and frequently by one or more of the practitioner ranks).

In addition to the above issues on the *practice of geriatric nursing,* certain closely-related questions were raised concerning the *geriatric nurse practitioner*. These questions have to do with some major rewarding and unrewarding aspects of working with the aged ill, with freedom for independent action for the professional nurse in geriatrics, and with the preparation of nurses for geriatric practice, especially for the care of terminally-ill patients:

10. What are some of the high-priority satisfactions nurses derive from working with the aged ill? Conversely, what constitute some of the greatest frustrations or dissatisfactions experienced in the geriatric work situation? Under what circumstances, if any, would it be desirable for the professional nurse to be granted greater freedom for independent action and practice in the care of the aged ill? (Chapter 15.)

11. A nursing home is frequently identified as a "place where the aged go to die." An axiom cherished by the nursing profession is that "the first duty of a nurse is to her patient." With these thoughts in mind, how may a nurse prepare herself (himself) to insure maximal nursing care to the dying? What conflicts and dilemmas confront the nurse, and how may she (he) cope with and overcome them in the interest of the patient? (Chapter 16.)

While the material in Chapters 15 and 16 is not unrelated to the issues on nursing practice discussed in Chapters 4 to 14, the data concerning the nurse practitioner did not lend themselves to an identical analysis as those on nursing practice; hence, they are cited here separately. The content on job satisfactions and dissatisfactions, on additional freedom of nursing practice, and on educational tools for nurses who endeavor to work more effectively with geriatric patients is analyzed in terms of priorities. Hopefully this material will provide some further challenge to individual nurses and to the profession for raising work standards and enhancing the field of geriatrics as a nursing speciality of merit.

Treatment of Aged Patients:
Adult or Childlike

For they say that an old man is twice a child.
SHAKESPEARE

The relationship that is established between nurse and patient is a primary element in patient care. This is no less true when the patient is old and the nurse is young. Indeed, a wide difference in age may have significant effects upon a patient's care, especially when reinforced by folklore idioms such as "once a man and twice a child."

Furthermore, nursing assistants make up much the largest proportion of nursing personnel in long-term care institutions, and it has been said that no one is quite as close to the patient in a nursing home as is the nurse aide—a rather sobering thought. Registered nurses are apt to number exceedingly few, and they usually occupy supervisory or administrative positions. Licensed practical nurses, on the other hand, may be either assigned to a leadership position, such as being in charge of a floor, or to giving direct patient care.

In view of this it would seem pertinent to inquire how nursing personnel regard their elderly patients. What is the nurse's approach when she talks with her patients? What is her behavior when attending them? Do nurses differentiate in their care and treatment on the basis of whether the patient exhibits regressive traits or is mentally alert and keen? Is there a widespread belief among nursing personnel that "childlike" patient behavior warrants childlike treatment? What effect does a professional nurse's insight into an elderly patient's condition and situation have on her attitude and behavior toward him, and to what extent, if any, is this communicated to the staff who is directly involved with the patient's care?

This is an important issue, for there is little doubt that a nurse's treatment and care of a patient reflects the attitude she holds toward him as a person. This is also a controversial issue, as is revealed by the four ranks of nursing personnel who addressed themselves to it: nurse aides, licensed practical nurses, registered nurses, and degree registered nurses.

THE NURSES' IMAGE OF GERIATRIC PATIENTS

The nurse practitioners who were interviewed often were quite candid in asserting that a person who lives much beyond the proverbial three-score-years-and-ten will, to a varying extent, exhibit characteristics reminiscent of childhood behavior. At the same time many of them stressed that chronological age is not the only cause for regression: one person may at the age of 70 exhibit childlike traits whereas another may remain remarkably keen at the age of 90.

Indeed, many individuals of venerable age live creative and fulfilling lives and go to their graves relatively free of regressive tendencies. Even the most superficial search for individuals who, though no longer young in years, lead productive lives reveals many illustrious names—consider de Gaulle, Pablo Casals, Marianne Moore, Stokowski, and Pope Paul. History tells of remarkable endeavors and achievements of men such as Churchill, who at the age of 81 won his last electoral victory in England; Adenauer, who at the age of 73 was elected Chancellor of the German Federal Republic, a post he held until he was 87; the sixteenth-century Italian, Michelangelo, who completed some of his finest masterpieces in painting and in sculpture when, chronologically speaking, he was already an old man; and on the American scene, Robert Frost, the poet, and Grandma Moses, who won fame with her paintings in her old age.

Many persons of advanced age, however, suffer mental deterioration, with the result that the individual may become confused and disoriented. These patients, some of whom remain in relatively good physical health, are apt to become increasingly dependent upon others for their daily needs. Often they are quite apathetic and withdrawn—they are the "quiet ones." To illustrate:

> It was lunch time when the nursing home administrator showed the visitor about the premises. The Home was attractively furnished, light and airy, with large windows overlooking well-kept lawns and beautiful old trees.
>
> In one corner of the dining room, seven people were seated around a table. The group included a former university professor and a former scientist of some renown. Each one seemed preoccupied with the task before him or her—eating with a teaspoon—and not a word passed among them. In front of each patient was a dinner plate containing finely chopped meat, mashed potatoes, and a pureed vegetable. The table was devoid of any other tableware. The administrator stopped momentarily at the table and, turning to the visitor, she commented, "See how well they are eating—like well-behaved children."

How much of this was understood by the persons about whom this remark was made, and how they and the other residents in the dining room—who could not help but overhear—reacted inwardly, remains a moot question.

Childlike behavior is variously interpreted, and regressive character- istics are seen as differing both in degree and kind, ranging from extremes of selfishness, with jealousy, pouting, sulking, and temper tantrums, to al- most complete passivity, accompanied by disorientation and excessive de- pendence upon others for almost every need, physical and psychosocial. These needs may include feeding, bathing, dressing, and protection from environmental dangers on the one hand, and a need for loving, humoring, and emotional support in countless ways on the other.

Nurses expressed diverse opinions concerning possible causes of re- gressive or childlike behavior. Some attributed such traits largely to men- tal deterioration, but others reported their prevalence also among elderly patients who are lucid and alert. The belief was voiced, moreover, that unmet emotional needs, such as the need for recognition, respect, love, and cravings for a sense of security and human worth constitutes a threat to the wellbeing of elderly persons. Any deprivation of these needs was seen as possibly hastening, even being a major cause of, regressive be- havior. The claim was also made—and there is considerable supportive evidence in the literature—that abrupt changes in the environment often precipitate such behavioral changes in the elderly. Nurses reported in- creased regression in situations where an aged person had been moved from a warm and secure environment, such as a harmonious family setting, to an institution ill suited to his needs and wants; or from one institution to another, where the patient found himself once more in an unfamiliar, and what was for him a nonsupportive situation. Conversely, when the change involved a patient's move from a nonsupportive situation to an environ- ment where he felt treated with warmth and respect and as a person of human worth, positive behavioral changes were noted, such as increased lucidity, restored continency, and renewed participation. Involving pa- tients in useful activity also was cited as an important element in bringing about positive changes in an elderly person's behavior.

Other relevant factors on the issue under discussion include certain characteristics associated with aging, as well as some particularities based on individual differences that are unrelated to age or aging. Thus, some nurses suggested that the elderly as a group may be more sensitive in some ways, and less so in others, than are persons who are younger, including children. Others pointed to the fact that the threshold of pain varies among individuals regardless of age. For example, a positively firm grip on the arm of a hesitant or faltering child may be overly firm for an aged hesitant or faltering person—and may have an entirely different effect, physically and psychologically, than would the hold on the child. It was further suggested that many elderly individuals are extremely sensitive concerning attitudes of others toward them, particularly in situations where they are no longer in control. Consequently, a nurse may be adding insult to injury by admonishing or shaming an elderly person who no longer has complete bladder or bowel control and wets or soils his clothes or bedlinens.

Elderly patients exhibiting pronounced regressive traits often are referred to by staff as *senile,* and the care of senile patients is considered by many of these nurses as the most difficult and disagreeable part of geriatric nursing. A director of nursing commented, "this is the hardest part. It is sad and tragic to see a person reduced to the level where there is little or no understanding left—where the personality is all but gone." A supervising nurse in another geriatric facility, however, declared that she finds all of geriatric nursing a tremendous challenge for "one has to apply all one has ever learned, as a nurse and as a person." And a nurse aide explained simply, "I am here because my children no longer need me. These [the aged patients] are now my children—they need me and I need them." Then she added that her elderly patients are a great deal more appreciative than a child.

There was considerable agreement, however, that it takes a great deal of personal motivation, patience, understanding, and fortitude to care for the aged ill, especially those with pronounced regressive characteristics, but that there are, nevertheless, the lighter moments—with some laughter and gaity—and many occasions for gratifying experiences.

INTERPRETATION OF CHILDLIKE TREATMENT

In contrast to the seemingly widespread agreement on the existence of regressive or childlike behavior in many persons of advanced age, the idea that nursing personnel resort to childlike treatment of their elderly patients appeared a point of controversy in all four ranks of nurses, particularly among the three groups of geriatric nurse practitioners—with certain confusing or ambiguous statements being made. From analysis of responses to the question of treating aged patients like children, the issue was certainly viewed as complex, very delicate, and frequently weighted with strong emotion. While nursing personnel of the four categories were ready to admit or even assert that the aged ill often take on childlike characteristics, to treat them as one would a child appeared to many of them a very dubious or objectionable practice. On occasion a defensive attitude came to the fore, or open resentment was expressed at the suggestion that any nurse would treat her elderly patients like children. It was alleged, also, that some aged patients strongly resent being considered as children, and several nurses related instances where elderly patients had registered complaints concerning childlike practices which they felt had been meted out to them by staff.

Furthermore, nurses were openly critical of co-workers or associates who resort to, even rely upon, childlike treatment when caring for elderly patients, and numerous instances of such practices were related. A degree registered nurse noted that while searching the literature, she had found almost no reference on the treatment of the aged ill as children, but that she had observed the practice during her many years of nursing; and she cited practices such as scolding patients for incontinence and diapering them with an attitude that carried degrading connotations which appeared to surpass in effects any merit that might have been anticipated. Others related similar experiences.

Several degree registered nurses suggested that nurses who engage in childlike treatment of the aged ill search within themselves for some of the reasons why they would resort to or rely upon such practices, or condone them on the part of their staff. One DRN proposed that a nurse examine her reasons for treating an older adult patient as a child, especially her subconscious motivations for it, and that she consider seriously whether she has failed to understand the real needs of the patient. Another raised the question whether resort to childlike treatment might be some indication of the inability of the nurse to deal with aged ill persons professionally.

The issue was further compounded by the differing opinions that were expressed on the meaning of "treating as children," reflecting perhaps the nurses' own background and culture with respect to child-rearing practices. To some it meant directing their patients—by persuasion, encouragement, and rewards when one can—and controlling them—by command, scolding, threats, or deprivations when one must. Others interpreted childlike treatment in a more positive and supportive sense. To them it meant encouraging patients to do for themselves whatever they can without excessive frustration or exhaustive effort, and then lending a helping hand or making suggestions—supporting them physically and psychologically in whatever they tried and failed.

Still others distinguished between tasks that need to be done and the attitude with which it is accomplished. A particular need of an aged ill person may be the same as that of a child (such as help with bathing, dressing, and feeding), but in attending to that need one must always remember that the patient is an adult whose self-reliance and self-respect are constantly threatened and ever need safeguarding. Again, limits may need to be set for his safety, but this should be done in a kindly manner. With a disoriented patient, the nurse may need to be directive, but this can be accomplished without having the patient feel any loss of dignity. It was pointed out again and again that, while a nurse may need to do things for an elderly patient as though he were a child, she must never forget that he is an adult and accord him the respect his years demand. These nurses found the idea of staff inflicting any physical or psychological hurt on their patients unacceptable and deplorable.

Behaviors that are related to the issue under discussion, yet appear to belong in a somewhat different category than the interpretations given above, include such practices as addressing elderly persons in casual or familiar terms, lavishing effusive affections on them, and dolling them up in childish attire.

Nurses and aides who engage in these practices defend them on the basis that the aged ill crave, and thrive on, such direct expressions of love and affection. Others frown upon such treatment but condone it because, as several RN's explained, some of their patients seem to enjoy the extra attention, and their aides seem to derive satisfaction from giving it. Still others, however, criticize and deplore conduct of this sort. According to these critics, such treatment perpetuates the concept of "once a man and twice a child" and, as is true of all practices connoting childlike treatment, encourages further dependency and promotes regressive behavior. In the words of a nursing supervisor, "Such practices undo what some of us try so hard to accomplish—to reach the mature person in our patients—to maintain an adult relationship with them.

AGED PATIENTS TREATED LIKE CHILDREN

The foregoing discussion attests to the variety of responses to the question on childlike treatment of aged patients on the part of the four ranks of nursing personnel. Their judgments and comments will be reviewed in terms of 1) an affirmative position, which indicates that aged ill persons should be treated like children; 2) a conditional position, which precludes a categorical answer and emphasizes that each individual is different and each situation unique, and that both must be evaluated before a care plan can be decided upon; and 3) a negative position, which holds that aged persons should never be treated like children.

A small proportion of the nursing personnel—mainly nurse aides—subscribed to treating aged patients like children; as one moves up the ranks from nurse aide to degree registered nurses, the proportion diminishes considerably.*

* NA's, 21.5 percent; LPN's, 9.4 percent; RN's, 6.2 percent; DRN's, 2.2 percent. See Appendix B, Table 1, Items 1 to 3.
NOTE: Statistical tests of "significance" were not used since each group of nurse informants was "handpicked"—not for representation of geriatric nursing, but as concrete instances and ideals in the improvement of patient care for the aged ill.

Of the *nurse aides* interviewed, one in five saw little difference between caring for an aged person and caring for a young child. According to them, childlike behavior calls for childlike treatment, no matter what the age. They explained that elderly patients often have to be taken by the hand and led, be coaxed to eat, and at times even be spoon-fed like children. Moreover, some of them indicated that aged patients need to be treated with firmness, and at times scolded. If, for example, a patient refuses to bathe, he may be told that unless he complies he will not be permitted to see his relatives when they visit. Rewards, such as candy, may be promised in order to secure a patient's cooperation. Some aged patients, especially those who are senile or very aged, are said to act not only like children, but like infants, and they must be "talked to like babies" in order to have them understand what is being said to them.

Some nurse aides enjoy dressing their patients up, much like dressing a child in his Sunday best—selecting the clothes a patient is to wear and tying bright ribbons in a patient's hair. They make a practice of addressing their patients by their first name, though this is not necessarily on a reciprocal basis. Pet names and endearing terms such as "dearie," and "honey" are widely used. They kiss their patients "good-bye" or "good-night" when completing their tour of duty and admonish them to be "good children" or to "behave" themselves until they, the aides, return to care for them. Their explanation is that their aged patients need and thrive on such direct expressions of affection; they want to be wanted. One nurse aide concluded:

> Yes, they must be treated like children. They behave like children—are dependent, need help with feeding and such. You must say very simple things, for in their use of words, many of them are like 2-year-olds. There is one difference, however. A child can be trained, but old people are set in their ways—still you talk to them as you would to a child. You must be kind but firm with them. You must treat them like children—it is the only way to handle them.

Of the *licensed practical nurses,* about one in ten admitted that they treat their elderly patients like children. Some of them stressed that the aged are often argumentative and need to be treated with firmness in order to quiet them. "You must let them know that you mean what you say, because often they cannot see where they are wrong." Other LPN's reported that they resort to small bribes or flattery. For example, if a patient has been refusing to take his medicine, he may be told that unless he does so, he won't be shaved. Another may be offered a piece of candy to prompt him to eat his dinner.

Registered nurses who believe in treating their aged patients like children constitute an even smaller proportion as compared with the nurse aides and licensed practical nurses. These RN's claimed that most aged patients love being treated like children, as it gives them extra attention which they crave. They enjoy having their hair combed, being helped with dressing, and having their bread buttered and meat cut at table, even though they are capable of doing these tasks themselves. It is said, also, that many elderly patients like to be called by their first names and with a variety of endearing terms, since this gives them a feeling of closeness and being wanted. But one RN cautioned that the more "intelligent" patients insist upon being addressed by their last names. One of these RN's commented:

> To the extent that they need to be told what to do, they need to be treated like children—the mentally alert and the confused alike. They behave like children and you must be firm with them as with a child; but only with those who are mentally impaired. With the confused you get more cooperation if you talk with them as you would with a small child—but you must be gentle and go along with their thinking.

The few *degree registered nurses* who took an affirmative position did so with some qualification. They supported the idea that certain patients do need to be treated with firmness, and some with extra affection, like children, depending upon the degree of regression. These sentiments were based upon the following premises, as expressed by one of them:

> Patients should be treated like children if they exhibit behavior indicating childlike patterns. For example, possession of some simple object may be of great significance to them. It is like a child with a favorite toy. Let the patient have the object. He may be associating it with some feeling of security in the past.

TREATMENT CONDITIONAL TO THE INDIVIDUAL SITUATION

As indicated above, those who believe that aged patients should be treated like children constitute a small minority of the nursing personnel. An opposite view was taken by a large majority of their co-workers, whose general position was that under no circumstances should a nurse treat an aged patient like a child. Another group, to be considered now, took an in-between position. This latter group supported the idea that neither an affirmative nor a negative decision should be made; that individual and situational differences abound; and that each patient must be considered in terms of the various factors involved.*

---

* NA's, 37.2 percent; LPN's, 15.1 percent; RN's, 24.7 percent; DRN's, 12.6 percent. See Appendix B, Table 1, Items 4 to 6.

The factors this group considered relevant include the personality of the patient, his background, education, life pattern, particular handicaps, state of mental health, and any physical and emotional debilities associated with growing old. There were also suggestions that any decision to play up to a patient's regressive behavior should be reached in a joint team or staff session and become part of the nursing plan for that particular patient.

Of the *nurse aides,* more than a third indicated that their approach to a particular patient is determined by his behavior. If a patient is extremely jealous or stubborn, requires help with dressing, must be coaxed to eat, and is persistently incontinent, he is treated like a child. Such treatment may run the gamut from humoring, pampering, pleading, teasing, hugging and kissing, talking baby talk, to rewarding and bribing, ridiculing, and threatening. If, on the other hand, a patient "acts his age," he is met on an adult level. One NA who was caring for two roommates claimed that she treats one of them like a child, the other as an adult. The one patient is bathed, dressed, diapered, and fed, and she talks baby talk to her—"this is the only way she understands." The other patient is able to care for herself to a large extent. She is treated on an adult basis—"I talk with her as I do with my mother." Furthermore, "she would not stand for being talked to as though she were a child."

The comments of other NA's, however, reveal more perceptivity and insight. One aide who finds each situation different, and who believes that some patients need to be treated like children, hastened to add that she treats all of her patients as human beings. For her, the important consideration is to be kind and understanding, and she stressed that each person has his dignity—"and that includes children as well as aged persons."

Licensed practical nurses who claimed that one cannot generalize asserted that the right decision lies in each particular situation which must be reviewed in detail and with understanding before one's approach can be determined. They expressed little doubt, however, that there are times when aged patients must be treated like children—and some even like babies—in order to handle them.

Registered nurses who took the conditional position on the question of treating aged patients like children, asserted that broad generalizations are unreliable and that each individual in his situation is unique and must be evaluated. They stressed consideration of such factors as personality differences, degrees of mental deterioration, aging effects on the particular patient and his family, and regressive traits, whether physical or psychological, or both.

Several RN's contended that each person-situation is different. One must observe, listen, try to decide, and then act accordingly. And always, one must remember the patients' adulthood, the persons they once were:

they had lives of their own—they have memories. A nurse has to deal with the patient's past experiences, and approach each one differently. Some are just tired, some have sustained brain damage and are incapable. They find their infirmities hard to take. The nurse should not try to force anything on them, but do things their way as much as possible—let them make their own decisions, for this is important.

These nurses pointed out that the basic personality stays with a patient regardless of age, but during senescence personal traits become exaggerated. Each patient should be listened to and treated accordingly:

> One person here constantly fondles a stuffed animal—it means a tie with his sister. Another carries a doll which she brought with her when she was admitted to the home. No one is going to reverse her senility; the doll gives her comfort, and she becomes almost violent when someone tries to take it from her. Another patient, almost 100 years old, fusses over a doll the staff gave her, but she is not silly with it; she realizes it is a doll. It is all very individual. What works with one may not work with another. Treat them as adultlike as the situation permits.

The relatively few *degree registered nurses* who declared that one cannot generalize on treating the aged ill like children also maintained that one's approach depends upon the particular individual and his special situation; that the nurse must be sensitive to the personality and the needs of her patient and take her cues from him; and that getting to know and understand the patient is really the first step toward deciding upon a course of action. However, in her relationship with him, there should be no doubt left in anyone's mind as to the nurse's respect for the patient as a person and the dignity which is the right of any individual:

> To 'treat like children' depends on what this quote means. As a quality of respect is equally important to a child as to the aged, its application to behavior at either age is appropriate. A child who is incontinent is usually embarrassed, and likewise the aged person has similar feelings if this occurs. Understanding of the person's feelings would be the thing that would determine the approach. (Steffen) *

MAINTAINING AN ADULT RELATIONSHIP

By far the largest proportion of nurses held that the aged ill should be treated on an adult basis.† Their general position is that *under no*

---

* See Appendix D, p. 358 for list of degree registered nurses.
† NA's, 40.2 percent; LPN's, 73.6 percent; RN's, 67.9 percent; DRN's, 84.2 percent. See Appendix B, Table 1, Items 7 and 8.

circumstances should an aged person be treated like a child. "What an affront to humanity!"

These nurses emphasize that aged persons deserve to be treated on an adult level, and that they respond better on the whole when they are accorded the dignity and respect that is their due. "It is their right and our responsibility," according to one of these nurses. Their thesis is that aging into senescence and illness take a heavy toll on patients. An elderly person may find that his world has shrunk, physically and mentally. He lives from day to day, thinks and talks of the past, shows little concern about the future, has no interest in current events unless they touch him directly, and loses his purpose and zest in life. Such a situation calls for genuine and purposeful interest in the patient as the person he once was, with special effort to learn about him, his makeup and life pattern, and what and how much is left of all this. They asserted also that therapeutic results are more likely to ensue for almost any aged patient who is treated as an adult instead of as a child.

Nurse aides who deplored and denied treating any of their aged patients like children made a good case for treating them with special kindness, affection, understanding, and respect—much as one would give one's elderly parents. The fact that a person is senile and more or less out of contact with reality does not diminish this obligation. The senescent person is dependent upon others and needs the kind of help that he once gave to his helpless offspring. He is an adult and must be approached on an adult level. "You take care not to demean them, no matter how their behavior appears." Good nursing means that the staff stand by, encourage, and direct the patients in activities of daily living—such as dressing, shaving, tidying up, eating—doing with them or for them the things that they would do for themselves, were they still able to accomplish them. But judgment needs to be exercised every step of the way, and it behooves staff to work closely with the patient, encouraging independence and self-help wherever any possibilities are left. If, for example, a patient is capable of selecting the clothes that he may wear, or can with help slip his arm into a garment held for him, he should be permitted, even encouraged, to do so.

But, several NA's cautioned that the time factor has to be considered because other patients also need care. When there is a shortage of help, one may have to do things *for* the patient in order to get on with the work, even if it would be better for him, physically and psychologically, to be given only whatever help he actually needs.

Special pains must be taken not to hurry in assisting elderly patients. Old age has slowed their pace; they resent being hurried or pushed, and overt haste in helping them may be self-defeating:

> Recently one of our patients was looking forward to attending a religious service in the chapel. The assisting staff member tried to hurry him and also began doing things for the patient, which he strongly resented. He became so upset that he refused to attend the service. His mood was affected for the rest of the day, which made caring for him much more difficult.

Of the *licensed practical nurses* interviewed, two out of three declared that it is demeaning and wrong to treat an aged ill person as one would a child. According to them, aged persons must be treated with dignity and respect, regardless of any childlike tendencies they may exhibit. Treatment on an adult level is imperative because this involves a question of human worth, and also because it has therapeutic value. An elderly person clings to a sense of self-identity and dignity, which one must be careful not to destroy. Moreover, aged patients do not like to be treated like children, and often resent childlike practices. Some of them come from fine homes and families, had positions of status and power, and were accorded respect. "A sense of culture and refinement stays with them, even if they become senile."

Staff should never talk *about* patients in their presence, but should include them in whatever is said, and with their personal interest in mind. Aged patients should not be made to do things, mimicked, subjected to ridicule, or pushed around. They should not be scolded or coaxed, but should be spoken to calmly and gently. They should have things explained to them before a treatment or a procedure is begun, and be informed of what may be expected at each step. For example, in applying alcohol to the skin before an injection, one should explain that it will feel cold for a moment. A patient should not be reprimanded for his previous refusal to cooperate when a nurse comes back a second time to give him his overdue medicine. Patients are apt to be more relaxed when the nurses go calmly about their tasks. "Getting patients upset usually can be avoided."

Some therapeutic results are likely to ensue for almost any elderly patient who is treated as an adult rather than as a child. If he is not treated as an adult, he may regress even further than he already has. Incontinence may worsen, for example, if an insensitive staff member shows harsh disapproval by severely scolding a patient for wetting his bed. According to one LPN, "If you treat an aged person as an adult, with respect, kindness, and understanding, and have patience with him, he may again behave like an adult—I have seen this happen." Another summed up her position this way:

> With a child, there is a person who is growing up. You teach him and he *learns for the future*. With an elderly patient you don't put as much for the future in what is being done. With him, it is kindness and understanding that is needed, and respect for him as a person in the present or for the person that he once was.

Of the *registered nurses,* more than two thirds objected to the idea that the aged ill be treated like children. Speaking with compassion of those who are no longer lucid or in control of themselves, these nurses supported the position that, regardless of regressive tendencies, it is far better to treat the aged ill on an adult level. They also were critical of their co-workers who treat elderly patients like children.

While acknowledging that persons of advanced age may be losing their mental capacities and the long-established disciplines in their lives, these nurses asserted that it helps no one to call them belittling names and to forget that they are adults with records of achievements that frequently surpass those of the nurses attending them. It is better to reach out to the adulthood still left in them and to treat them like the gentlemen or gentlewomen they once were and now relive in their memories. Any kind of derogation is considered inexcusable. To illustrate:

> An aged physician seemed to find it difficult to adjust to the nursing home to which he had recently been admitted. He was withdrawn, ate poorly, and exhibited a negative attitude in general. The patient's son expressed concern about his father's behavior which he said was very different from what it had been before he entered the institution. The patient voiced no complaints. When after some weeks the director of nursing looked into the situation, it was learned that an orderly was habitually addressing this elderly gentleman as "Pop," which he deeply resented.

The aged ill find their infirmities hard to take. Some are weary and worn out; others have been neglected and all but forgotten, beaten down into the role of "the quiet ones" by circumstances beyond their control; others have mental impairment and are almost totally incapable of helping themselves. "What is to be gained by forcing them down to a level beyond their pride and dignity?" asked one RN who summed up her position as follows:

> Don't treat them like children, whatever you do. As human beings we all have early-established traits that don't leave us—but *we* cover them up more than those who are old. Remember their adulthood and try to meet them on their maximum level as a person. We must go beyond their external behavior to get anywhere with them, though this is hard to do at times, especially when a patient is depressed or full of complaints. Let us not forget for a moment that they have had lives

of their own; attempt to reach them through their experiences, and try to rebuild in our own minds the kind of person that they once were.

We cannot afford to ignore or dispose of their interim years.

Another RN commented:

> They are not like children—a child does not know what his future is, but the old do. I hear them mention death often and they talk about this nursing home as being their last place. Their own home is gone and *this place* is not what they had planned or hoped for for the rounding off of their lives. Again and again they will say, "I should have died long ago."

The *degree registered nurses* in positions of leadership who addressed themselves to this question were the most vocal of all four nursing ranks in protesting the idea that the aged ill be treated like children. Commenting in considerable detail on the meaning of "treating like a child," they elaborated upon the diverse aspects and connotations involved in the term. Distinctions were made between dependency needs of elderly patients and the condescending attitude with which these needs are often met. The importance of providing means for keeping the aged person in touch with reality was stressed, as was respect for the individual, whether child or octogenarian. It was also implied that the professional nurse's attitude and actions—indeed her whole approach—should be toward effecting possible therapeutic results within a setting supporting such a relationship:

> If by treating aged patients like children is meant "talking down" to them, it is never justified. But providing bodily contact to a frightened patient, as one would to a frightened child, may sometimes be a supporting communication.
> I think of a woman dying of lung cancer who coughed until she had not the strength to cough again. And the only way I knew to provide some comfort in such a coughing spell—when drugs are ineffective—was to sit next to her on the edge of the bed and "splint" her chest with my arms around her as one supports with one's hands the chest of a child with whooping cough. With tears in her eyes she finally spoke—not of the reduction of pain provided by the splinting—but of the fact that no one had put an arm around her for many years and that it gave her a feeling she had not hoped to have again. (Schwartz)

All activity and communication that may promote regressive behavior is frowned upon, it being the responsibility of the nursing staff to bring the patient back to reality, even if he is mentally impaired. "If his only sense of reality comes through cuddling a doll, then this doll is *his reality* and a form of therapy in maintaining him at his highest level." If a patient is in a state of dependency that requires the almost total care that would be given to a small child, then the nurse tries to meet these needs in a way that does not degrade a person's self-esteem as an adult with creditable accomplishments in his background.

Regardless of the presence of regressive traits, treating aged patients like small dependent children is to be deplored and opposed. Such treatment is viewed as adding insult to injury, being an offense to one's esteem as an adult, and doing no one any special good. Indeed, it tends further to promote the regressive traits themselves, makes for increased dependency, destroys self-reliance, intensifies false feelings of helplessness, and mars as well as undermines any remaining sense of strength, power, and adult dignity. Moreover, it casts a blemish on the image of the nurse, magnifying an authoritarian role on her part and interfering with her goals of returning the patient to some degree of independent wellness; it is entirely unbecoming to her as a professional.

A Catholic Sister put the matter this way:

> I have a strong feeling that many patients' dependency needs can be met by the nurse by being well-mannered and courteous. This kind of idea may lie behind the fact that although I can put on my coat without a gentleman's assistance, even do it with more ease, and I can adjust my chair when sitting down to table—when a gentleman helps with these things graciously, evidencing a sincere interest in me as a lady, then I respond more as a lady. (Kerrigan)

Comments another Sister:

> It is most unbecoming for nurses to treat aged patients like children. The keen observer may read in the wrinkled face a reflection of painful annoyance when his self-image and self-respect receive the blow. . . . Not only the mentally clear, but also the partially confused geriatric patient may feel deeply hurt by such treatment. (Frenay)

Discussion

Any axiom connoting the concept of "once an adult twice a child" suggests a critical issue in geriatric care. The nurses in all four ranks manifested a like-mindness on the meaning of the term "childlike behavior" and its presence in most aged persons who linger long in their decrepitude; but they differed sharply concerning the meaning implied in "childlike treatment" of elderly patients and, also, in their proposals for the application of such treatment in rendering care to them.

The question of nurses treating aged patients like children appears to be both a critical and controversial issue and one that needs more concerted attention. The person who is ill or infirm is, to a greater or lesser degree, dependent upon others for his basic needs and wants. The often degrading and second-class status which the elderly are accorded in our society, coupled with the enforced dependence upon others, tends to undermine the dignity of the individual; this situation becomes magnified even further when those who extend whatever help is needed accord him little or no respect. Further studies would seem to be called for if we are to become more fully aware of the extent and seriousness of the problem and what can be done about it.

It is often said that Americans venerate the young and tolerate the old. In a youth-oriented culture such as ours the aged and infirm are all too often placed in institutions and more or less forgotten. Government and private organizations are beginning to attempt to cope with this problem more realistically, but major changes are required in order to better meet both the fundamental and instrumental needs and wants of elderly Americans, and especially those who are ill or infirm. Furthermore, a philosophy would need to be developed which sees all segments of our population—the young as well as the old—as being mutually supportive and as individuals of human worth. Some of the nurses pointedly raised the question of whether it is too much to ask that a small share of the veneration, economic resources, and supportive care expended upon the youth of America go to the aged who are no longer able to fend for themselves? And one of these nurses categorically stated that the image of the elderly in our culture as useless and spent individuals and as second-class citizens will need to change substantially before the nursing care of geriatric patients can reach high standards of genuine compassion and quality service.

SUMMARY

Three major positions on the issue of childlike treatment of geriatric patients emerged from these findings: 1) Aged patients should be treated like children for they behave like children; 2) the decision would depend upon circumstances and the kind of patient involved; 3) under no circumstances should an aged patient be treated like a child. The relative proportions of nurse respondents and the percentages represented by the positions they take is reflected for each type of nursing rank in the following figures:

	NA's %	LPN's %	RN's %	DRN's %
Affirmative position	21.5	9.4	6.2	2.2
Conditional position	37.2	15.1	24.7	12.6
Negative position	40.2	73.6	67.9	84.2

A comparatively small proportion of the nursing personnel subscribed, in a sense, to treating aged patients like children; and most of these were nurse aides, of whom about 1 in 5 took the affirmative stand on this issue. As one moves up through the nursing ranks, there is a progressive decline in representation. The justifications for treating aged patients like children, whenever any were given, are for the purpose of making them feel wanted and of gaining their cooperation. Others supported the childlike treatment proposal without explanation other than, "As you find them so you treat them." Here are the figures on the affirmative position:

	NA's %	LPN's %	RN's %	DRN's %
Treating aged patients like children is a means of making them feel wanted	0.0	1.9	1.2	1.1
Treating them like children is a means of gaining their cooperation	7.8	0.0	2.5	0.0
They behave like children and hence must be treated like children	13.7	7.5	2.5	1.1

Nurses who were disinclined to commit themselves to a generalized course of action and declared that the approach depends upon the particular circumstances and the kind of patient involved, also reached the highest proportion among the NA's and the lowest among the DRN's. The conditioning factor most often cited was the mental health of the patient:

	NA's %	LPN's %	RN's %	DRN's %
A nurse's approach concerning childlike treatment would depend upon the patient's state of mental health	32.3	11.3	21.0	6.3
Deciding factors would depend on the patient's background and personality	4.9	3.8	3.7	4.2
Personality of staff is a factor	0.0	0.0	0.0	2.1

On the negative side, the proportion of nursing personnel disclaiming or protesting the childlike treatment of aged patients reached a pronounced majority in all nursing ranks except the NA's. Disclaimers among the DRN's constitute more than 4 out of 5. Respondents who repudiated the idea of childlike treatment of aged patients did so by either an emphatic denial or by adamantly stressing that aged patients be accorded the respect and dignity that they deserve. The figures on the negative position are as follows:

	NA's %	LPN's %	RN's %	DRN's %
Aged patients should never be treated like children	7.8	0.0	12.3	77.9
They should be treated with respect and dignity	32.4	73.6	55.6	6.3

It seems apparent from the statistical information that all four ranks of nursing personnel hold contrasting positions on the question of treating aged patients like children. The divided opinion can be said to be more equally balanced and perhaps more of a controversial subject among the nurse aides and least among the degree registered nurses, who overwhelmingly take the negative stance and who are followed more closely in their general position by the licensed practical nurses than by the registered nurses.

No meaningful correlations were possible on the different interpretations of childlike treatment by nursing personnel and endorsement of such treatment for geriatric patients. However, a perusal of the pertinent material reveals that relatively much larger proportions of the nurse aides and licensed practical nurses equate childlike treatment with rewards and punishment than do the registered and degree registered nurse groups, who interpreted such treatment in a more positive and supportive sense. Furthermore, a relatively high percentage (1 in 5 of the NA's and 1 in 10 of the LPN's) hold the affirmative position, claiming that their patients are, and should be, treated by them as though they were children. The fact that nurse aides and licensed practical nurses are, also, most directly involved in the care of geriatric patients suggests significance for those concerned with nursing care of the aged ill. Moreover, with almost 10 percent of the LPN's taking the affirmative position, it should be noted that, of the LPN's interviewed, more than half occupied charge or higher leadership positions in the geriatric institutions.

For full statistical details, see Appendix B, Table 1.

5 Humor in Nurse-Patient Relationships

Humor is the saving grace—there is but a frail line between misery and humor.
ORIGIN UNKNOWN

It is generally recognized that patient care can be enhanced by mutually trustful, responsive, and supportive nurse-patient relationships. Since an essential element in productive person-to-person verbal encounter is free and effective communication, and since humor is widely used in human relations, the question of its use in geriatric nurse-patient relations may well be considered.

Simmons (unpublished), who has collected data on humor and aging from many different primitive and historical cultures, found that humor played an important part in a great many, if not all, of them. He observed further that humor was initiated by comments from elderly members as often as it was by their younger associates within the group. Usually within these cultures, however, old age was an honorable state, and, also, rarely did an aged member linger long into decrepitude.

It is acknowledged that the effects of humor can reach extremes of not-too-veiled derogation on the one hand or a "saving grace" on the other; and the line of division between these two can, indeed, be frail.

Since the question of whether or not to use humor or jocularity in nurse-aged patient relations is not unlike the earlier issue of treating aged patients like children, these two topics were explored side by side. Even as the idea of treating aged patients like children brought about sharp differences in nursing opinion, so the question of utilizing humor aroused considerable controversy.

INTERPRETATIONS AND IMPLICATIONS

Diversity in nursing opinion was encountered also with respect to the meaning of the terms employed: kidding, joshing, humor, which were used interchangeably by the interviewer when the issue was explored with nursing home personnel. On the questionnaire mailed to the nurse leadership, no definitions were given.

A few nurses regarded humor and kidding or joshing the aged to be analogous to treating them like children; a few others questioned the equating of kidding and joshing with humor. Still others pointed to ambiguities contained within each of these terms which permit the user to construe them either in a positive, constructive way or in a negative, destructive manner. Nursing home personnel, however, would most often stress the positive and wholesome effects sought when using humor in the care of aged patients. Many of the degree registered nurses, on the other hand, emphasized the destructive effects when nursing staff resorts to the use of kidding and joshing.*

However, both the practitioners and the leadership group stressed that an important difference exists between saying or doing something with the intent of its being mutually amusing and in poking fun with someone as the target. It was also emphasized that with humor and banter carelessly bandied about, or when the nurse has insufficient rapport with, or knowledge of, the patient as a person, there exists real danger of misinterpretation by the patient and hurt to him, even though this humor may be expressed with the best intent on the part of the nurse.

The possible constructive effect of a lighthearted relationship or humorous encounter between nurse and patient is seen by many nurses to hinge upon numerous factors, such as that kidding with an aged patient must be done as one would with one's contemporary, the concept of equal status being important; the type of humor must be such that can be mutually enjoyed; and the nurse must consider the fact that among the infirmi-

---

* Following are the definitions of these terms as described in Webster's Dictionary:

Kidding: to deceive as a joke: fool; to make fun of: tease; to engage in good-humored fooling or teasing: joke;

Joshing: to make fun of: tease; to engage in banter: joke; a good-humored joke;

Humor: that quality which appeals to a sense of the ludicrous or absurdly incongruous; the mental faculty of discovering, expressing, or appreciating the ludicrous or absurdly incongruous; something that is or is designed to be comical or amusing.

ties of advanced age are slowed comprehension and reactions. The
patient, instead of enjoying a joke with the nurse, may feel left out and
become more acutely aware of his afflictions. Similarly, the elderly are
apt to be more sensitive than those who are younger, and sometimes suspicious as well; so that special care must be taken, lest the patient sense
sarcasm where none was intended.

Others who see pitfalls in the employment of kidding and joshing
with elderly patients point to the wide age gap which often exists between
nurse and geriatric patient and which they view as a distinct barrier to
entering upon a jocular relationship with the patient. Some of these
nurses suggested that kidding or joshing is a technique difficult to em-
ploy across lines of authority, and that it works best within a single
status group.

The implication would seem to be that the nurse who would embark
upon a lighthearted or jocular relationship with her aged patient should
be very circumspect or even wary; it would be far better to "err on the
side of sobriety" than to convey to the patient the idea that he is no
longer a person of human worth. A very few of the registered nurses, but
a relatively larger number of degree registered nurses contend that much
humor skirts misery; that it tends to carry hidden barbs; or that there is
always some potential threat to self-pride and dignity.

It was suggested that one must allow for individual differences not
only among aged patients, but among nursing staff as well; and that it is
essential to remain "true to oneself." Some nurses are not the "kidding
kind." According to one nurse, if a staff member is endowed with a jocular
nature that is characterized by kidding, then usually neither the patient
nor the staff member is traumatized; but for a staff member deliberately to
pursue a kidding approach would suggest certain deficiencies within
herself.

Practitioners as well as nurse leaders deplored any kind of kidding or
joshing which contains within it derogation of the patient. But certain
practitioners revealed, either directly or indirectly, that destructive kidding and joshing does occur. Thus, a licensed practical nurse commented
that one must be subtle with patients who are lucid because they are
quick to recognize when one is insincere—when "you are putting on."

Degree registered nurses repeatedly hinted, and at times openly
charged, that the reason for resorting to kidding with aged patients
might lie within the nurse herself. They cautioned against the use of
jocular relationships when it is mainly, or only, to relieve the nurse's own
discomfort over a situation; the nurse must be sure that she is not using
this to sidestep a problem that requires a more serious approach, even
when the patient welcomes and appears to enjoy the lighter talk. Others
bluntly suggested that a nurse may resort to the use of humor because she

is unable to cope on a professional level with the real needs and wants of the patient.

Finally, the geriatric nurse was admonished to examine her reasons for kidding and joshing—she should make sure that her use of humor is not an expression of hostility (as might be her reason for treating aged patients as though they were children): a method to thwart the patient in his endeavor to make his needs and wants known or a way of denying him the truth that he is seeking about his condition.

In contrast to those who would be adverse to humor, kidding, and joshing in nurse-patient relations in order that the dignity of, and respect for, the patient be preserved at all times, there were others who singled out the practice as an important means of bringing warmth and cheer to the aged ill. These nurses viewed the practice in a wholesome, constructive sense. "When humor is mutually enjoyed by patient and nurse, it can be a useful way of raising the patient's self-esteem and promote his overall comfort." The point was also made that kidding and joshing need not necessarily be therapeutic or purposive—advocating kidding for the sake of kidding.

Some practitioners saw the institutional setting at times as actually "calling for" humor and lightheartedness. According to them, humor can be a tool to relieve the inescapable monotony so often experienced in institutional milieus, and individual staff and patient may find humorous interchange a welcome relief from the monotony and tension that are concomitants of the many hours, days, weeks, even months or years, spent in close proximity. Some of them also pointed out that it need not be restricted to the individual nurse-patient encounter but that it may be as aptly employed in group situations. While recognizing many of the risks involved, there was considerable agreement within all four ranks of nursing personnel that the judicious use of humor can and does benefit many aged patients and staff members as well.

To what extent do nurses resort to, or recommend, the use of kidding, joshing, or humor in communicating with their elderly patients? The exploration of this issue revealed some close similarities between the nurse aides and licensed practical nurses on the one hand and between the registered and degree registered nurses on the other. Some sharp differences also appeared between the three practitioner groups and the nurse leadership, and others between the registered and the degree registered nurses.

ENDORSING THE USE OF HUMOR

Of the nurse practitioners, more than a third of each rank favored and indicated the use of humor in their interface relations with their elderly, and even seriously ill, patients. This contrasts quite sharply with the mere 7 percent of the degree registered nurses who supported the affirmative position.*

The *nurse aides* and *licensed practical nurses* who endorsed the use of humor with aged patients argue somewhat as follows. Every human being possesses a potential sense of humor, but background, personality, and the present mental state determine the kind of humor. Nearly all patients will respond favorably when the fun point is aptly and timely put. Nurses' use of humor should be relevant to the particular situation and to the patient's mental state. One may kid to good effect even patients who are confused or suffer mental impairments somewhat as one might with a child, for in a nursing home, the patients respond to just about any sort of attention—it perks them up and shows them that someone cares. Kidding and light humor help to put the patient in a better frame of mind or at least help him to get over something that is unpleasant or disagreeable. For some of these patients, kidding and a little joshing seems to work "better than all the medicine they take." An example was related by an LPN:

> One of our patients, Mrs. S., had a permanent colostomy, a condition she found most unpleasant and hard to live with. She complained of feeling unclean and was very reluctant to help take care of it. One day when Mrs. S. was particularly depressed, I said to her, "If Miss —— (a well-known theatrical personality) can go through life with a colostomy, so can you." That made her smile. She also seemed impressed when told that this actress had continued her career despite the colostomy. Thereafter, I would address Mrs. S. by the actress' name which she thought amusing. It never failed to bring a smile to her face, but even more important, she seemed to be more accepting of her condition. The idea of associating her name with that of a famous person must have been pleasing as well as amusing—it surely boosted her morale and made taking care of her much easier.

Others reported that a kidding relationship with their aged patients helps them to get their work done. One nurse aide commented:

---

* NA's, 39.7 percent; LPN's, 35.9 percent; RN's, 35.4 percent; DRN's, 7.1 percent. See Appendix B, Table 2, Items 1 to 3.

Many old people are selfish. With them it is often 'monkey see, monkey do.' When you get a glass of water for one of them, the others want one also. One day I said to a 95-year-old patient who kept asking for whatever the others had, 'If you keep this up, you will wind up an old maid.' She laughed lightly and retorted, 'Oh, worse things could happen to me.' For quite a while after that she was a little less demanding.

Another nurse aide contended that there are times when one can tease patients out of their depressions.

The *registered nurses* who held that humor has an important place in geriatric facilities expressed the belief that a real need exists for a light, cheerful, hopeful, and perhaps even playful spirit and atmosphere on the part of the staff in their relationships with patients; and that such qualities, along with deep personal commitment to the welfare of their patients, cannot help but make it easier for the patients to accept their infirmities. It also makes the work easier for the staff.

Mutual kidding and joshing are regarded as important means of bringing warmth and some cheer into the lives of the aged ill; it is a good way of letting them know that they are still loved and wanted. Some nurses also feel that kidding tends to get patients "out of themselves" when nothing else seems to accomplish this.

The following is a brief digest of RN views of those who attested to the value of humor in the nursing care of aged patients: You kid and josh with elderly patients mainly to convey to them that you love them and want, in an informal way, to reassure them. It gives them some extra attention, which they crave, and brings special warmth into their lonely lives. They realize that their health is failing; they feel themselves losing out in life—time is running out for them. They see their roles with their relatives regressing or being reversed; this increases their feelings of dependency, physically and emotionally, and they sense being abandoned in one way or another. Humor becomes a saving grace for many of them. They enjoy some jokes, like to laugh occasionally, love some kidding, and welcome young people around them, especially those who can give them a sense of closeness and belonging.

But kidding, banter, and fun-play must be done carefully, respectfully, and kindly. The nurse should always try to approach an elderly person with a smile, if possible, and watch the tone of her voice; for old people are quick to sense whether one is angry, fooling, or serious. Don't joke with them when they are really suffering or show any callousness toward them. Take special care to be as truthful as possible and try never to tell a very ill person, "Oh, things will be better soon," if you know that they won't. Almost all aged patients will respond to some form of humor when the situation is right; but the level of kidding differs, depending, among other things, on the patient's state of well-being and his capacity to comprehend and to retain the points in humor that are conveyed.

The relatively strong endorsement which the NA's, LPN's, and RN's gave to the idea that humor has an important place in geriatric nursing contrasts sharply with the mere 7 percent support of the *degree registered nurses*. Moreover, the DRN support seemed, in general, to be more qualified.

Those who took the affirmative position on the subject did so because humor may serve as a morale builder, put patients at ease, and promote relaxation. But they cautioned that kidding and joshing must be done in good taste and the tone must be right. Its success depends on good nurse-patient rapport. Under conditions such as these, "A little blandishment or foolish cajolery accomplishes far more than do commands and insistence."

OPPOSING THE USE OF HUMOR

Relatively much smaller numbers of the nurse aides and the licensed practical nurses opposed and deplored the use of humor in geriatric patient care than did the registered and degree registered nurses.

The difference in the relative strength with which each of the four categories of nursing personnel supported the affirmative position discussed above, and the negative stance being considered now, is noteworthy. Whereas the positive stand was taken by more than a third of each of the practitioner groups (NA's, LPN's, and RN's), but by less than 10 percent of the degree registered nurses, the negative position was endorsed by less than 10 percent of the NA and LPN groups but by approximately a quarter to a third of the RN and DRN groups.*

Not only were the *nurse aides* and the *licensed practical nurses* close in their negative representation, but they also expressed similar comments. A few in both ranks said that they never resort to the use of humor in relating to their aged patients. Some pronounced such behavior as undignified and disrespectful; and a very few remarked that such a practice could reflect unfavorably on both the patient and the nurse.

The *registered nurses* who rejected the use of humor in geriatric patient care agreed in general with one of their peers who had remarked, "I don't kid, its not professional." Others equated the practice with disrespect and lack of dignity. A few RN's claimed that kidding and joshing

---

* NA's, 6.8 percent; LPN's, 9.4 percent; RN's, 28.1 percent; DRN's, 33.6 percent. See Appendix B, Table 2, Items 4, 5.

cannot be of much help to patients and is likely to carry for them a touch of sarcasm or a sting to their pride and self-esteem. It was said also that staff members should look up to older persons and accord them the respect that is rightfully theirs.

The strongest disapproval of humor in nurse-aged patient relations was expressed by the *degree registered nurses.* Wrote one of them, "Never, never, never—what a question." The position of DRN's who strongly oppose kidding and joshing within a geriatric milieu is that any resort by the staff to humor is unacceptable in dealing with the aged ill. Some granted that it might be helpful for the nurse to possess a "saving sense of humor," but that all too often, when she uses it in face to face encounters with an aged patient, she does so—either wittingly or unwittingly—in a derogatory manner. They preferred that humor be ruled out of nurse-patient relations, and that dignity and respect toward the patient be preserved at all times. However, they considered a smile between nurse and patient to be in order, "since it makes certain conditions more bearable and no patient wants to see his nurse with a starched face."

Kidding, joshing, in fact any jocularity is viewed by these DRN's as indications that the staff may be incapable of coping effectively with the real needs of the aged ill on a professional level. Some, however, temper this implication with the idea that a bit of humor that arises spontaneously may be acceptable, but to pursue such an approach suggests "certain discrepancies" in the nurse herself.

The overriding concern of those who rejected the use of humor and of jocularity in geriatric patient care appears to be their professed respect for the aged ill and the desire that the patients' real needs be met, that the aged be regarded as of intrinsic worth, and that they be treated with the dignity that is their due.

CONDITIONAL ENDORSEMENT

A majority of the nurse respondents in all ranks except the registered nurses declined to make a clear-cut decision on the issue of humor and jocularity in geriatric nurse-patient relations. They considered it a perilous practice to generalize on the question and took the position that a judgment concerning the use of humor rests upon a number of factors and how these relate to each particular situation. Among such factors listed were: a patient's personality, background, previous pattern of life and his present state of mental and physical health; his ability to see and hear, the keenness of his reaction to external stimuli, and the length of his attention span. Included also were the nurse's sensitivity, her knowledge and tact, and the rapport that had been established between nurse and patient. All of these were considered critical bases upon which to decide whether or not to resort to the use of humor.*

Nurse aides and *licensed practical nurses* again expressed similar sentiments when qualifying their conditional stand. According to them one can joke and josh with more ease and greater safety with some aged persons than with others and it is usually not difficult to sense how a patient likes it or takes it. They thought most aged persons amenable to kidding, but they recognized that much depends on the mood of the patient. If, for example, a patient is bent on going home, and denied the opportunity, it is a poor time to kid with him. In the opinion of some of these nurses, more women than men enjoy kidding, and women particularly welcome being complimented. Others suggested that joking be geared to the mental level of the patient and associated with immediate events and surroundings, but that to some extent the use of humor nearly always depends on the particular individual. One nurse aide commented, "You are always dealing with individuals; you don't put people into typed groups—as for kidding, with some I do, with some I don't."

The purpose of humor and kidding according to these NA's and LPN's is to make patients forget what is on their minds, but they caution that one must always be sensitive to their moods. Sometimes when you joke with them, they will tell you, "That's not funny," or "Don't be so fresh." They find it hardest to joke with patients who are depressed and those who have lost their purpose in life and have nothing "to hang onto."

In addition to the ground rules mentioned above, the LPN's emphasized personal relations: the patient and the nurse must come to know and to trust each other before a wholesome joking relationship can be established. Some of them also mentioned good timing, expressing the caution that not just any time is propitious for kidding. According to these nurses there are times when the patients are sensitive to, and resent, laughter. At other times, they enjoy staff members being light-spirited and gay: then kidding cheers them up, brings the extra bits of sunshine into their lives, and makes them feel a little more wanted. And with a little coaxing, they cooperate in getting things done—even if they have previously been difficult to work with. But when a patient is critically ill, or is senile and does not understand, kidding may be neither right nor useful, and can even become cruel.

The *registered nurses* who contended that the question of kidding

---

* NA's, 53.3 percent; LPN's, 52.9 percent; RN's, 36.6 percent; DRN's 57.1 percent. See Appendix B, Table 2, Items 6, 7, 8.

with aged patients is conditional to the particular situation stressed how complex the issue can become. They seemed to feel strongly that the decision depends upon knowledge of the individual-situational context. Among the criteria cited by them for making a judgment were: information on the personality of the patient, his established pattern of life, and any predisposing experiences that have special meaning for him. These interests were followed by emphasis upon the patient's physical and mental condition, such as degree of physical debility and suffering, extent of brain damage, state of senility, and prevailing mood.

These RN's pointed out that it takes two to engage in kidding. Behaving in a jocular manner within situations of major illness and disability may greatly disturb the patient and, also, ill-fit the personality of the nurse. There are nurses who find it impossible to use humor effectively, especially in the face of suffering, just as there are patients who find themselves unable to reciprocate or appreciate it. Furthermore, in stressful situations it is much easier to offend and hurt by whimsicalities than to console and sustain the patient. Special importance was placed upon the ever-present need of the nurse to retain flexibility and to temper her mood and attitude to that of the sufferer. These RN's seemed to say that, "When in doubt about the use of humor, don't use it, unless it is introduced by the patient himself." However, they do not seem to deny or doubt that a judicious use of humor can serve the patient well as a supporting agent.

The *degree registered nurses* representing the conditional position expressed more caution and qualifications in their endorsement of the use of humor than did the other three groups. A major concern of these respondents also appeared to be whether or not resorting to humorous nurse-patient exchanges might be regarded as a professional compromise. In other words, these DRN's responded somewhat as though they were confronted with a possibly unpopular, but potentially practical proposal for the improvement of patient care for some of the aged ill.

To illustrate this apparent dilemma for the truly professional nurse, one DRN commented that the old folk-saying, "Every man to his own poison," seemed inappropriate within a therapeutic setting; however, the idea of bits of humor introduced into nurse-patient relations on the basis of individual differences is important. She went on to recognize that a person usually needs a feeling of security with himself, within his family, and in his relationship to this "world." With many patients, light and humorous nursing exchanges boost their sense of security, while others might be harmed by the same approach. (Shaffer) Another admitted freely that good-natured teasing can be pleasing and supportive to some, and perhaps most, patients, and cited a German proverb to the effect that "those who love each other, tease each other"; but she hastened to add that teasing is not to everyone's liking, and that some patients are hurt, rather than helped, by it. (Frenay) Still another DRN made the point that whether or not a patient can be kidded and joshed effectively depends upon an aged person's makeup and interest; but she cautioned that the nurse needs to be very sensitive and alert to a teased patient's hidden reactions, knowing well that "there is a time to josh and a time not to." She warned moreover, that joshing should not be overdone, lest the patient become wary and defensive, interpreting the nurse's jocularity as an indication that she does not really care to listen to his needs and wants. (Aiello) Several DRN's wondered whether joshing and kidding is ever quite appropriate unless mutually enjoyed by the josher and the joshed; and it was noted that ever so often humor starts out pleasantly but turns into pain for one or the other or both parties. Also, a few of them asserted that the use of humor as a policy on the part of a professional nurse might be challenged by certain of her colleagues and viewed by them as a lapse in, or substitute for, the full exercise of her professional skills and prerogatives.

According to the DRN's, justifying criteria for the relevance and value of touches of humor in geriatric nursing are discernible mainly in predisposing characteristics and circumstances associated with the immediate situation. A very few cited qualifications of the nurse(s) responsible for the care of the patient as criteria to be considered.

As reflected in a condensed summary of DRN statements on the subject, it was recommended that each patient be considered separately, in staff conference, if feasible, and within the context of an overall patient plan of care. They also cautioned that the use of humor is unlikely to be effective unless the nurse's rapport with, and knowledge of, the patient is sufficient for reliable appraisal of his welcome of, tolerance for, and potential gains out of, the playful give-and-take. It was held that the prospects can be viewed as more favorable where the use of humor has been an accustomed life-style in the patient's past. The resort to humor was believed to be safer and more strongly indicated when the initiative comes from the patient, and he sets the tone. Some reasoned persuasively for tentative feelers or tryouts, allowing the patient's reaction to be the guide. It was suggested that a certain levity in relationships can be maintained by references to former amusing incidents and bits of humor that patient and nurse have previously shared. Some DRN's cautioned that humor should not be used as a substitute to cover over or conceal from the patient the nurse's readiness to attempt to understand and face seriously with the patient any aspect of the gravity of his plight. In fact, geriatric nurses repeatedly were urged to beware of reliance on lighthearted or jocular relations to relieve the nurse's own discomfort over a disturbing issue or situation. A nurse can ill afford to use humor to sidestep problems that require a more serious approach. On the other hand, the same respondents cautioned against keeping the nurse-patient relationship on a continuous serious and sober plane, with, again, each situation requiring continuous appraisal in terms of the therapeutic goal. For instance, if kidding and joking creates misleading situations in which the patient escapes and stays out of touch with reality, the therapeutic effects could be worse than nil. Again, occasionally an aged patient will respond to the kidding by an attractive young nurse in ways that can "backfire" so disturbingly as often to prove detrimental. The risks of such unplanned effects led one DRN to propose that if frequent and spontaneous use of humor is to be encouraged by the professional staff, a certain amount of control and guidance should be provided to guard against the occurrence of mishaps and to insure maximum gains to the patient.

That humor does have a place in nurse-patient relations in geriatric nursing and that positive good can, and often does, ensue from it is attested to by the experience shared by a DRN:

> Humor is a useful human defense. If observation of the patient and assessment of his needs lead the nurse to recognize that for this patient humor which is initiated by him is a supporting defense which he finds of value, then, in certain circumstances, a kidding relationship may be useful.
> I have had a joshing relationship with a dying incontinent patient in which mutual kidding about my need for work and his anxiety to see me well-employed helped both of us through innumerable bed changes which were a source of great dismay to him and would have been almost impossible for me to have a neutral or reassuring attitude about, if humor had not provided a straw at which to clutch.
> There is no rule for this: it is a question of sensitivity and, once again, "What—all things considered—should be done." But no nurse has a right to inflict *her* humor on a sensitive patient. In this, the lead is provided by the patient. The nurse's leadership role, in contrast, is the provision of a good-natured environment. (Schwartz)

That any resort to humor, kidding, and joshing is conditional to the individual patient and the particular situation is also succinctly commented upon by another DRN:

> Certainly there are some patients with a ready sense of humor who find relief in some "joking." In any case, the dignity of the patient, the timing, and the situation are determinants of the validity of joshing. The nurse needs to be sensitive to the individual patient and to take her cues from him. The joshing should never impinge on an utterance leaving doubt in anyone's mind as to the nurse's respect for the patient as an individual and the dignity, which is the right of any man. (Quinlan)

SUMMARY

Because of the relatedness of the issues of childlike treatment of aged patients and the use of humor in staff-patient relationships, these two topics were explored side by side, and identical code guides were used. The three major positions on the use of humor and kidding are 1) humor has a definite place in staff-patient relationships; 2) joshing and kidding should never be resorted to in geriatric patient care; and 3) the use of humor, kidding or joshing is conditional to the particular situation and the kind of patient involved. The statistical details on these positions are as follows:

	NA's %	LPN's %	RN's %	DRN's %
Affirmative position	39.7	35.9	35.4	7.1
Negative position	6.8	9.4	28.1	33.6
Conditional position	53.3	52.9	36.6	57.1

Slightly more than a third of each of the practitioner groups advocated the use of humor, whereas the degree registered nurses endorsed this position by less than 10 percent. A majority of those favoring the use of humor did so because of beneficial results anticipated, such as giving the patient a feeling of belonging or gaining his cooperation on some aspects of his care. Others endorsed this position without amplification. The nursing responses on the affirmative position are reflected in the figures below:

	NA's %	LPN's %	RN's %	DRN's %
Kidding or joshing is a means of making aged patients feel wanted	18.4	20.8	25.6	5.1
Kidding is useful in gaining a patient's cooperation	2.9	3.8	6.1	0.0
Kidding is appropriate, without amplification	18.4	11.3	3.7	2.0

Some nurses, however, took a contrary position. A small minority of the nurse aides and licensed practical nurses disclaimed that they resort to humor and kidding when caring for their aged patients. Registered and degree registered nurses, on the other hand, opposed the use of humor by considerably larger proportions. Respondents who rejected the idea of humor in staff-patient relationships did so either by their strong emphasis that aged persons be accorded respect and dignity, or their unqualified opposition to this idea. Following are the figures on this negative position:

	NA's %	LPN's %	RN's %	DRN's %
Humor or kidding is never appropriate in staff-patient relationships	3.9	1.9	6.1	26.5
Accord aged persons respect and dignity	2.9	7.5	22.0	7.1

However, a majority of all except the registered nurses asserted that the question does not lend itself to absolute positions of either "yes" or "no." They maintained that such a decision is conditional to the individual patient within his particular position, with factors such as the patient's personality and background, his present state of mental and physical health, and the attending nurse's personality to be considered. They claimed, furthermore, that the decision of whether or not to use humor or kidding can shift for the same person with changing circumstances, times, and moods. The figures on the conditional position are:

	NA's %	LPN's %	RN's %	DRN's %
This depends upon a patient's health, mental, and physical	11.6	5.7	4.9	2.0
It depends on the patient's personality and background	38.8	45.3	29.3	52.0
Personality of the staff is a factor	2.9	1.9	2.4	3.1

It is apparent that the use of humor and jocularity by nursing personnel in their relationships with geriatric patients is favored more by the nurse practitioners than by the degree registered nurses. This is indicated by the fact that more than a third of the former and much less than a tenth of the latter support the practice; and the ratio is largely reversed when the respondents register their disapproval of the practice. However, when the use of humor is made conditional to individual personality characteristics and appropriate circumstances, there appears to be more common and favorable agreement among all four ranks of nursing personnel, but with the DRN's tending to express much more caution and encouraging greater safeguards in its use. Finally, the question remains as to whether the findings would have been different if the interviews and the questionnaire had been prefaced with a generalized and arbitrary definition of the terms used (humor, kidding, joshing). The analysis of the data lead the authors to believe that the diversity of opinion expressed by the nurses on the subject goes deeper than the issue of semantics.

For full statistical details, see Appendix B, Table 2.

6 The "Hostile" Patient and the Nurse

No attempt will be made here to catalogue and classify in any comprehensive way the types and varieties of problems that are confronted in the care of aged patients. From preliminary exploration and reviews of published reports, three particularly disconcerting problems that prove difficult for nurses to deal with have been singled out for special consideration: 1) mistrust and aggressive behavior expressed by aged patients toward those who care for them; 2) breakdown in conventional proprieties on the part of patients; and 3) hallucinations and other delusory phenomena. They will be discussed, in that order, in this and the following two chapters.

These behaviors are known to occur frequently in aged persons within institutional settings, and the symptoms may last over varying lengths of time—sometimes even months or years. Underlying causes no doubt are complex and varied, but it is recognized that behavior disorders such as these are not necessarily caused solely by mental deterioration; they may constitute for the aged person adaptive efforts to various stresses, whether these be of a physiological, psychologic, or social nature. Even if they constitute adaptive efforts, they may still be aggravated by organic factors such as brain damage. But, whatever the cause, for some patients the move into an institutional setting may bring on, or aggravate existing behavior disorders. In others, they may not manifest themselves until long after the patient's admission to the institution, if they develop at all.

THE NATURE OF THE PROBLEM

Mistrust* and aggressive or hostile behavior of aged patients are viewed by many of the nursing personnel as frustrating and time-consuming problems in geriatrics. Factors involved in such patient reactions are undoubtedly intricate in background and build-up as well as in the immediate aggressive or suspicious expressions. They often lead, admittedly, to nursing treatment of symptoms without getting at causes. The problem would be complex enough if the sources of mistrust and aggression could be confined to the immediate bodily discomforts and personality conflicts of the individual patient; but rarely can they be so confined. They build up and can be triggered by long-standing and unresolved disappointments and stresses that reach back into the past life of the patient; they may be provoked unintentionally by inept and ill-prepared members of the nursing staff; or they may arise out of conflicts, contradictions, and inefficiencies built into the institution which provides the setting and regulates the procedures for patient care and therapy. More often than not, they spring out of a combination of such determining forces and may become further complicated by intervening relatives and friends or associates of the patient.

The realities of the situation may be viewed somewhat in this light: An aged person entering the institution finds himself ill-prepared for what lies ahead of him; the attending staff is usually poorly prepared to deal sensitively and expertly with a long life nearing its completion; and the institution has been planned and constructed for, and is committed to, sustaining and prolonging dwindling lives rather than to the enriching, fulfilling, and rounding off of them. Is it any wonder that for a given patient the situation may engender distrust and frustration, and the adaptive efforts of the patient may find expression in aggressive responses or withdrawal, which can become as effectively aggressive as open hostility from the viewpoint of the nursing staff? To face the realities bluntly, the typical hospital or nursing home is not always a *good* place psychologically or socially in which an aged person can live out his life. Many of the nurses undoubtedly are aware that elderly patients frequently would prefer to remain and die within their own home or family setting—if such places still maintain tolerable ties in kith and kinship relations. And even

* In this context mistrust and distrust are treated as synonymous terms.

though some elderly persons have few social ties left, they would very probably choose to stay on in their own home, rather than be confined to an institution with its congregate living arrangements. The challenging task of exploring and understanding the varied conditioning causes of patient mistrust and aggressions cannot be adequately examined here; but neither can it be overlooked.

Mistrust, aggression, and other hostile behaviors are interpreted by a few of the registered nurses and by a great many of the degree registered nurses as natural survival assets to the patient. In unfamiliar and bewildering or disturbing situations, many persons are known to exhibit hostile behavioral traits in routine living, either openly or covertly, and often to their obvious advantage. Within the therapeutic milieu such as a hospital or nursing home, aggression, mistrust, and other hostile behavior may be said to be natural survival assets to the patient. A few RN's and a considerable number of DRN's deemed it important and helpful for the patient, as well as for the geriatric nurse, that she understand and be prepared for such symptomatic behavior on the part of the patient. Frequently, an elderly person feels angry about his fate, even though he tries to be resigned and accepting. Or he may feel frustrated because of his impaired mental capacity or because of his uncomfortable and uncooperative body and take these frustrations out on the staff as an available target. One of the DRN's regarded this issue as an excellent and timely topic for review and for some soul-searching on the part of geriatric nurses, especially as to whether they possess the knowledge about human behavior, the skills in the area of interpersonal relations, and, perhaps, the sense of humor to deal adequately with patients who engage in distrustful and aggressive behavior.

Factors underlying aggression or similar behavior problems exhibited by geriatric patients are conveniently divided by some nurses into *internal* and *external* bases. Examples of internal grounds for legitimate mistrust and aggression include: effects of drugs prescribed, inadequate blood supply to the brain, sensory deficits in sight and hearing, and mental deterioration. A patient's rebellious disposition may also have its roots in personality characteristics and defensive patterns internalized and hardened through long years of use. A perceptive nurse who properly understands these internalized factors will realize that the patient cannot help himself in his misbehavior and will look toward situational factors within the institutional setting to solve some of these problems. Exclaimed one DRN, "How can one possibly place value judgments on such behavior of elderly patients in their terminal desperation?"

There are times, however, when a patient's mistrust seems externally grounded. It may be brought on or intensified by the care provided by members of the nursing staff who leave much to be desired in their ministrations to, and understanding of, their aged patients. Attitudes within the therapeutic setting, pressures of time, interest in getting the work over and done with, and diversified or devious job satisfactions (or lack of them) may all play a part in inadequate care. Elderly patients are said to sense readily the attitude of those caring for them; and mistrust and aggression are natural defense mechanisms available to the patient who considers himself shortchanged where the stakes are high. Moreover, it may actually be true that a particular nurse or aide cannot or should not be trusted. Some nurses hold to the principle that when a patient becomes distrustful, it is better to search first for some realistic grounds for his belief that his trust has been betrayed until it is proven otherwise. (Aiello, Declan, Patrick, Santorum, Steffen, Wolanin)

Lack of trust, at least to some degree, may also be attributed to a feeling elderly persons often acquire toward the nurse because she represents to them the embodiment of authority, power, and control over matters in their daily lives concerning which they are most sensitive: their pride, privacy, and personal prerogatives acquired over a lifetime. The patient may resent being in an institution because it separates him in his last days from so much that he has come to treasure and which for him represents achievement, prestige, comfort, and safety. A person's ability to adapt to change lessens with age, and when he finds himself permanently in strange, impersonal, and apparently indifferent surroundings, he is understandably distressed and frustrated. Then, when frightening treatments are forced upon his person, often without prior notice, in unprivate fashion, and with inadequate explanations, why shouldn't his tried and tested defense mechanism come to the fore to sustain him against his adversaries?

It should be remembered that aggressive behavior is generally believed to be a response to frustrations—a response which helps to sustain a person from lapsing into a state of powerlessness. Moreover, within a patient-nurse relationship, such aggressions may not be without backlashing penalties, for they are likely to arouse in the nurse anxieties or even some hostility reducing the effectiveness of her ministrations and partially blocking her further communications with the patient.

Where the institutional system and the lines of communication are laden with frustrations of omission and commission, mistrust and aggression can present serious obstacles to constructive patient care. If, on the other hand, the social system is well organized and coordinated with smooth operations and harmonious relationships, and if the administration is intelligently committed to, and supportive of, exploring and devising creative approaches to the care of elderly ill and dying persons, a climate can permeate the organization, resulting in a minimum of suspicions and aggressions and in superior care.

NEGATIVE ACCEPTANCE

The reactions of the four ranks of nursing personnel on the issue of hostile patient behavior varied from attitudes of *nonacceptance* and patient control at one extreme and of *positive acceptance* and treatment at the other extreme. A major approach of nurses supporting nonacceptance was to more or less ignore the presence of the hostile behavior or to shift the responsibility for coping with it to someone else. A major approach of those supporting positive and constructive acceptance of such behavior was for those ministering to the aged ill to give priority to reassuring their patients. Several of the RN practitioners and a substantial number of the DRN's went beyond mere acceptance of the behavior and cited the importance of the underlying cause or causes of hostile behavior exhibited by aged patients.*

The negative or nonacceptance stance was supported by a minority in all four nursing ranks. In the case of the nurse aides, however, this rate amounted to about 2 in 5. The degree registered nurses gave this position the least support.†

The nurse aides, licensed practical nurses, and registered nurses who supported the negative position expressed great similarity in their views and the treatment of their offending patients. Their methods of coping with mistrust, or any other patient behavior they consider hostile to them, are reminiscent of the negative childlike treatment practices discussed in an earlier chapter. They run the gamut from scolding or withholding to bribing or rewarding. The degree registered nurses who supported the negative position suggested more positive approaches.

If an aged patient cannot be reasoned with or be persuaded to desist from a particular act of hostility or aggression, some of these nurses and nurse aides would report the incident to the person next highest to them in the nursing hierarchy or, in the case of the nurse in charge, to the attending physician. Should the staff encounter extreme difficulty with a patient, medication or restraints might be prescribed by the physician; or, in some of the selected institutions, if the staff considers the patient "unmanageable," he might be transferred to a mental hospital.

Several practitioners reported that it is a good practice to leave an

---

* The nursing responses on the three issues (mistrust and aggression; improprieties; and hallucinations) permitted the use of identical categories for coding.

† NA's, 40.2 percent; LPN's, 32.6 percent; RN's, 17.0 percent; DRN's, 7.2 percent. See Appendix B, Table 3, Items 1 to 5.

offending patient alone for a while; often when they return they find that the patient's behavior has changed. Thus a patient who for some reason refused to eat will do so now; and one who before "lashed out at you with her tongue" will now desist—in short "if a patient has had time to think, his mood may change."

Others would bargain with a patient; but according to one nurse aide, "This does not always work." She then related a recent incident:

> We have a 92-year-old patient, a former university dean, who often refuses to eat anything we give him. When I bring him food, I take different things such as milk, eggnog, and fruit juice. One day when he would not take anything I said to him, "If you drink something for me I'll help you get into bed." He just looked at me for a while and then said, "don't you bargain with me."

Several nurse aides reported giving tit for tat, and some of them reported the following example of this:

> One patient kept pulling my hair. When I asked her why she did this, she answered, "because I want to." Then I told her that if she would stop pulling my hair, I would not pull hers.

She then added that it is important to get through to patients, but if she finds that she is not able to, she just ignores the behavior; or she tells them, "don't you dare do that."

Still another spoke about a situation which involved a patient who would not let the floor nurse do anything for her, and she commented:

> And I tell the patient that I agree with her. Then when the patient is to be given an injection, I talk with her and keep her interested while I turn her on her side. The nurse then comes quietly into the room, crouches so that the patient does not see her, and quickly gives her the injection.

An LPN, in charge of a floor, declared:

> You can't reason with them. One patient kept accusing me of stealing her dresses—and I am three times her size. When I explained that to her, she just said that I was taking them for my children. She was finally transferred.

One of the RN's who took the negative position commented that she falls back on tranquilizers. She also stressed that it is important to divert the attention of the other patients when one of them engages in some hostile act so that the incident does not turn into a situation that upsets all of them.

In some instances, an objectionable behavior is modified and the patient assuaged by means of trial and error, as illustrated in the following situation:

> Mrs. L, in her eighties and slightly senile, was continually clutching a large handbag in which she had the few treasured keepsakes she had brought with her to the nursing home. When she first arrived in the home, a staff member suggested that she keep the bag in her bedside table or in a bureau drawer, whereupon she became extremely agitated and abusive.
>
> Mrs. L. kept misplacing her bag and when she did she was quick to accuse the staff of having taken it. In the beginning, the staff ignored her accusations and told her that she no doubt had misplaced it and would find it again. When Mrs. L. became so agitated that she finally refused to take her medicines and, at times, refused to go to bed, the nurse in charge requested that a staff member go and help Mrs. L. find the bag whenever it was missing.
>
> The bag was always found—in the bath room, in a bureau drawer, under the bed-pillow—wherever Mrs. L. had placed it and forgotten that she had done so.
>
> Very slowly a trusting relationship between Mrs. L. and a few of the staff members was built up. In time, Mrs. L. seemed more accepting and more cooperative—she was also misplacing her bag less often.

There was no intimation among those who supported the negative or nonacceptance position that behavior such as that of Mrs. L. might have been symptomatic of her stress upon being admitted to an unfamiliar environment. Their concern appeared to be with symptoms—with the behavior exhibited by the patient—and not with underlying causes.

Positive Acceptance

Compassion, patience, and understanding was stressed by many of those who would cope with aged patients' aggressions and suspicions in more positive ways—a position that was supported by a majority in all four nursing ranks, and which among the degree registered nurses amounted to about 90 percent of the group.*

A nurse aide spoke for many of her co-workers when she said that "kindness means everything to them," and she contended that one gets further with sugar than with vinegar. Another suggested that a patient's hostile behavior may be an attention-getting device; that the aged are

---

* NA's, 55.8 percent; LPN's, 50.0 percent; RN's, 76.8 percent; DRN's, 89.4 percent. See Appendix B, Table 3, Items 6 to 9.

quick to realize when a staff member does not like them or is afraid of them; and that in situations like that they are apt "to bite."

Some licensed practical nurses claim that it is important not to go back on one's word, for trust is all important. Not keeping one's word might trigger a patient's abusive behavior, and if the staff does not have a patient's trust, it is a "lost battle." One LPN expressed this as follows:

> We have one patient who "goes off" at times. She often thinks the food we bring her is poison, and when she does, I taste it—and she realizes it is not.

Many of the registered nurses emphasized continued reassurance, honesty, kindness, and acceptance. A few of them also attested to ascertaining underlying causes, so that the behavior may be diminished or eradicated, thereby bringing greater comfort to the patient.

Several of the practitioners voiced concern lest the staff should court aggressions of their aged patients, or to arouse their suspicions. A nurse aide who raised this question commented that on her floor the aides habitually put bedlinens into the patients' bureau drawers, to which some patients object—even to the point of accusing the staff of taking their belongings. She added that often she has to take the linen back to the linen closet. Another aide related instances where nurses had, unbeknown to the patient, mixed medicine in the fruit juice or coffee only to have this "snowball" with the patient making accusations of being poisoned.

An LPN observed that in her previous place of employment the patients' accusations mostly involved being poisoned, whereas in the present work situation most of the patients' suspicions have to do with stealing. She then added, "I have never found out how to handle this."

An RN cautioned never to borrow from an aged patient, lest their suspicions be aroused.

GUIDELINES

Possible guidelines for the improvement of geriatric patient care which are derived from nursing comments on behavioral disorders include the following:

1. Some unconventional behaviors, particularly aggressions and suspicions, are bound to arise in the care of aged persons within institutional settings; and understandably so. In brief, they can be regarded as natural to the situation.

2. The nurse shares responsibility to safeguard the patient from injury to himself or to others which might result from his aggressive or other improper behavior.

3. Maintaining patient-nurse rapport, reassuring the patient, and rebuilding his trust, self-confidence, and sense of security are essential functions of the nurse.

4. To identify and understand the basic cause or causes of particular behavioral problems of the patient would provide the major key for coping with them.

5. Knowledge and understanding of the main reasons for behavioral problems of the patient, such as aggression, provide the nurse with strong reinforcements in her own professional endeavors.

6. Corrective improvements in the institutional environment in which the patient is treated appear fundamental to optimum therapy and care of the patient.

While the following elaboration of these guidelines represent a composite of the ways in which nursing personnel in all four ranks would cope positively and constructively with aged patients' behavioral problems, such as mistrust and aggressions, the concepts and themes to a very large extent are drawn from the degree registered nurse responses.

Reinforcement for the Patient

A major objective for the geriatric nurse is the rebuilding of the patient's self-confidence, trust, and feelings of security with the staff and within the institutional setting. How this can be accomplished will depend largely on the nature of the stress problem, the illness and personality of the patient, the specific frustrating situation, and the particular nurse; her own previous conditioning, personality, knowledge, and skills.

With so many variables to be considered, it would be inadvisable to prepare a standard procedure to be used or to attempt to outline the conditions which would warrant this use. With the potential backgrounds and complexities of frustrating factors being manifold, it becomes mainly a matter of sensitive listening for and taking note of the clues that are provided through observation and communication with each separate patient.

The art of listening is not infrequently called the communicative skill. It also seems to be an invaluable means of "reaching" the elderly and improving relationships with them. So few people take time to listen to the aged, especially those whose thinking is slowed, whose sight and hearing are impaired, and whose conversations may be difficult, repetitious or dull, touching frequently on topics out of a distant past. It was found by Schwartz and her associates that the thing that meant most to the aged patients they interviewed was that someone cared enough to listen.

Getting to know the distrustful elderly patient and gaining some understanding of why he feels and behaves as he does toward those caring for him may be very helpful in planning his care. Initially, the nursing task may be to accept the patient as he is and try to adjust to him and to reassure him as much as possible, making every act and attitude indicative of respect for him and a sincere desire to understand and help him—and above all, to convey trustworthiness. A nurse might well provide opportunities for the patient to unhurriedly voice his feelings as much as he will, explaining to him whatever seems appropriate with respect to what is or will be happening around him or to him, and by frequent visits, kind words, and perhaps an occasional touch, convey to him a feeling of being cared for. Also considered important is attempting as much as possible to anticipate the patient's nursing needs and, if he is extremely upset, to ask his physician to prescribe a medication to impose enough quiescence for getting in closer communication with him. (Carlton, Maliepaard, Shaffer, Smith, Windeler)

Often some sense of security can be built up in the patient through adhering to routines, being consistent and, thus, predictable in time of appearance and attendance to his needs, and spending frequent extra bits of time with him. A nurse often can, by being reassuring and timely in her suggestions, gain the cooperation of the patient, so that even a pill that is "poison" at one moment will be swallowed without question at another time. Continued faithfulness and thoughtful consideration will often convince the patient that he was mistaken in his distrust. (Damon, Sr. Gabrielle, Schwartz, Travelbee)

Further buildup of trust has a better chance of success when one nurse adapts to the patient, fits into the situation, and cares for him day after day—rather than subjecting him to a different nurse every day or so.

It is also reported that an empathetic head nurse can often work wonders on a particular unit. Her particular way of working with people sets the tone and determines largely whether the atmosphere will be of reasonable harmony or of emotional stress and strain.

When confronted with distrust and aggressions of elderly patients, a nurse who can view these like any other symptoms, organic or psychologic, is apt to make a more constructive approach. And a nurse has a head start when she realizes that the patient is usually using the best coping behavior of which he is capable at that particular moment. The question is raised by one DRN whether it is not better for the patient to attempt to protect himself in any way that he can against what he perceives to be a threatening situation than for him to give up and do nothing—to vegetate. (Schwartz)

Since distrust and aggression in elderly patients may spring from a variety of complex causes past and present, if the key factors can be sifted out and effectively formulated, they are apt to provide useful clues for planning constructive courses of action. For instance, a patient may have suffered deep frustration in some real or imaginary ambition of his life, and this may become a constant irritant for him. For a nurse with insight, this frustration may become the most effective point of her intervention in order to reconcile the patient to some extent to the realities of his past. If a patient is angered and resentful because he has become hopelessly ill, his nurse may help him, perhaps more by her manner than by her words, to achieve some positive implication from, or reconciliation to, the apparently inexplicable. Or a patient may exhibit aggressive behavior as a result of a traumatic illness, such as cerebrovascular accident or other pathology, and his contentious attitude may be a cry for help for regaining some sense of identity and reality. To illustrate:

> Mr. R. had only recently been transferred from a general hospital to the nursing home, having suffered a cerebrovascular accident several weeks prior to his admission to the home. The medical record revealed extensive brain damage. His speech was slurred, and he was incoherent at times.
>
> Seventy-four-year-old Mr. R. had been a prominent citizen in his community. As a successful politician he had held considerable power in the affairs of his city. He was said to have been a very autocratic person and a most difficult patient in the hospital.
>
> When Mr. R. arrived in the nursing home, he was belligerent and used loud and abusive language. He also kept rattling the side rails that had been fastened to his bed for protection. Giving him his medicines proved a trying experience for the staff, for he kept pushing the nurse's hand away; and when finally persuaded to open his mouth, he would refuse to swallow the medication. Though he was too weak to get out of bed, he had considerable strength in his extremities and, on a number of occasions, had tried to hit particular staff members. He forever seemed to be pushing his bed covers to the foot of the bed, leaving him exposed, except for his brief nightshift.
>
> A few days after Mr. R. had been admitted to the home a new head nurse arrived. Mr. R. was one of the first patients she visited. Upon entering his room, she bade him a friendly and calm "Good-morning" and asked him how he felt. She then stood quietly by his bedside, remaining silent. After several minutes, during which Mr. R. looked at her with apparent puzzlement, he responded with, "Oh, so today you have time for me." With the comment that it was a little chilly in the room, she took the bed covers which Mr. R. once again

had pushed to the foot of the bed and covered him gently and unhurriedly.

Drawing upon her knowledge of Mr. R.'s background and his present restive nature, she asked, "What about writing some letters, since you cannot get to your office today." His eyes lighted up as though he remembered, and he vigorously nodded his head. She then asked a co-worker to assist her in helping Mr. R. to a more upright position, produced some paper and a pencil, placed this in front of him, and sat down near the bed.

For the first time since entering the home, Mr. R. remained quiet for any length of time and he appeared engrossed in his activity—an activity which perhaps represented the only element of reality in his present situation and condition. The "letters" which Mr. R. produced consisted of some childish scrawls such as might have been made by a 3-year-old. Despite the very considerable brain damage Mr. R. had sustained, it seemed that the head nurse was able to "reach" him as a person and her therapeutic interventions perhaps restored some sense of human worth in him.

Following a case conference attended by all involved in this patient's care, including the physician, a detailed nursing plan was developed. The care plan prescribed that extra time be spent with Mr. R., that staff attempt to converse with him, and that whatever care was given be attended to slowly and with deliberation. Mr. R. also was to be given his morning care as soon as possible after breakfast, and then be provided with writing paper and pencil.

Mr. R. did not become a model patient, but the changes in his behavior were noticeable. He appeared much less agitated than he had been, resorted to emotional outbursts much less often, and in general became more cooperative than he had been when he first entered the home.

While Mr. R.'s condition did not improve, he apparently was more at peace with himself during the final weeks of his life than he might have been without the intervention of the nurse.

If, beyond her routine duties, the nurse succeeds even in a modest degree to assist the patient to gain some sense of inspiration and achievement in the way that he meets and copes with his problems, does she not add some significant reinforcements to the terminal phases of a long life? (Maliepaard, Travelbee, Whidden)

The need to initiate some change in a stressful situation—such as relieving, allaying, fighting against, or seeking to gain some benefit from, or at least to do something about an aggression- or suspicion-arousing predicament—is a well-known trait of great survival value and a human propensity that does not pass easily with aging. Indeed, most prognoses for the aged probably would be weakened by their loss of such self-defense potentials. It is recognized that the means of self-defense of elderly ill and institutionalized individuals are very limited. "Pure cussedness" may become one of their last resorts and may, on occasion, prove to be "an incredibly good defense." (Schwartz) It is a valuable nursing

insight to recognize this and to learn to adapt its potentials in constructive ways.

Whenever a nurse discovers persistent aggravations that arouse the
distrust and ire of her patient—whether having a basis in fact or only
appearing valid from the patient's point of view—certain possibilities
usually remain open to her. She may attempt various modifications in
staffing, institutional arrangements or routines, or in her approach to the
patient. If, upon trying whatever appears promising, no changes for
the better occur, she is then at least in a better position to share with the
patient a realistic or plausible explanation for the disagreeable elements
and to communicate thereby a sense of her appreciation of his problem.
She has become, also, better prepared to commiserate with him, to encourage his tolerance, or even to support his "right" to feel as he does.
It can then, also, become opportune to attempt some diversional interests
and activities to sidetrack the patient's preoccupation with his frustrations. (Aiello, Baziak, Nagy, Shaffer, Steffen)

The particular way of coping with each situation will vary with the
knowledge, skill, and ingenuity of the nurse, but it is considered important that she at all times give the best possible care and try to allay
mistrust through constant attention, gentleness, and thoughtfulness of
manner and kindly ministrations. The soundness of such advice is attested to by a nursing home administrator who writes:

> Even in brain-damaged patients the treatment must be gentle and
> unhurried. They can be retaught toilet habits, though it might take
> some time. Tranquilizers ordered by the doctor are carefully given so
> that the patients are not kept in a drowsy state, but can respond when
> spoken to. They are praised when they do the right things, but never
> scolded for mistakes. A nurse who provokes such a patient unwittingly
> is removed from the situation. We have seen the most violent and
> noisy patients respond to this treatment and become docile and lov-
> ing. They have a tendency to walk a great deal in the hall, but never
> disturb anyone. They will look up at a passing nurse and smile. They
> have a sense of security. They now recognize their families. Unbe-
> known to us, some of these patients had been put out of other nursing
> homes and are on the waiting list of a mental hospital. The families,
> through fear that they will not be accepted by us, do not tell us the
> truth. They are greatly relieved when they find that their patient does
> not have to be committed. We think that senile patients should not
> be sent to state hospitals if it can possibly be avoided. (Mrs. E. S.
> Brown)

Certain changes in the environment or interpersonal situation may
produce good effects. Placing the patient in a different room; requesting
that family members visit more often or at more favorable times;
changing routines to avoid particular incidents and procedures or to alter

their effects; being more alert and prompt in meeting a patient's request or, even better, in anticipating his needs; and making other similar modifications in the nursing plan can and may soften or alleviate some of the patient's sullen or belligerent behavior. Occasions may arise, also, which require dealing more directly with the problem. (V. Brown, Damon, Dixon, Hagen, Palmer)

If the patient-nurse relation continues to worsen, with the former gaining few or no reinforcements, some change in staff probably should be made. At this point it is generally viewed as a waste of time and effort, and a sidetrack of the main issue, to begin to blame either the patient or the nurse for the problems that remain unsolved. New patient-nurse combinations—such as shifts in sex, level of nurse training, personality characteristics, or even age ratios—are usually available and are often quite simple and effective changes. A young nurse or aide may be able to attain more harmonious and trusting relations with an elder patient than a nurse who is older—and *vice versa*. Sometimes a nurse aide relates better to an aged patient than does a registered nurse. Although occasionally every effort and patient-nurse combination fail to improve the situation, the general nursing consensus seems to be that persistent effort will usually produce someone who can obtain a more congenial and rewarding joint relationship. (Aiello, E. S. Brown, Bixby, Lindstrom)

In general, the nursing comments strongly imply that an aged patient's feelings of security may be substantially reinforced by his receiving concerted staff attention to his problems and by being constantly assured that certain basic living conditions are being met. These would seem to include the obvious provision for the fulfillment of such instrumental needs as a fairly comfortable and "accepting" environment; opportunities for engaging in suitable activities for decreasing idleness and for affording a sense of useful participation; adequate therapy whenever indicated; and whatever personal attention is required for promoting optimal mental health as long as life lasts.

Reinforcement for the Nurse

Mistrust and aggressions can be difficult for the nursing staff to deal with, partly because the nurse is so often the most direct target within the patient's range. But a nurse's recognition that the patient's "obstreperous conduct" is largely caused or conditioned by his illness or by the readjustments required of him in a disciplined and unfamiliar environment can temper her irritations of the moment and reinforce her continuous efforts and tolerance. Moreover, the better she comes to understand the patient and why he behaves as he does, the more realistic will become her goals in therapy for him. In nursing, as in other professional endeavors, overly idealistic goals can become the foremost pitfalls for discouragement and defeat.

Furthermore, the prime solution may prove to be a surprisingly simple step. Perhaps all that the upset patient wishes is to be left more alone; or he may crave more time in interpersonal exchanges. And either reason may have been the basis for his institutionalization in the first place. Simple, and almost artless solutions, examples of which have been cited above, are often difficult to get at because the patient and his relatives may not be willing or able to disclose them. The professionals who care for the patient are challenged to find them—and to spot a simple, workable plan. (Corona, Nagy, Wolanin)

While searching for a solution to a patient's suspicious and aggressive responses, the nurse should realize that he is probably doing the best he can at the moment. Increased understanding of the problem may provide her with renewed incentives to search for intermediary measures for bringing about positive changes. She should remember, also, that often staff-shared—and sometimes patient-shared—decisions on planning a course of action can be jointly reinforcing. (Nagy, Schwartz, Shaffer, Steffen)

The nurses frequently mentioned the gratitude of many patients whose institutional existence had been plagued for a time by misinterpreted distrust and irrational acts of aggression—and how such patients find ingenious ways of conveying their appreciation, even into the extremities of their lives.

Caution should be expressed, however, that deserving reinforcements for the nurse are not always forthcoming. It is worth repeating, perhaps, that, more often than not, nurses bear the brunt of patient distrust and aggression, no matter from what cause the behavior arises. It can be set off by circumstances of ill-kept or inadequate facilities, breaks in the continuity of services, overly rigid administrative rules and regulations, common misunderstandings or personnel affronts, and the like. It is true enough that the nursing staff generally gets the frontal attacks and that these greatly interfere with nursing routines. The nurse tends, thus, to view herself and her staff as subject to multiple jeopardy—from her own defaults and those of several allied categories of specialized or job-assigned personnel. It seems very possible that such a plurality of exposure and personal risk promotes in the nurse, of whatever rank, a certain overcautious, self-protective attitude which, though not intentionally at the expense of the patient, is not entirely without cost to him. It is also possible that much of this is due to systems of dynamics determined by the institution which provides and regulates the patient care.

SUMMARY

Behavior disorders are fairly common occurrences in geriatric institutions; and it comes as no surprise that they present some of the most frustrating problems for everyone involved in the care of the aged, especially for the nursing staff who are charged with their care on a continuous basis.

The attitudes and reactions of the four ranks of nursing personnel to behavior problems such as mistrust and aggression divide into two broadly defined contrasting positions: negative or nonacceptance or even denial of the presence of such patient behavior at the one pole, and positive acceptance at the other pole. Nonacceptive attitudes and reactions were reflected by a minority of nursing respondents ranging from a high of 40 percent for the nurse aides to a low of 7 percent for the degree registered nurses. On the side of positive acceptance of hostile patient behavior, all four ranks showed strong or approximate majority representations, led by the DRN's with a near 90 percent, and with a low of 50 percent for the LPN's. The relative positions of the nurse respondents and the percentages represented by the positions they take is reflected for each type of nursing rank in the following chart:

	NA's %	LPN's %	RN's %	DRN's %
Nonacceptance	40.2	32.6	17.0	7.2
Positive acceptance	55.8	50.0	76.8	89.4

The categories of negative acceptance of mistrust and similar hostile behavior by nursing personnel are reflected in the following chart:

	NA's %	LPN's %	RN's %	DRN's %
Denying or ignoring the presence of such behavior	15.7	7.7	6.1	0.0
Shifting responsibility for dealing with it to others	10.8	3.8	2.4	3.6
Use of medication or restraints	0.0	1.9	1.2	2.4
Use of diversional tactics	5.9	7.7	4.9	0.0
Resorting to reasoning and persuasion	7.8	11.5	2.4	1.2

On the side of positive acceptance of patient mistrust and aggression, the nursing responses divide into four categories. These are the respective figures:

	NA's %	LPN's %	RN's %	DRN's %
Change of staff with supportive attitude	18.6	9.6	30.5	17.9
Acceptance with attempts to reassure	34.3	38.5	24.4	2.4
Support to extent of not permitting suffering	2.9	1.9	14.6	28.6
Acceptance and attempts to ascertain basic cause	0.0	0.0	7.3	40.5

It should be noted that while the nonacceptive stance represents a minority position, it is most strongly supported by those more directly involved with direct geriatric patient care—the nurse aides and the licensed practical nurses, in that order.

On the positive acceptance position, category 9: acceptance of the hostile behavior with attempt at ascertaining the underlying cause or causes has no NA or LPN representation. The RN representation was 7.3 percent. The finding that the NA and the LPN representation of this most professionally orientated category is nil, comes as no surprise, but that only about 1 in 14 of the RN practitioners would express concern about the cause of hostile patient behavior raises the question why—particularly when it is recalled that more than three fourths of the RN's interviewed occupy head nurse or higher leadership positions in the geriatric institutions. Of the DRN's about 3 in 5 would ascertain the underlying cause. Little or no reference was made to possible cause when the question on patients' behavior problems was posed, though it is conceivable that some of the practitioner respondents presumed that the underlying causes were known. On the other hand, many of the DRN's discussed possible causes in some detail and relative to possible modification or disappearance of the symptomatic behavior.

From the detailed discussions of the problem and the statistical tabulations, it appears reasonable to conclude that nursing attitudes and proposals, and probably nursing practice—at least as represented by these respondents—is moving toward greater toleration and acceptance of such disconcerting and disturbing behavior on the part of aged patients—and with positive endeavors to understand and treat it.

For full statistical details, see Appendix B, Table 3.

7 Breakdowns in Conventional Behavior

Our endeavor is to search constantly for the meaning of disturbed behavior.

ELIAS SAVITSKY

Another major problem for the geriatric nurse involves violations of conventional proprieties on the part of aged patients, a problem not very different from the one of mistrust and aggression that was discussed in the foregoing chapter. It is not always easy to distinguish between manifestations of disturbed behavior such as distrust and improprieties; and it is recognized that there may be a causal relationship between these two types of symptomatic behavior. Different individuals react to stress in different ways, depending upon diverse factors, such as personality, temperament, and the kinds of stress-producing elements. Some of us are said to "overreact," and others to "underreact" to stress; and the overt behaviors associated with these reactions differ accordingly.

Many nurses referred to patients' hostile acts, such as distrust, as "something that is meant to inflict hurt," and breakdowns in conventional proprieties as "something that embarrasses or annoys others." The differences in interpretation of these two kinds of behavior problems as well as the differences encountered in nursing reactions when attempting to cope with them were sufficiently great to warrant their being considered separately.

THE NATURE OF THE PROBLEM

Breaches in propriety are fairly common occurrences within the institutional milieu and range over wide areas of behavior. General categories covering what nurses regard as conventional proprieties frequently

83

broken by aged patients include: any pronounced violation of what is customarily considered to be proper conduct between two or more persons; behavior that would cause great embarrassment to the patient himself in his more lucid moments; offensive eating habits and toilet practices; uncovering or handling the genitalia before others; engaging in intimacies of any kind that stimulate interpersonal sexual activity; or any other behavior that clearly crosses the conventional boundaries of what is acceptable conduct, and particularly within a therapeutic context.

The breakdown of conventional behavior, even by a dying person is often viewed as unacceptable by nurse and relatives alike. However, improprieties which the staff considers to be willfully engaged in by their patients are generally viewed more harshly than are violations by patients who are seriously ill and who may not realize the offensive nature of their acts. Thus, an alert patient who is up and about and seen walking along the hall in his nightshirt may be severely reprimanded by a staff member, marched to his room, and told that he should "know better," whereas, in the case of a critically ill patient, bedfast and semiconscious, who keeps pulling at his bedcovers and overly exposing himself, the nurse may arrange them without a word or other sign of disapproval. The *kind* of infringement also has a close bearing upon the nurses' method of coping. There is considerable evidence that the most tabooed improprieties are those which in any way hint at sexuality.

Substantial numbers of the DRN's take it for granted that improprieties are bound to arise in institutional settings and tend to regard them as normal occurrences. They consider it their obligation to tolerate them matter-of-factly—up to a certain point—as "part of the game," but to stand firm and gentle as possible, with minimum emotional involvement, when preestablished limits in improper behavior are crossed by their patients. Objectivity, positiveness, and firmness should not give way to pity, although each nursing approach should be made reassuringly in order that the patient at no time be left with a sense of insecurity in the relationship. Ways of coping admittedly vary with the knowledge, skill, and ingenuity of the nurse. In the words of one DRN, "It is questionable whether any categorical answer can be found to the infinite variety of these complex problems." (Duxbury)

One of the nurses pointed out that with long lives, it is *natural* that changes occur in all aspects of the physiology and psychology of the individual. A nurse working in the field of geriatrics should anticipate breakdowns in conventional proprieties among her aged patients and be prepared to cope with these failings; and, at the same time, she must sustain in each patient a sense of self-worth and dignity, even though the individual can no longer function on the level to which he was once accustomed.

Conventional breakdowns in the aged ill are attributed to several factors: mental deterioration, failing physical capacity, specific illnesses or disabilities, and emotional disturbances such as anger, fear, and frustration. Attempts at early recognition of conventional breakdowns as symptoms of an illness, an organ damage, age debilities, or other causes and the recognition that they call for procedures based on the assumption that the improper behavior may be reversible until proven otherwise, is considered more effective than the imposition of sharp restrictions on the breakdowns. There are times when a little ingenuity is required to discover the cause of unbecoming or improper patient behavior, as the nurses who cared for Mrs. C. discovered to their chagrin:

> Having found it increasingly difficult to maintain her own home, Mrs. C. entered a nursing home. The staff was very fond of her and considered her a woman of refinement and culture. A fastidious person, she took pride in being able to attend to her personal needs.
>
> Mrs. C. had recently celebrated her ninety-third birthday. For several months prior to that she had been exhibiting signs of senility, had had lapses in memory, and physically was beginning to be less active than she had been. But she remained "the lady she has always been" according to one of the nurse aides who took care of her.
>
> Then came the breakdown. When she thought no one was looking, Mrs. C. would keep her hand in the pubic area and gently rub through her dress. When she was asked why she was doing this and she responded with an embarrassed laugh, the nurse reprimanded her and told her that her actions offended others. Instead of desisting, however, her offensive actions became more noticeable as the days went by.
>
> When the aide who cared for Mrs. C. noticed a redness in the pubic region, the aide cautioned her that she was irritating the skin by rubbing. But despite admonitions and Mrs. C.'s promises to desist, her behavior continued. When a fellow patient complained to the head nurse, the physician was contacted and asked to speak to Mrs. C. about the situation.
>
> The physician visited, examined Mrs. C., and discovered that the redness of the tissue was not caused by the manipulation of the tissue by the patient, but that Mrs. C. had engaged in the objectionable behavior in an attempt to ease the itching that was caused by a medical condition.
>
> The condition responded to medical treatment, and Mrs. C.'s "improper" behavior stopped.

A perceptive nurse would no doubt have been alerted when Mrs. C.'s unconventional behavior was first noted and upon observing the irritated tissue, would have recognized the problem for what it was—a medical problem in need of medical treatment. The physician would have been called in sooner, and Mrs. C. would have been spared much discomfort and embarrassment, as would her fellow patients and the staff.

A provocative issue raised by some DRN's is the question of nursing tolerance of conventional improprieties committed by aged ill persons. Serious attention was focused upon *whose* proprieties are offended and who usually takes the initiative in enforcing restrictions on them. It is recognized that the nursing staff exercises a major role in such situations. Nursing personnel reflect or represent middle class mores, morals, and standards of decency and propriety; they tend to establish and impose the limits on improprieties and sometimes penalties as well. The question then arises of whose sensitivity needs shall be accorded priority —the offending patient's, his fellow patients', his family's and friends', or those of the attending staff? The question is *not* whether any proprieties have been violated or even whether warm and supportive care should continue to flow from nurse to patient; the issue is *who should become flexible and tolerant* toward the violations and to what degree? As one nurse phrased it, "Whose world of proprieties should come to the fore?"

There is considerable agreement among the DRN's that the patient's world should be considered first with respect to both its background and the consequent effect on it of any intolerance exercised against him as a person. If the impropriety existed in the patient's pattern of behavior prior to his illness and institutionalization and was accepted by his associates at that time, it should be tolerated as much as possible *now* in the end stages of his life.

The observation has been made that residents in a nursing home or similar institution are often able to tolerate certain behavioral improprieties on the part of their fellow patients to a greater degree than are the attending staff. The aged, in general, tend to be less inhibited than those who are younger. At the same time, their senses are apt to have become dulled. This combination may account for some of their behavior; for quite often they do not seem to realize that a certain behavior is considered objectionable by the staff and others.

NEGATIVE ACCEPTANCE

The question raised with respect to improprieties was similar to the one asked concerning patients' suspicious and aggressive behavior: "How do you cope with a situation in which there is a breakdown of conventional proprieties on the part of an aged ill person?" In the questionnaire mailed to the degree registered nurses the question was worded: "Suggest and appraise possible ways of coping with. . . ."

As with the problem of mistrust and aggression, the nurses' reactions to improprieties on the part of aged patients divide into two broad categories, with negative acceptance and even particular objectionable behaviors being ignored at the one extreme, and with positive acceptance and attempts to get at underlying causes and therapy at the other extreme.

In all four nursing ranks a large minority spoke out for nonacceptance of patient behavior which violates common decency or cultural mores. This position received its strongest support from the nurse aide group of whom close to one half supported nonacceptance, and the least from the degree registered group with one fifth taking this position. *

Repeatedly, the point was made that mental deterioration is an important variable to be considered when coping with objectionable patient behavior. Concerning this, one nurse commented that "some don't realize what they are doing." Others declared that some patients are well aware that they are engaging in improper behavior which cannot be condoned.

Nonacceptive *nurse aides* and *registered nurses* place diversional tactics high on the list of methods of coping with improprieties; *licensed practical nurses* would resort to persuasion and reasoning first, but they also rate diversional activities high. *Degree registered nurses* adhering to the negative position suggest the use of medicines and restraints first, then reasoning and persuasion.

While the relative strength with which the three practitioner groups support the negative position varies, much less variation is encountered on approaches to such problems and ways in which they treat their offending patients. Coping devices such as diverting patients' attention in an effort to have them desist from doing whatever is considered offensive may require keeping the patient busy with some kind of handwork; walking with a patient; having him join others to watch television; and the like. Reasoning and persuasion is considered effective when, for example, a patient appears in the public rooms dressed only in his pajamas, or when a patient habitually takes off or tears at her dress. These patients often respond when it is explained to them that their attire is not proper, or when one appeals to their "better instincts" by telling them that "it is not ladylike" or that there are others around. They can usually be persuaded to return to their room and dress or be helped with dressing properly. Some staff members consider humor helpful in coping with objectionable patient behavior; others would resort to "gentle scolding" or "scaring them just a little." To illustrate some of the more common ways in which nurse practitioners cope with patient behavior which they consider deviant:

* NA's, 45.6 percent; LPN's, 44.1 percent; RN's, 33.0 percent; DRN's, 20.7 percent. See Appendix B, Table 4, Items 1 to 5.

> If patients are confused, you put slacks on them or put a dress on backwards so that the patient cannot undress without help;

> I remind them that there are others around who don't like it; or, as a last resort, I will say to a patient that "Father So-and-so will be here," and that scares them;

> One patient keeps putting her dentures in her milk. I explain to her that it is not nice to do that and ask her to go and wash the glass— and she does;

> We have one patient who is almost 100 years old. She masturbates when she is in bed, so we keep her up as much as possible;

> If a patient is not properly dressed, I'll say, "you are grown up now— let's go back to your room and put something on you."

According to these nurses, some patients need to be handled with gentleness; others, with firmness. One NA, who reported using humor quite often, offered the following example of the type humor he uses: "I'd say things such as, 'I may have to spank you if you keep this up.' Another related that scolding sometimes backfires—"Some, when you scold them, rebel against you."

Several staff members commented that deviant behavior such as engaging in improprieties indicates reversion to childhood. Several LPN's declared that they treat their offending patients as one would one's children, and one LPN related that:

> If it is a masturbation problem, I tell them to stop. If they don't realize what they are doing, just gently pull their hand away and distract them. If indecently exposed, cover them up and talk with them. If they are too noisy, they should have sedatives for the benefit of the other residents. If it gets very bad, we have to lock them in—we have rooms with Dutch doors for that.

If a particular behavior is very objectionable, the physician is apt to be called in. This is how an RN coped with a situation she felt needed to be handled by the physician: "Two male patients kept exposing their genitals—I asked the M.D. to talk with them, and they stopped." Another RN, who gets "very angry inside" when her aged patients engage in improprieties, said that she tries not to have her anger get in the way when she talks with them and added that she tries to reason with the patients if they are alert and know what they are doing.

The nurses' approach seems to depend largely on what a particular behavior consists of. The thinking and doing of some of the RN practitioners is reflected in the following comments made in different geriatric institutions:

> Often they go back to childhood and masturbate. Most of them do it without realizing it. I cover them up, but if it gets bad, I call the psychiatrist;

> If the behavior hurts no one, neither themselves nor others, let them live in their own world;

> Don't make a point of it, if they know what they are doing—just ignore.

If a particularly offensive behavior continues, physical restraints or isolation may be resorted to. Some of the institutions have special sections and others have special rooms with Dutch doors where patients may be kept "for their own protection and the protection of others." So it was with Miss Y.:

> The upper half of the Dutch door leading to the patient's room was wide open and fastened securely to the wall behind it; the lower half locked with a key. The head nurse, who was showing the visitor the facilities of the unit cautioned her not to go too close to the door as Miss Y. "may spit at you."
> She then explained that Miss Y. is quite senile and in the habit of expectorating indiscriminately. She refuses to use the paper tissues that are provided. Since Miss Y. "cannot be reasoned with and made to stop" this offensive behavior, she is kept locked in her room for her own protection and that of others on the floor. The home hesitates to transfer their patients to a mental institution "unless it is absolutely necessary."
> With the upper half of the door open, the staff is able to "watch Miss Y., and she in turn is able to see what goes on outside her door." Miss Y. could be seen in the dimly lighted room sitting quietly at the edge of her bed, fully dressed, staring at the half-open door, hands folded in her lap. When the nurse spoke to her through the open half of the door, she never answered.

There was no opportunity to ascertain her medical diagnosis, or what methods had been tried to induce Miss Y. to desist from her offensive habit.

In another institution, another patient was observed in isolation:

> A woman's screams and a loud pounding on a door could be heard at the nurses' station. The nurse in charge and her visitor walked toward the room from which the sounds emanated and found Mrs. S. rattling the lower half of a Dutch door in an attempt to get out of her room.
> The head nurse spoke to Mrs. S. and asked her to be more quiet,

to which the patient did not respond. The nurse then explained to her visitor that Mrs. S. was senile and to control her agitation required medication which was to be given on a p.r.n. basis. But "I don't like to give it to her so often and she'll have to wait for a while yet," the nurse commented. The screaming continued.

These two incidents bring to mind some very urgent questions such as, is this kind of treatment fairly common or exceedingly rare; what were some previous treatment methods that were tried, and failed; on what basis did the nurse make her judgment with respect to the frequency of the medication; how close is the working relationship, including communication, between nurse and physician; and what was the reason for such confinement—what dangers warranted such confinement for the protection of the patient and the protection of others on the unit?

POSITIVE ACCEPTANCE

Acceptance and constructive care to counter improper patient behavior was supported by a majority of all four nursing ranks. This position was most evident among the registered nurses, and especially the degree registered nurses, who strongly emphasized supportive and constructive acceptance of deviant behavior, coupled with searching for causes and therapy.*

Many of these nurses advocated acceptance of the unconventional behavior matter-of-factly, as in the course of nature, and assistance of the patient in accommodating himself to it. An attempt to understand the basis for the behavior is regarded as a necessary step on the part of the nurse. Identifying the cause and using it as a clue for making changes in the patient's environment or in the nursing plan, or perhaps in both, is emphasized as all-important.

Several nurse aides declared that their patients would not engage in improper conduct if they realized what they were doing *or* were not asking for something. One NA suggested that:

> Patients may engage in improper conduct because they are angry with someone. Maybe they think their family will take them back if they misbehave—it's a way of getting back at their family. I try to calm them. . . .

* NA's, 53.5 percent; LPN's, 53.8 percent; RN's, 67.1 percent; DRN's, 73.1 percent. See Appendix B, Table 4, Items 6 to 9.

Some of the licensed practical nurses also contended that a patient's misbehavior may be an indication that he needs or wants something:

> There's always a reason—the way they act may be the only way they can express themselves.

Many of the registered nurses concurred with this idea, and several of them went a step further and alleged that it is important to find the reason *and* "to act accordingly." One RN worded her concern this way:

> Don't condemn them; talk to them quietly and try and find out why they do it and take this into consideration when attempting to cope with the behavior. Something may be troubling them; they may be asking for something—expressing some need. It may be their way of asking for more attention than they are getting.

Many of the degree registered nurses who would cope with unconventional patient behavior in positive and constructive ways responded at length and in considerable detail to the question. Their major themes are contained in the following discourse.

To begin with, geriatric nurses are cautioned not to place any value judgment on the behavior of the offending patient; and it is suggested that they view the outlandish behavior calmly, quietly, and without any apparent shock, in order to preserve the patient's dignity. He should be neither ignored, scolded, or ridiculed. An attempt should be made to guard and maintain his self-respect by overlooking or offsetting any offensive behavior that may be embarrassing to any others present. A critical point was also made of how much the incident involves others beside the patient and the nurse; if none, it may be simpler to pay no special attention to minor breaches in propriety. When other persons are involved, efforts should be made to control the situation, but without criticism or censure of the patient. Rather, in coping the nurse should endeavor to leave no doubt in the patient's mind that she is on his side in his plight.

It is advisable for geriatric nurses to acquire any available knowledge of the patient's pattern of conduct before he became ill or misbehaving; to try and identify any discernible excitants for the breakdowns; and to use these preliminary insights as a basis for retaining rapport with the patient and sustaining his dignity and sense of security despite his unbecoming habits. Relatives and friends who are upset about a patient's misbehavior should be given information that is brief and to the point. Often these explanations serve to safeguard the patient from some of the anxious concerns, criticisms, or even ostracism by them.

Other approaches proposed were for geriatric nurses to consider making adjustments to minimize the impact of the offending behavior upon staff, fellow patients as well as family; changing or revising elements in the environment wherever potential advantages appear; changing or rotating nursing personnel on the one hand, or stabilizing it on the other, wherever indicated; suggesting to the physician that outside help such as a psychiatric consultant be called in when needed; and undertaking some self-examination with respect to personal coping capabilities and patterns. It was advocated that nurses learn to deal with such matters in a relaxed, routine, matter-of-fact, and self-reliant manner, and with minimum of dismay—and that liberal allowances be made whenever these seem to improve the physical and mental comfort of the patient.

It was recommended, also, that whenever feasible, any discussion and decision-making on the course to be followed be shared with the patient. Such sharing could become an important step toward solution of, or learning to live with, the problem. Moreover, an important differential might exist in age itself. When the affected person is relatively young, management of the behavioral problem is justifiably designed primarily to stimulate a return to fully normal behavior. In the case of the very aged, ill, and spent person, however, management and care can justifiably be directed toward *protection* of the patient from the consequences of his infringement on proprieties.

It was recognized, however, that there comes a time when nursing staff must set some limits to socially offensive patient behavior. If the patient is rational, it may be best to discuss the problem gently, but frankly, with him and with definite authority describe to him the permissive limits to such behavior. If more severe restraining is needed, it should be done with dignity and explanation. "Distinguish in thought and action between the disturbing behavior of the patient and the person behind it." One's focus should be on the behavior and not on the person exhibiting the behavior. Under no circumstances should the nurse react in such a way that communication with the patient is jeopardized. Anger and force have no place in such situations; but neither has excessive permissiveness.

Some nurses hold that staff intolerance of improprieties which backfire in the form of disturbed and disrupted patient-nurse relationships are rarely if ever justifiable. One DRN raised the question *why*, in the face of imminent death, should certain lapses in conventional proprieties be treated as so very significant, especially when considered in the context of previous decorum and contributions that characterized the individual whose life happens to linger into the stages of personal irresponsibility? (Olson, Prock)

The attitudes and recommended actions of the DRN's who would deal constructively with the problems of unconventional behavior on the part of aged patients are succinctly expressed by one of them:

A breakdown of conventional proprieties on the part of an aged ill person would indicate, or at least suggest, that he has either forgotten what they are or desires to rebel against them. If the former is believed to be true, the nurse of any rank would and should make direct efforts to reclarify for the patient what the rules are and why they exist.

It seems rather natural for the person who, for the most part, is uninvolved and nonparticipating within his setting to become confused, say, after a nap. No one expects him to do anything, and no one seeks his advice, although he has had a wealth of life experiences which seem somehow meaningless in his present environment. In such a state of nebulous existence, it is possible for a patient to forget he is in the hospital and even momentarily confuse his nurse with his wife who died a few years previously.

The nurse can help this patient by creating additional involvement for him in his present setting. She must provide frequent cues, cues that help him define his relationships within the environment and provide some participating activities.

Part of the nurse's task is clarifying her own role for the patient in terms that are meaningful in the situation of the moment. She cannot expect the aged ill person clearly to remember explanations intended for a future time but, rather, should be willing to repeat directions and limitations until feedback from the patient indicates understanding has taken place. Scolding the aged person will not promote his learning but, instead, will increase his feelings of inadequacy and render him less able to make decisions for himself. I have seen an aged person become physically more shaky and mentally more confused from being scolded for mistakes.

If it seems that the patient is rebelling against hospital conventions, the nursing team should discuss what his rebellion is accomplishing for him. Likely it raises his self-esteem by providing him with power in an organized institutional setting which all but removed his very identity upon admission to it. Displaced from his safe, secure home environment at a time when physiological imbalances are acute, he may have heightened needs for love and affection. If instead he finds merely tolerance, he may become so frustrated that he rebels against the authoritarian proprieties, crying, "I command you to notice me."

Having lost his capacity for adaptation, he may use hostile rebellion, if he has developed this coping pattern, because he lacks skill in developing new interpersonal relationships. In other words, he is doing the best he can to meet his needs at this time, but he needs nurses who will go more than halfway with him. He needs nurses who will provide him with a clear framework for adapting to a strange and fearful situation and who support him with a clear "I am with you" attitude. (Nagy)

SUMMARY

The statistical profile of nurse respondents' reactions to patient breakdowns in observing conventional proprieties resembles that of their reactions to mistrust and aggression. This probably should be expected since the latter also result more or less in conventional violations. Again, a minority of the respondents of all four nursing ranks reflected negative acceptance, which decreases progressively from a high of 45 percent for the nurse aides to a low of 20 percent for the degree registered group. This pattern is identical to that for mistrust, but the percentages for mistrust are substantially lower, ranging from a high of 40 percent for the nurse aides to a low of 7 percent for the degree registered nurse group.

On the side of positive acceptance of patients' violations of conventional proprieties, the majority representations increase progressively through the nursing ranks from the nurse aides to the degree registered nurse group. The exact figures are given below:

	NA's %	LPN's %	RN's %	DRN's %
Negative acceptance	45.6	44.1	33.0	20.7
Positive acceptance	53.5	53.8	67.1	73.1

On the negative acceptance side of improprieties, the tabulations present a diffuse pattern. When the percentage representations for the five procedural choices are combined and averaged for the four nursing ranks, two procedures vie for top choice: use of diversional tactics and resort to reason and persuasion. Following are the figures:

	NA's %	LPN's %	RN's %	DRN's %
Denying or ignoring the presence of such behavior	7.9	1.9	8.5	0.0
Shifting responsibility for dealing with it to others	4.0	1.9	4.9	2.4
Use of medication or restraints	1.0	9.6	4.9	8.5
Use of diversional tactics	17.8	11.5	11.0	3.7
Resorting to reason and persuasion	14.9	19.2	3.7	6.1

Among the four coded categories on the positive acceptance side for coping with breakdowns in conventional behavior, the foremost representation is found in the acceptance of it with simple attempts to reassure the patient and possibly correct his misbehavior. This position is supported by large proportions of the nurse practitioners led by the NA's with 40 percent, but it is supported by very few degree registered nurses. The largest proportion of DRN respondents accepted such improper behavior of aged patients to the extent that suffering does not occur (28 percent), and this group is followed by those who recommend acceptance with attempts to ascertain the cause (22 percent). The respective figures are:

	NA's %	LPN's %	RN's %	DRN's %
Change of staff with supportive attitude	5.0	1.9	7.3	20.7
Acceptance with attempts to reassure	40.6	36.5	28.0	2.4
Support to extent of not permitting suffering	6.9	13.5	22.0	28.0
Acceptance and attempts to ascertain basic cause	1.0	1.9	9.8	22.0

See Appendix B, Table 4, for figures used in this chapter.

The Hallucinating Patient

Your old men shall dream dreams.
BIBLE

The aged patient who hears voices and sees visions of absent or dead persons, or who is subject to sound, time, place, or object illusions, tends to be more acceptable to the nursing staff than is the patient who shows mistrust or violates conventional proprieties. This propensity is reflected in the attitudes and actions of the participants of this study, of whom a substantial majority favored acceptance of the illusory experiences of aged patients with their accompanying irrational or unrealistic behaviors.

THE NATURE OF THE PROBLEM

There appeared to be no uncertainty in the minds of nursing personnel as to what is meant by hallucinations, but considerable concern was expressed in regard to possible underlying causes of the delusions as well as to what the particular experience means to the patient. The wide range in conditions and factors which may bring on hallucinations and other illusory phenomena was repeatedly touched upon. Distinction was made between a so-called normal elderly patient who hallucinates and one who is psychotic. The question was raised, also, whether a "psychotic" patient can adequately be cared for in a geriatric institution, or whether this diagnosis warrants a patient's transfer to a mental hospital. In one of the selected geriatric facilities, an RN who held a supervisory position declared that rarely do their nurses or aides encounter such behavior disorders, since, upon the initial appearance of behavior problems, the patient is transferred to a mental hospital. However, another facility claimed that with proper medical attention and skilled nursing care, even patients with obvious mental illness are "manageable," and that, in their particular institution, it is rarely necessary to transfer such patients to a mental hospital. The administrator of another home reported that his experience has shown that with proper medical and nursing provisions, such patients *can* be cared for adequately.

Relative to this, a few of the RN practitioners and of the DRN's contended that, for the provision of skilled and effective nursing care of the aged, it is essential that the geriatric nurse have knowledge of the normal processes of aging and be aware of the particular illnesses to which an elderly person may be subject more often than would be a younger person. A background in psychiatric nursing also was considered to be helpful. The point was made that while elderly persons may be more considerably afflicted with illness, it is a fallacy to equate old age with disease. Mental symptoms in aging persons may be closely associated with any number of organic causes, such as oxygen deficiency in the tissues (anoxia), severe vitamin deficiencies due to faulty nutrition, cumulative effects of drugs, and acute infections; but, particularly in an older person, his general personality integration and the vicissitudes to which he is exposed are influencing elements in the way he reacts and behaves.

Another variable to be taken into account when coping with a patient's delusions is the way in which a patient interprets what he sees or hears—the meaning his illusory experience has for him. For example, one patient may hear the voice of a long-deceased parent who is expected to take him or her home or "is coming to take care of me," and the anticipation of this may engender a sense of comfort; whereas, another patient may express anxiety or stark fear because of "that man at the window" or "the snake in my bed."

NEGATIVE ACCEPTANCE

The contention that a patient's unconventional behavior is to varying degrees consciously engaged in may have influenced some of the nurses in the ways in which they cope with elderly patients' illusory experiences. Perhaps this accounts, to some extent at least, for the smaller minorities of nonacceptive nurses on this issue, as compared to the number who took the negative stand on the two issues discussed previously: mistrust/aggression and improprieties. Concerning the present issue of hallucinations, the negative acceptance position received its strongest support from the

nurse aides with 37 percent and the lowest from the degree registered
nurses with just under 10 percent.*

Of the nonacceptive *nurses aides,* the largest proportion reported that
they try to reason with patients and persuade them that their illusory experiences are not real. Others report that they "just listen—don't answer." If
a patient talks about an illusory experience as having happened "last
night" or in the past, it is easy to tell them that they probably had been
dreaming. One NA related a recent experience as an example of how she
handles such problems:

> One patient from time to time sees worms crawling along the wall. I
> tell him that he was dreaming, or that there are no worms on the
> wall. If he does not believe me, I walk him to the wall and let him
> run his hand over it—but sometimes even that does not work, and then
> I report it to the nurse.

Still others would change the subject or just ignore what the patient
is saying.

Licensed practical nurses who took the negative position seemed
more divided on the ways in which they handle such problems. Some
would reason with the patient; others prefer to use diversional tactics.
Still others believe it best to report the incident to the supervisor or the
physician. According to one LPN, "It's all part of the aging process—
when they say those things you just listen; you might say 'is that so' and
then go about your way." Another declared, "I want to be truthful—I say,
'Oh, there is nothing there'—most of them don't seem upset when I say
this."

Several of the nonacceptive *registered nurses* also claimed that such
phenomena rarely upset patients and that it is best to ignore the behavior
—"If they enjoy it, let them be." These practitioners stressed, however, that
if, despite their methods of handling such problems—ignoring the behavior, denying the illusion, diverting the patient's attention, or resort to
reason and persuasion—the patient continues to hallucinate, then it is time
to report the condition to the head nurse or to the physician.

Of the four ranks of nursing personnel, the *degree registered nurses*
constituted the smallest nonacceptance minority. Of these, one or two
would listen to the "visions" and merely accept them. Others suggested
that some aged patients are quite content with their delusions and see
no need for disrupting or dispelling them. Still others intimated that,
when the situation involves an aged psychotic person, the nurse may
have to play along in a role for a while and may only at times be able

---

* NA's, 37.0 percent; LPN's, 17.3 percent; RN's, 15.9 percent; DRN's, 9.6 percent.
See Appendix B, Table 5, Items 1 to 5.

to persuade the patient that she is not "Aunt Lucy." One DRN added, however, that it is important to get through to the patient and attempt to reorient him to the reality instead of continuing to play the role.

POSITIVE ACCEPTANCE

It bears repeating that minorities, though of varying proportions, in all four nursing ranks spoke out for the nonacceptance of hallucinations or other delusory experiences of aged patients. Conversely, majorities in the four ranks would deal with such behavior disorders in more positive and constructive ways. Nearly 60 percent of the nurse aides and almost 90 percent of the degree registered nurses took the positive acceptance position.*

Most of these respondents took a firm stand both on the importance of the nurse giving special attention to the illusory experience and of reorienting the patient to the realities of the situation. Of the four categories denoting specific behaviors, the two most preferred were: the nurses' acceptance of the behavior, with simple attempts to reassure, and her support of the hallucinating patient to the extent of not having him suffer.

Nurse aides gave the following representative examples of how they cope with illusory behavior:

> I have two patients, a husband and wife, who occupy one room. The husband is blind and hard of hearing. Quite often the wife "sees a prostitute" where a coat hangs, and she tells "her" in a firm and loud voice to get out of the room. When the wife indulges in this behavior I ask her to explain more of what she sees, and I let her feel the coat to show her that there is no one there. Sometimes the husband hears what his wife is saying and he starts "hollering at her." Then I take her out of the room and walk with her.

> I go along with them for the moment. One patient at times refuses to be bathed because she sees someone at the ceiling. When she says this, I look at the ceiling and say, "Mister, please go away so Miss C. can have her bath"—and the patient is reassured.

> Patients often tell you that they saw or heard something during the night. I usually say to them that perhaps they were dreaming, that there is no one in the room now, and they have nothing to be frightened about. This morning one of my patients "saw a man in a white

* NA's, 59.3 percent; LPN's, 73.1 percent; RN's, 82.9 percent; DRN's, 88.0 percent. See Appendix B, Table 5, Items 6 to 9.

coat"—I told her that I did not see him and put my arm around her, and she felt better.

Yesterday a patient told me he saw a man coming through the ventilator. I said, "Oh, you did?", and then explained that it must have been the painter—and we both laughed.

It happens often when a patient is very old and confused. We have a patient who is almost 100 years old. She tells me that she sees nude men and women in the tree outside her window—and I keep telling her that I do not see any. Then she makes no further comment —apparently this does not have much meaning for her.

One patient insists her father is out there in a tree—and she will insist that I leave food for him. I go along with her, and when she asks whether I see him, I tell her that I do—otherwise she gets upset. Sometimes she won't eat unless I tell her that this food is for her and that I'll get other food for her father—she is very confused.

One patient keeps calling for her mother, and when I ask her why she does that she says, "I want her to come after me—maybe she will and take care of me." I just let her talk, but keep telling her that we will take care of her.

Some of the *licensed practical nurses* who took the positive position reported that extra attention often helps. One of the LPN's explained that she gets someone to stay with a patient who is upset by what he sees or hears and reassures him that nothing will happen to him. Others stress the importance of ascertaining how real the experience is to the patient; sometimes patients get very set in their ideas and one may have to go along with them for the time being. One of them declared that sometimes they really do see something: "A patient recently had a vision, and when I checked, it was a reflection in the glass door."

Another LPN seemed to be in somewhat of a dilemma when she spoke of a patient who keeps calling for her dead sister:

Then she starts crying and looks for her. I tell her her sister is no longer here—I can't tell her that her sister is dead—"I should ask the doctor what I should say to her."

One of the *registered nurses* reflected the attitude and approach of many of her peers to the problem when she said that one must feel one's way: with one patient you must go along; with another, not. The important thing is to keep the patient from becoming agitated. Many of the patients—particularly if very old—call for their mother or father; others see animals on the light fixture or on the ceiling; some forever want to go home. It is important to find out how real a vision or a sound is to them:

do not try to reason, but change the subject to one that is realistic for the patient and the situation. The following examples are illustrative of some of the ways RN's cope with illusory phenomena:

> One patient seemed frightened by what he saw. I reassured him by saying that I could see it frightened him and asked whether he thought he might have been dreaming, for I could not see what he saw. One should never reenforce the vision—that way you do not bring the patient back to reality. But it is important to listen to them and to let them know that you are there to help and care for them.

> We have a patient with Parkinson's disease who sees and feels rats and snakes in her hair. This began after she had had a very traumatic experience one night: Her husband "dropped dead" and fell on her, and she was alone with him all night and could not move. Their doctor found them in the morning. By repeated persuasion and reasoning we were able to convey to her that there was nothing in her hair and she seemed more at ease. Not long thereafter she fell and broke a hip—after that she had a real breakdown.

> Another patient becomes very agitated and she sees things. This morning she told me that the devil was in her room. I just put my arm around her and "rocked" with her, holding her arms all the while. With her it goes in cycles—I change the subject after a while—one must find out whether a patient wants the illusion, finding it a comforting experience, or whether it frightens them.

The consensus of RN opinion seems to be that if a patient is frightened, you reassure by word and deed; if the patient is not frightened, you may find it best to go along for the moment—but without reinforcing his illusions. "It is all very individual." The point was also repeatedly made that some of the patients may have a psychiatric problem, in which case the various disciplines get together and a care plan is worked out—and, according to at least one RN, "if at all possible, we keep the patient here where he knows he is wanted."

GUIDELINES

As with the problems of mistrust and improprieties discussed in the two previous chapters, the testimonies of the *degree registered nurses* who spoke out for positive and constructive approaches in dealing with patients who experience hallucinations are reviewed in considerable detail. This is for the purpose of providing clear-cut portrayals of patient-nurse relationships and of identifying certain specific guidelines, supported by nursing opinion and experiences, for those who must cope with the problems of aged patients who are subject to illusory sensations. These nurses indicate five possible guidelines for sustaining and improving the nurse-patient relationships:

1. Listen consistently to the patient's accounts of his illusory experiences and note the interpretations that he puts upon them. Listen purposefully, with attention, concern, respect, and an accepting and supportive attitude—seeking understanding, in order to be helpful.

2. Guard against any contradictory, argumentative, disparaging, or indifferent responses to the patient's illusory claims. Simply make it clear that, though they are apparently real to the patient, they are not real to the nurse and that she wishes to understand why.

3. Endeavor to identify the reality factors within the situation that can be shared by patient and nurse, and attempt to keep the patient in contact with as many of these factors as possible; for they constitute anchor points for sustaining or restoring perceptions of reality.

4. Deal directly with any underlying cause or causes that can be identified which intensify the illusory sensations. If they cannot be removed, seek ways for helping the patient live with them.

5. Appraise the effects of illusory symptoms upon future prospects and welfare of the particular patient, and exercise a permissive, or even sharing, attitude toward the less harmful symptoms in the patient's situation.

An overriding admonition that appears relevant to all five suggested guidelines is a constant assurance for the patient of his full acceptance as a person of potential dignity and respect in spite of any or all of his symptoms, no matter how extraordinary or pronounced they may become. Another recurring theme is the avoidance of any appearance of surprise, shock, incredulity, or rejective attitude. Other strongly supported ideas were that the nurse maintain a natural, comforting, and supportive position; to permit the patient to do most of the talking, but to speak up at suitable points in calm, inquiring, or reassuring tones; and to make it a point to return to the patient at brief but frequent intervals, whenever circumstances permit.

Nurses who took a positive and constructive approach in coping with illusory phenomena of aged patients included in their elaborations the following: Never pass over or pass off the illusory episode as unimportant; nor ignore, belittle, or make fun of the patient or embarrass him in any way for having them. Some patients become really terrified by what is happening to them and can be in desperate need of reassurance and understanding. There are situations in which a patient needs to hear, with the confidence inspired by someone he can trust, that he is not losing his mind.

Another recurrent caution is: Never under any circumstances make use of the delusions to gain an immediate advantage over the patient, such as to suggest to him that it is God's voice that he hears, or the voice of a long lost friend or relative, telling him to eat his food, take his medicine, get up, go to bed, or to do anything else that is required of him by the nursing staff. Moreover, in critical periods, the patient should not be left to cope all alone with the voices, visions, or other illusory sensations. Since a patient may act impulsively under the stress and harm himself or others, there is also need for protection. In short, be prepared to do whatever it takes to let the patient know for sure that you respect and care for him, and that you or another understanding nurse will try to be there with him when he needs you most.

A further strong admonition is that the nurse should neither deny that the voices or images can be real to the patient nor confirm or "feed into the situation" any supportive inferences for the delusional system. In other words, do nothing to aggravate the patient over his deceptive sense of present reality. If one adds anything to support and perpetuate belief in the sounds and sights, one may be putting oneself in a compromising and untrustworthy light during any recurrent moments of lucidity on the part of the patient when he has had an opportunity to check reality for himself, as is illustrated in the following incident:

> A 90-year-old patient told her attending daughter that her own mother, who had actually passed on more than 50 years before, had sent a mutual friend with a message that she was on her death bed and wished the patient to come to her. A few days later the patient said to the daughter and her son, "Now I want you both to know that I was mistaken the other night. It has come back to me that it was not my mother who was sick and sending for me, but another woman. I remember that my own mother died many years ago."

The daughter was then glad that she had not "played along" with the illusory experience.

It is regarded as very important to help the patient by every possible means to hold onto and exercise his remaining functional links with, and his self-checking sense for, the concrete realities in his current daily existence, no matter how limited these may be. To direct the thoughts and activities of the patient *around* the illusory sensations and toward the existing unchallenged realities appears to be a much more useful procedure than to try to talk the patient out of his imaginary sights and sounds. The idea is to find and present for the patient's consideration as substitutes to his unrealistic views, selections out of his own presently acknowledged realistic perceptions within his immediate environment. The goal is to fortify his existing realities as a bulkwark against his recurring unrealities. That such a course may be beset with difficulties is acknowledged by one of the DRN's:

> A difficult and terribly tough problem lies in the reassurance of the elderly patient who hallucinates intermittently, knows that he does this, but during the episode is unable to recognize it as an unrealistic recurring experience. . . .
>
> I have sometimes, but only sometimes, been able to move such a person away from such an illusory episode by talking softly to him about a topic he is intensely interested in—literally disengaging him from an unwanted experience by engaging him in a more desirable one.
>
> This tends to work more successfully with a patient who: 1) trusts me; 2) has strong interests of his own; 3) can have his interests caught up by repetition of something very familiar: a simple poem, a Bible psalm, and the like.
>
> With a question or comment fired at him at the right moment in the recalled interference, he will at times reply to it in normal conversation, as though the illusory episode has not occurred. . . .
>
> This is an area needing further exploration. (Schwartz)

Another DRN testified to the value of similar procedures from her personal experience:

> When an aged person hallucinates, has visions or other illusory experiences, again the nurse's knowledge of the patient and his background are necessary for effective action. . . .
>
> In my father's terminal illness, he referred to absent or deceased persons. I was able to recognize the names and calmly and quietly make relevant and corrective comments without causing him anxiety. I found a brief response in kind to his questions and conversation was calming to him. . . . When he voiced that someone was coming into the room and then showed anxiety when, in fact, no one came, he was accepting of my quiet but firm statement that no one was actually entering the room and that probably he misinterpreted the sound of the treatment cart through the corridor just outside his door.
>
> A few calm and quiet queries regarding the patient who is hallucinating, applied with the nurse's knowledge of the patient's background, will help her to respond to the patient within his frame of reference and keep him calm until his instance of hallucination diminishes or passes. (Quinlan)

It is advocated that opportunities be routinely provided for the patient to test and reinforce his sense of reality along the lines of his accustomed interests by exploring a nonthreatening environment in company with his nurse or some other trusted person. The idea is to begin where the patient is and try to bring back to him recognizable bits of reality. For example, getting the patient up in a chair; keeping him in contact with other persons and in contact with radio and television; telling him where he is and what you see and don't see in his environment; and keeping him "oriented"—repeat and repeat—until, hopefully, he fits himself into a self-orienting pattern of tested and reinforced reality. There was Mrs. J., for instance:

> At 82 years of age, Mrs. J.'s only complaint was failing eyesight, and she looked forward to having eye surgery which was to restore her sight. A widow, she lived alone and managed her home without outside help.
>
> Three days following her eye surgery, Mrs. J. recognized no one who came to her bedside, and neither did she remember where she was or what had happened to her. Her disorientation encompassed seemingly "everything." Her reality was her early childhood. Though there was no apparent reason for her not to be up and about, she could not walk, was not able to dress herself, and needed to be fed like a child. She kept calling for absent or deceased brothers and sisters and for her mother, who had died some 50 years before.
>
> When this condition persisted, her children decided to take their mother home, where she would be cared for amid familiar surroundings and where one of her daughters would be in daily attendance.
>
> Day after day, and week after week, when Mrs. J. would dwell on the distant past and talk as though she were still a small child, those who cared for her would gently remind her of some element in her present "world" and try to have her recognize a particular person who was in the room or an article she used to cherish.
>
> Very slowly the mantle of darkness lifted from her mind. After some 6 months Mrs. J. began to recognize the daughter who had been with her constantly and also a son who had been visiting frequently and regularly. She began to dress herself and show an interest in her surroundings. Her illusory episodes recurred intermittently, however.
>
> When another daughter came to visit, Mrs. J. did not recognize her, though she had been prepared for the visit and seemingly looked forward to it. The daughter had been cautioned beforehand and, realizing her mother's predicament, greeted her with, "Mother, I am Anne, your daughter—I have come to see you," to which the mother answered, "Yes, I know," but falling silent then and looking at her daughter as though not certain of her identity. After a while she asked, "Are you really Anne?"
>
> A week passed, during which time this dialogue was repeated many times, until one morning Mrs. J. said, "You are Anne—how good of you to come and see me."
>
> With the coming of spring, Mrs. J. began to take an interest in the out-of-doors once more. She would sit quietly in the garden or

take a brief walk, with someone accompanying her. Her reorientation to the present increased. She would recognize a neighbor who stopped by, a favored tree in the garden, a flower she had planted before her surgery. If a person spoke quietly and slowly with her, using simple phrases, Mrs. J. would respond.

Occasionally Mrs. J. would appear puzzled, as though not sure what had happened to her. At times she would say that she knew she had been very ill but could not remember. From time to time her illusory world became apparent to a perceptive observer. Most important, however, Mrs. J. appeared to find once more some joy in living.

She died peacefully the next winter, following a brief illness.

Whether under different circumstances and a different treatment plan the outcome would have been different is a moot question. When the children discussed with the physicians their plan to take Mrs. J. home, they were cautioned that caring for her would be extremely difficult and a burden, for she would require constant care, day and night, until the end of her days. They held out no hope for improvement in her mental condition, and recommended that she be placed in an institution for the mentally ill. Her family physician, however, was not so positive in his prognosis. Throughout he was a pillar of strength, closely supervising Mrs. J.'s care and giving moral support to those who cared for her. A neighbor called Mrs. J.'s recovery "a miracle."

Nurses also called attention to the fact that when aged persons can no longer see or hear, they tend to create their own sights and sounds, and that it may be difficult to "get through" to them and help them to know what is real and what is not. Yet, these nurses insist, it is well to be alert to the few lucid and clear moments and use these to reorient the patient to reality points in his life. It may help to focus his attention on some specific point in space and time, such as an important event in his life, a flower, a jigsaw puzzle, playing checkers or some other game, a treasured memento, or even the view looking out the window at currently transpiring events, such as moving traffic, a familiar person, a bird in flight, or anything that fixes attention at a point or on an event or object of immediate and concrete reality. Such concerted attention on the present situation may give the patient some confidence and stability and certain concrete anchor items to which to direct his thinking. It is possible for almost anything of interest to become the core of a reality situation for the patient. Within a situation such as this, with groping to grasp hold of reality items, the inadvisability of leaving a person alone to come to terms with and find control over his illusionary tendencies becomes all the more apparent.

One DRN expressed some of these ideas succinctly from her professional experience:

When a person calls attention to a recent illusory experience, I usually ask him to tell me about it—what he sees and what he hears—and I display interest in what he says. It has come to my attention that blind patients very often experience seeing other persons or objects which are not there, and that this is a great torment to them. . . .

After exploring the sights and sounds as far as possible, I try to find out what this person or thing has meant to the patient in the past. There are often significant observations around which a nursing care plan may be constructed. In other words, it is often a very caring person whom the patient "sees" and who is not really in the picture. Occasionally, however, it is a frightening person. I would approach this problem by saying that although his loved one—perhaps his son —is not really with him, that I am there and that I care about him.

On the other hand, I have had experience with an older person who was entertaining herself by living through again and again certain experiences which apparently once were real but are no longer within her environment at all. In this situation, I took the approach of thoroughly enjoying the visits into the past with her.

But I have found that if we can make the present more interesting, the patient generally tends to stay more in contact with the present reality and makes fewer references to sights and sounds that are no longer real. (Knowles)

The uniqueness of each individual and the complexity of each situation was frequently commented upon by nurses when coping with a patient's illusory experiences. So was the difficulty of "getting through" to a patient in terms of reality factors when there is little or no reality left in a patient's world, as happens with some of the very senile patients. Is there, after all, any difference between a patient of very advanced age who clings to a doll—her only touch with reality—and the senile patient whose present reality includes a deceased relative? One DRN touched upon this problem when she commented:

I find this question almost too "iffy" to package a reply. When an agitated, senile person climbs out of bed to hunt for a relative dead these 20 years, I have found her energy self-limiting. By gently walking with her the length of the ward and looking for "Mother" with her, she has used up physical energy that might otherwise have been spent in climbing over the bed rails again. And by the time we had opened closet doors to look and had walked the equivalent of a street block, she readily went back to sleep without sedation. (Schwartz)

Another DRN reflected the views of several of her peers when she declared that she did not think that "a categorical answer to the infinite variety of these complex individual problems can be developed, except to say that they must be met as the individual problems demand." (Duxbury)

It bears repeating perhaps, that when the affected individual is a relatively young ager, or when there is no obvious mental impairment, management of the problem is designed to stimulate a return to normal behavior. On the other hand, in the case of a very aged or senile patient, who has little or no sense of reality left, emphasis should probably be directed toward protecting him.

DISCUSSION

In conclusion, it may be important to point out that the general and somewhat elusive query remains with respect to the prevailing nursing attitudes toward the three behavioral problems of aged patients that have been discussed; namely, what are the differences in staff attitudes and reactions to patients' symptoms and needs—whether they manifest them in hostile behavior such as mistrust, improprieties, or hallucinatory behavior? From the viewpoint of the nurse respondents, this question seems to hinge on the issue of the aged ill person's awareness of, and capacity to measure up to, expectations held for him by staff, family, and friends as they view and appraise him.

The reporting nursing personnel imply that the mistrusting and aggressive patients *know* what they are doing and *could* better control their behavior; that the patients who violate conventional proprieties *may or may not know* what they are doing but *should* behave; and that the behavior of the hallucinatory or delusional patients is largely *beyond their understanding and control.* Whether there is any basis in fact for such differentiation is difficult to say. Whether there are pertinent clues in these points of view for further useful exploration—either on better understanding of nursing attitudes and reactions, or on the behaviors of aged persons, or both these areas—remains to be seen and challenges further examination.

Whatever the complexities in coping with the geriatric patient behavior disorder problems considered in the foregoing pages or the varied causes underlying particular behavioral problems such as these, it may be useful to quote the words of Overholser and Fong who, in their discussion on the relationships of mental disorders to the aging process and the impact of internal and external stress on the individual, describe the symptoms of gradual transition into senile psychosis:

> These begin as a decrease in alertness; slowing up and narrowing of interest span; loss of memory (particularly spontaneous recall and memory of recent events); absentmindedness; a tendency to over-

talkativeness, circumstantiality, and irrelevancy; disturbances in sleep rhythm (daytime drowsiness and nighttime prowling about the house); some periods of confusion; some ideas of persecution; untidiness progressing to carelessness of eliminative functions; irritability and feelings of inadequacy; reduced sexual activity but sometimes increased sexual interest; nocturnal deliria with noisiness; anxiety; fear; loss of orientation; illusions and hallucinations; impaired judgment. The progress of these symptoms may be spotty, with brief temporary improvements in the early stages.*

The distinguished psychiatrist Dr. Alvin I. Goldfarb, well-known for his work with the aged ill, sheds some further light on the problem in the following statement:

> The aged with mental disorders are a heterogeneous group who may differ in ages by 30 or more years and who vary markedly in their physical, emotional, and social status . . . because they have distortions in social perception, in goal, in activity, and in self-understanding, we find it difficult to see what they want or are trying to get—it is hard to understand and to help these people. Difficulty in understanding them may be met to some degree by the recognition that certain needs are universal; the special needs of the person may be grasped by catching onto the themes that appear to underlie and hold together what must otherwise be disconnected and meaningless behavior. . . . In dealing with older people, one of the most difficult problems one encounters is that of bringing home to the family, friends, and attendants that disordered behavior is a way of making known certain needs.†

SUMMARY

As with mistrust and aggressions and with improprieties, the statistical profile of nurse respondents to patients' hallucinations or other delusory experiences shows a minority pattern of negative acceptance which, again, is led by the nurse aides and trailed by the degree registered nurses.

The converse is found with respect to positive acceptance of such behavior. Here the DRN's lead and the NA's trail. The exact figures are contained in the following chart.

---

* Overholser, A. B., and Fong, T. C. In Stieglitz, E. J., ed. *Geriatric Medicine.* Philadelphia, J. B. Lippincott Co. 1954.
† Goldfarb, Alvin I. Patterns in planning a psychiatric program for the aged. *Bull. N.Y. Acad. Med.* Second Series, 34:818-819, 1958.

	NA's %	LPN's %	RN's %	DRN's %
Negative acceptance of patients' hallucinatory behavior	37.0	17.3	15.9	9.6
Positive acceptance of such behavior	59.3	73.1	82.9	88.0

Within the five coded categories of negative acceptance, the percentages of representation were all relatively low and were widely dispersed, rather than clustered. In the categories of positive acceptance, however, pronounced clustering appeared. *Change in staff with supportive attitudes* was especially low in representation, as was the proposal to *accept the symptomatic behavior with attempts to ascertain the basic cause.* But *supporting the patient to the extent of relieving suffering* and *acceptance with simple attempts to reassure* were both strongly represented. It seemed clear that, although a great many of these nurses are deeply puzzled about what to do for such patients, they were ready and willing to take a firm stand in their tolerance for and general support of them.

The evident similarities within certain aspects of the three behavioral problems (mistrust, improprieties, hallucinations) which were discussed in the two foregoing and the present chapters would seem to warrant the juxtaposition of the figures representing the negative and the positive positions on these three problems for easy comparison. They are given in the chart below.

	NA's %	LPN's %	RN's %	DRN's %
NEGATIVE ACCEPTANCE				
Mistrust/Aggression	40.2	32.6	17.0	7.2
Improprieties	45.6	44.1	33.0	20.7
Hallucinations	37.0	17.3	15.9	9.6
POSITIVE ACCEPTANCE				
Mistrust/Aggression	55.8	50.0	76.8	89.4
Improprieties	53.5	53.8	67.1	73.1
Hallucinations	59.3	73.1	82.9	88.0

As revealed by these figures, the statistical profiles of nurse respondents show a similarity in pattern. In every instance, though with varying proportions, the negative acceptance stance is supported by minorities in each of the four ranks. In each instance, also, the minority support consists of descending representations, from relatively high representations for the NA's to low for the DRN's.

With minorities supporting the negative acceptance position, it follows, of course, that majorities in the four ranks support the positive stance, and with descending representations reversed. In each instance, the highest support comes from the DRN's and, with one exception, the lowest support is provided by the NA's. The exception occurs in connection with the problem of mistrust, which is given the lowest support by the LPN's, and followed by the NA's.

The figures reveal also that, in general, the nursing personnel seem *most* accepting of patients having hallucinations or other illusory experiences, and *least* accepting of those which violate conventional proprieties. These differences, and especially the proportion of differences between the four ranks of nursing personnel in the ways in which they cope with these behavioral problems, may justify delving into the literature of medicine and other related disciplines in order to gain further insights into, and perhaps some clues for, improving the care of the aged ill.

For full statistical details, see Appendix B, Tables 3, 4, 5.

Loss of Consciousness:
Implications for Patient Care

Most patients are unconscious at the moment of death and some drift into this state unaware of what is happening.

CICELY SAUNDERS

Nurses entrusted with the care of aged patients in the select geriatric institutions frequently expressed the belief that most patients are unconscious at the time of dying. They maintained, also, that there is a wide variation in time span, as well as in depth, of a patient's unconscious state prior to death, especially senescent death. A director of nursing, who has devoted most of her professional life to the care of the aged ill, commented that Nature tends to be kind to very old people—many of them just "fall asleep"—and she judged that about half of those who closed their lives in the home drifted into a sleeplike coma days, weeks, or even months, before they died. So it was with Mrs. E.:

> Mrs. E. was in her late eighties when she died, having been a resident in the home for the aged about five years. She had been admitted to the institution following a hip fracture from which she recovered sufficiently so that she was able to walk and be independent in her activities of daily living. As the years passed, however, Mrs. E. became progressively more dependent, needing help with dressing, bathing, and the like. She also began spending more and more time in her wheelchair.
>
> Then, for no observable reason, Mrs. E. began to loose ground more rapidly. She grew weaker and needed to be fed. Her appetite was poor. Her usual cheerfulness gave way to a noticeable quiet. Several weeks before her death, she drifted into a "deep sleep"; however she could be sufficiently aroused to take the food and drink that were offered. As the days went by, Mrs. E.'s coma deepened, until one morning she quietly breathed her last.

112

DEGREES OF CONSCIOUSNESS AND UNCONSCIOUSNESS

The periods of drowsiness of varying lengths which may precede an aged patient's final sleep have significant implications for nursing care of seriously ill geriatric patients. So has the relative degree of patients' conscious or unconscious mental state. The range between a high level of consciousness and a deep coma is wide. Indeed, awareness differs greatly among aged patients as well as at different times within the same individual.

In order to provide optimum care, it is important that the nurse ascertain the relative degree of consciousness and responsiveness of a seriously ill patient. This is crucial for any participating involvement of the patient in his care, to whatever extent he desires and is capable of so doing. There can, of course, be no active involvement, physically or psychologically, without some sort of communication between nurse and patient. When a patient is very ill, it is rarely ever easy to become aware of all his needs, for some of them may only be covertly expressed. Even a very alert and conscious patient may not verbally make many of his needs known, but the unconscious state of a particular patient makes a nurse's task considerably more difficult, regardless of the depth of unconsciousness. Indeed, there are times when it may not be easy to judge when a patient is conscious and when he is not. Moreover, incidents have been reported where conscious, very ill or depressed aged patients more or less withdraw into themselves, refusing to respond to further stimuli around them. This also confuses the issue.

The problem is further complicated by the routine use of heavy sedation for control of pain or disturbing patient behavior. This sedation is sometimes administered to patients to relieve staff of some of the pressures and responsibilities of providing more supportive, but time-consuming care. Medical directors in two different geriatric facilities categorically stated that, among institutionalized aged persons, many more are over-, rather than undermedicated.

The unconscious state commonly preceding death may vary in its duration considerably more than nature decrees because of modern medical devices with which respiration and circulation can be prolonged "almost indefinitely." This may have been so in the following experience:

> The patient was an octogenarian whose condition had steadily worsened since being admitted to the hospital, and the doctors held out no hope

for her recovery. Because of a severe shortage of hospital beds she was transferred to the nursing home. The hospital physicians assured the family that the patient would be given the same kind of care in the home, and they reluctantly agreed to the transfer. The doctors predicted that death would occur within a matter of days.

In the nursing home the patient came under another Doctor's care. This physician informed the family that his philosophy was that "where there is life there is hope" and he instituted treatments such as regular nasogastric feedings, infusions, and various medications given by injections. These had not been part of the treatment plan in the hospital.

More than two months went by, during which time the patient's body was meticulously cared for. Then urinary complications set in, which did not respond to medical treatment and the patient died without ever regaining consciousness.

When, several days following the burial, a family friend made a condolence call, the patient's daughter said: "The hospital doctors had given mother just a few more days to live—they told us that she would never get over this. We should never have taken her to the nursing home; we should have brought her back home where she could have died in peace. We did not mind the expense, though we had to take out a bank loan to pay for her care; but I shall never forget how mother would lie there with tubes sticking out all over—never saying a word. I wonder sometimes whether the doctor ever thought of mother in human terms."

The particular illness afflicting the elderly person also affects his state of consciousness, as does the patient's general state of health. If stricken with a catastrophic disease such as cancer while still in the fullness of life and health, the person is apt to remain conscious and alert until a relatively short time before his death, whereas the advanced ager with no apparent organic disease, but weary in mind and body and slowly dying of "old age," may sink into a coma for a relatively longer period before death comes.

There is the possibility that some nurses tend to feel more comfortable by assuming "black or white" positions when caring for a conscious or unconscious patient and do not bother with uncertainties within the grey zones of partial loss of consciousness. Certain nurses behave as though communication is not possible between them and a patient unless they get clear evidence of his awareness. At any rate, a conscious and alert patient is treated more as a *person* than one who is semi- or unconscious. When a patient does not respond, he is apt to be viewed more as a "thing" or a "vegetable" and to be treated as though he were already dead. This is how nurses seemed to regard Mrs. D. when she was critically ill and unconscious:

Dr. and Mrs. D. had spent all of their married life in the big, rambling house, several rooms of which also served as the doctor's office. They were in their seventies when Dr. D. died. Though the house was quite large for one person, Mrs. D. continued to live there because to her it was "home." She was glad, however, when the physician who took over her husband's medical practice took over Dr. D.'s office as well. While she lived quietly, Mrs. D. said that she led a full life, keeping up with friends and neighbors, continuing with some of her community activities, and keeping house. Her children were married and lived elsewhere, but they kept in touch regularly and visited occasionally.

One day, when she was in her early eighties, Mrs. D. fell. Though she did not hurt herself, her children expressed concern about her being in the house alone much of the time and prevailed upon her to give up her home and enter a nursing home in the city where her eldest daughter and family resided. While admitting that age was beginning to take its toll and that she did not have the strength and endurance she once had, Mrs. D., nevertheless, opposed the idea of giving up her home; but after several months she yielded to her children's wishes.

No single room was available in the nursing home, and Mrs. D., who had always prized her freedom and her privacy, was asked to share a room with a person about whom she knew nothing. She had never been an outgoing person, and upon entering the nursing home, became quite withdrawn. Though the staff encouraged Mrs. D. to join the other residents and participate in some of the social activities, she preferred to spend much of her time in her room. Her daughter's questions about her well-being were usually answered with, "I am all right."

Two years passed, during which time her daughter and granddaughter visited regularly. On Sundays and holidays, Mrs. D. would often have dinner with her daughter's family. They also kept her supplied with her favorite jam, cookies, and other tidbits she liked. These she kept hidden in her room, since the rules did not allow food being brought in. Late at night Mrs. D. would eat a cookie or two, for at that time she would feel "a little empty"—the evening meal in the home was served some two hours before the dinner hour to which she had been accustomed. So was breakfast.

Mrs. D.'s health had never been very robust, but during her stay in the nursing home her health seemed to decline gradually but steadily. She became quite frail physically, but mentally she remained alert and very keen. She was bedfast for nearly 2 weeks before she died, and in a deep coma for about five days. During her final illness, Mrs. D.'s daughter spent a great deal of time with her. When Mrs. D. became unconscious, the daughter remained at her bedside almost constantly, going home late at night and returning early in the morning.

Mrs. D. did not regain consciousness, but the daughter was certain that her mother continued to have some understanding and was aware, to some extent, of what was going on about her. As evidence, she cited an occasional flicker of her eyelids and responses she felt when holding her mother's hand and talking assuringly to her.

After her mother's death, the daughter related that she was glad that she had kept vigil at her mother's bedside, for she was convinced that her mother had derived comfort from her presence there, even though she could not communicate verbally. The daughter felt strongly about this, particularly since the nurses and aides "would come into the room, bathe mother, move her from side to side—but never address a word to her, though talking among themselves." She also contended that during the many hours she sat at her mother's bedside, various staff members would come into the room from time to time to check whatever paraphernalia was used: to make sure that the clysis solution was running as it should be and that the indwelling catheter was draining. She expressed some bitterness when she said that the staff seemed more concerned about the mechanical apparatus that was used than about her mother as a person. In her words, "They treated my mother as though she were a lump of clay."

She also expressed some doubt that a nursing home had been the best possible solution for her mother, and she reminisced about her mother having always been a "gentlewoman," who invariably treated others with kindness and respect and who had devoted a great deal of her time to "doing for others."

Concerning such impersonal behavior of nursing personnel in their care of unconscious patients, a nursing instructor writes:

> Unfortunately, the semi- or unconscious person is frequently talked over and ignored while physical care is being given. This is violating the right of the person to a sense of dignity and worth. No one has the right to do this to another human being. Awake, asleep, conscious or unconscious, the person has the right to our attention and respect. He must not be ignored, or talked about as if he were not there. (Declan)

To be sure, loss of consciousness does not necessarily result in the death of the person. Nurses recalled a number of incidents in which aged patients had regained consciousness and recovered from the particular illness or accident which brought on the comatose condition.

It is quite generally recognized that one cannot dependably estimate the depth of consciousness or unconsciousness. Experiences have been cited by nurses in which an unconscious patient may at intervals be hearing and feeling out of proportion to his outward manifestations of awareness. Patients, upon rallying from a coma, are said to have commented upon matters discussed in their presence when they appeared unconscious. An experienced and dedicated nurse aide told of a patient who, when left alone, kept moaning, but who would relax and be quiet when someone went into her room and talked with her. A registered nurse related how one of her patients, an 87-year-old woman, had been in a semicoma for several weeks. She could be aroused with effort to take food and drink, only to return to a stuperous state.

Although unconscious patients may be hearing and feeling out of proportion to their outward manifestations, the margin on which to reach a decision may become very fine, as reflected in the story of Mrs. T.:

> Following a cerebrovascular accident, Mrs. T. was hospitalized. She was aphasic and utterly dependent. During the several weeks Mrs. T. was in the hospital, her condition remained quite static. She would take liquid nourishment when this was put to her lips, but in general appeared unresponsive to outside stimuli. She was also an "old diabetic" who, several years prior to her recent illness, had had both legs amputated because of gangrene.
>
> When Mrs. T.'s condition did not improve, her family arranged for her admission to the nursing home. Shortly after being transferred to the home clyses were started because the staff had difficulty in getting the patient to swallow. She offered no resistance when care was given, but neither did she give any sign of awareness when asked by the nurse or aide to help in turning or otherwise assisting in her care. She gave no recognition when spoken to, but from time to time would open her eyes and gaze about the room, seemingly bewildered.
>
> She died eight days after admission. The nursing staff were not sure whether or not they had at any time "reached" Mrs. T.

Voluntary withdrawal may partially explain why Mr. G. remained unresponsive from the day he entered the institution until his death several days later:

> Until his final illness, Mr. G. had been very active. A chemist by profession and a specialist in his field, he had kept working until his late seventies. During retirement he enjoyed and kept up with community activities and world affairs. Then he became ill, and his wife found it difficult to care for him at home and arranged to have him admitted to the hospital. Mr. G. pleaded with his wife and the physician to leave him at home where he had lived for so many years. His pleas were to no avail.
>
> From the moment he was removed from his home by ambulance until his death in the institution, Mr. G. was not heard to utter another word, though his wife, his physician, and the nursing staff tried in various ways to converse with him. He gave the appearance of someone in a coma, kept his eyes closed most of the time, gave no sign of recognition when spoken to, and refused to swallow when food and drink were offered to him. His physician stated that he could find no physical reason for Mr. G.'s lack of response.

Significant though causal factors and their relevance to patient needs may be, our present concern is directed largely toward the intrinsic condition and its effect, if any, upon care provided for the afflicted person; specifically, in what ways, if any, does or should a nurse's care differ depending on whether the patient is fully conscious and mentally alert or unconscious or under heavy sedation?

No Differentiation in Patient Care

When this topic was explored within the different ranks of nursing personnel, sharply opposing positions concerning the main issue emerged. More than half of the nurse practitioners: nurse aides, licensed practical nurses, and registered nurses, declared that no difference is made in the care they provide for their aged patients: no matter whether a patient is conscious or unconscious, responsive or unresponsive, each one is cared for alike. The degree registered nurses, on the other hand, endorsed this position less strongly, with only about one fourth of the group declaring that no difference should be made in patient care on the basis of his mental awareness.*

The justifications or explanations these nurses offer are similar regardless of nursing rank. In essence, their reasoning is that it is almost impossible to estimate the depth of consciousness or unconsciousness, and no one can be certain of the extent to which the semi- or unconscious person is aware of his surroundings. These respondents were unequivocal in supporting the idea of "sameness" of care for conscious and unconscious patients in all aspects of nursing care, from technical procedures and physical care to meeting psychosocial needs.

Their contention was that basically there can be no difference in the care of a conscious and an unconscious patient because their needs are the same, physical and psychological. The needs of all aged, critically ill patients must be anticipated, regardless of their mental awareness. Even if alert, an aged patient may not always make his needs and wants known. Both categories of patients require close attention for such needs as food and drink, elimination, positioning, and the like. Neither are differences made in medications and treatments which the physician may have prescribed—these are continued regardless of a patient's mental awareness.

Moreover, the semi- or unconscious patient may have lucid moments and be able to hear more than his outward behavior indicates. Therefore it behooves the staff to treat an unconscious patient as though he can hear or feel something of what is being said to him or done for him. Irrespective of a patient's mental state, the utmost care must be exercised, lest an untoward word be spoken in his presence that might throw him into a depression or otherwise aggravate him.

---

* NA's, 51.0 percent; LPN's, 54.7 percent; RN's, 54.3 percent; DRN's, 26.7 percent. See Appendix B, Table 6, Items 1, 2.

In brief, both the conscious and unconscious patients have the same needs, and no differences are, or should be, made in their care; both need protection from physical and psychosocial environmental factors; both need close supervision with respect to airways, nutrition, elimination, and assurances of safety; both should be given explanations concerning ministrations, whether these pertain to changing his damp pillow, a treatment to be given, medication being administered, or a visitor to be introduced. In the words of a DRN, "The unconscious patient deserves as much consideration and respect as the conscious patient—and vice versa."

Care Differentiation According to Degree of Consciousness

The idea of equal care for critically ill patients irrespective of their mental awareness is challenged by a substantial minority of the nurse practitioners and a strong majority of the degree registered nurses. According to this group, important care differences do exist for conscious and unconscious patients.*

Regarding the *nature* of these differences, however, many divergencies are encountered. The practitioner groups once more are sharply split, with roughly one in six supporting the concept of care differences, claiming that they give more care to the patient who is mentally aware and conscious. A similar proportion asserted that they provide more care for an unconscious patient. Among the DRN's who hold that loss of consciousness is a basis for care differentiation, approximately one in six also would give more care to a conscious patient; but a much larger number of them express the conviction that it is the unconscious patient who needs more nursing care and attention. A relatively small number of respondents who supported care differences did not indicate what these differences might be. Particular stances and counter stances are revealed by the figures in Table 6, but the very considerable divergences in the nature of care differences inherent in the nurses' practices described, and favored by them defies systematic analysis.

Nurses endorsing the concept of care differences variously view these in terms of kind, quantity, and patient involvement, among others. The more definitive of these differences will be briefly discussed.

---

* NA's, 40.4 percent; LPN's, 45.3 percent; RN's, 43.2 percent; DRN's, 73.3 percent. See Appendix B, Table 6, Items 3 to 9.

More Care for Conscious Patients

Those who held that a conscious and mentally alert aged patient requires more nursing care than the patient who is semi- or unconscious or heavily sedated reasoned more or less as follows: Anxious and fearful about his condition, the seriously ill person needs someone with him to share talk or just to listen. The mentally alert patient may be aware of his prognosis, be despondent about his recovery, and question the value of therapeutic measures prescribed by the physician. Such a situation may be more difficult for the nurse to manage than are the various technical aspects of care of a patient who is semi- or unconscious.

Extra time is also needed for his physical care. Old age does not appreciate being hurried, and the aged patient who is conscious will be less fretful if the nurse is deliberate in her talk and gives care without haste. This applies even to little things, such as changing the patient's pillow and offering nourishment. The feeling must be conveyed to him that he is still included in the living world around him. He may not have the strength or the interest to be a very active participant; yet it is important that efforts be made to involve him in decision-making and in his care—to whatever extent he desires and is capable, though this may take additional nursing time as well as patience. To guide his hand with a face cloth so he may wash his face, and to allow and assist him to drink out of a cup or glass instead of a drinking tube may be insignificant tasks as far as the nurse is concerned, but they may matter to the patient as a person. "It is the patient's right and prerogative as a person who has dignity and human worth."

Furthermore, though very ill, the patient may continue to be interested in the larger world outside and appreciate it when those who care for him share some newsworthy item with him or ask his opinion on a subject other than himself. On the other hand, he may appreciate having in the nurse an attentive and understanding listener who affords him an opportunity to express his feelings about himself or his condition. However, one DRN cautions that this should not be overdone: "It is important that the attention be given him in frequent but brief doses. Because of his limited strength, he is not to be subjected to lengthy discourses by long-winded nurses." (Russell) A religious Sister writes:

> When the patient is fully conscious and mentally alert the challenge is greater, because the patient is more aware of his needs and thus usually demands more of the nurse. The great challenge of death is more acute to him. One must have strong personal convictions about death to help this type of person. . . . I strongly object to medica-

tions used to make the patient unaware of his state. I do believe in the proper use of medication for relief of pain and anxiety, etc., but not to the point of cheating the person out of his opportunity to prepare himself to meet his Maker. (Frenay)

More Care for the Unconscious Patient

The idea that the needs of semi- or unconscious patients are greater as compared with the needs of patients who are conscious and alert is supported by less than 1 in 6 of the nurse practitioners. However, slightly more than half of the degree registered nurses endorsed this position.

Those who hold the "more care for unconscious patients" concept maintained that, while the mentally alert patient may be more demanding of attention and care, the semi- or unconscious person actually requires more intensive care, physical and psychological. They suggest that the physical risks of these patients are greater because they cannot verbalize their wants. Pressure sores and other complications may develop unless the patient is positioned frequently and regularly. Dehydration may result unless he is given sufficient amounts of fluids, which, in the case of a patient who is more or less unresponsive, requires more expert skill as well as a great deal of patience, understanding, and perseverance. Indeed the claim is made that often these patients fail to receive certain kinds of physical care because their needs are not recognized by the nurse.

Detection of all types of needs are, of course, far more difficult for the nurse when the patient is unconscious, for he is unable to convey the nature of his needs, thus leaving the decision to guesswork. A dedicated and very experienced geriatric RN declared that many patients with loss of consciousness are given nourishment or fluids artificially, because it is more expeditious or the nursing staff lack the skill or patience, or both, to give it to the patient by mouth.

These respondents contend that the care of a semi- or unconscious patient demands extra attention from the professional nurse, extra sensitivity, observational skills, and judgment, so that no avenue be neglected in order to reach him in any flickering moment of awareness. For the truly comatose patient, the nurse must take over for the patient's senses. Some nurses see this as a situation that calls for one-sided communication—much like a mother trying to perceive and interpret the needs of an infant. But regardless of whether or not the patient can be aroused, nothing should ever be said or done in his presence that would not be said or done were he obviously aware. All the senses should be utilized in an attempt to convey to him the feeling that he is still being cared for and wanted. It is a widespread belief that the sense of hearing and touch are the last to go and these particularly should be used freely up to the end with the hope of making the patient's dying a little less lonely. "The need for human contact remains, even though the person is unconscious."

A nurse aide related how she uses a "special language" with her unconscious patients. She explains what she is going to do and asks the patient to indicate his response by blinking an eye, nodding or shaking his head, or squeezing her hand. "It is surprising how often you can arouse them," she commented, adding that just because a person is dying does not mean that you should no longer communicate with or do for them.

Kinds of Care Differences

A fairly obvious, yet significant, difference pertains to a patient's participation in his own care. When a person is mentally alert and conscious, his care ideally is accomplished *with* him. Admittedly, critically ill aged patients often are weary to death and have very limited strength. Yet it is important that they be permitted, even encouraged, to share and assist in their care—to whatever degree this is possible in view of the particular patient's condition and desires. With a comatose patient, the nurse essentially does *for* him. He is more a passive, rather than an active, participant. The difference in nursing care for critically ill patients with mental alertness and those in semi- or unconsciousness would seem to lie largely in the communicative behavior utilized by the nurse.

Individual quotations may convey to the reader a more realistic and vivid conception of how these nurses feel about their opportunities and responsibilities in the care provided for seriously ill aged patients, whether mentally alert and conscious, semi- or unconscious, or under heavy sedation:

> There is the possibility that the patient who is conscious may be able to help the nurse identify his problems and his capabilities more clearly so that she can try different approaches for their solution or in assisting the person to strengthen his assets. For a patient who is semi- or unconscious or under heavy sedation, the nurse is more dependent upon her "standbys" of devices or instruments, such as thermometers, to assist her in getting "readings" of the patient's condition. If she is talking to the semi- or unconscious person, she can only hope that he may understand through tone and touch that she cares about him and is taking responsibility for everything, literally everything, in his life. She has to make observations and decisions on less available data, takes greater risks of making errors, and finds the evaluation of her nursing care more difficult. (Knowles)

> I feel that care for the semiconscious or heavily sedated patient needs an added time factor for arousing the person and explaining

what is going on. . . . This is why I think the professional nurse should work with subprofessional nursing personnel. The technical procedures, such as personal hygiene, fixing dressings, etc., can be done by these ancillary workers while the professional nurse expertly and gently turns and holds the patient in position and at the same time conveys verbally her interest and concern for him. She can show her concern, also, by stroking or wiping the forehead or holding a hand of the patient in expressing, "we care for you. . . ." In the area of sedation for suffering, I feel that if the patient is given nursing care that reaches a high level of personal interest and concern, less sedation is necessary.

For the care of the unconscious person, one of the most important things is to be continually making sure that the person cannot be aroused. This is important, whether or not the unconscious patient can actually "know" what is happening to him; for perhaps it is not so much that the unconscious person can "know" as that the patient's condition fluctuates from unconscious to semiconscious without being detected. For both the semi- or unconscious, I would expect some "family" to be around; and the professional nurse has to spend some time with them. To be in a room with some member of your family who cannot respond may be both dull and frightening. I am sure some family members have the urge to escape and at the same time feel an obligation to stay. The professional nurse should help in this situation. (Kerrigan)

For the conscious and mentally alert sick old person, one always gives *anticipatory guidance* to help him understand the next step in a plan of nursing care. . . . "I would like to turn you on your side, Mrs. C., and put a rectal tube in, to try and help you get rid of those gas pains. It will feel like having your temperature taken. May I?" I think the "May I" is important before undertaking any intrusive procedures with the conscious patient. It implies that she controls the situation; and although she seldom uses that control, I have often heard patients speak with relief of appreciation in their feeling that, "If I said no, you would not do it." In any event, it helps to keep the nurse aware of what otherwise may be the patient's mounting passive resentment. . . .

With the semiconscious or heavily sedated patient I would use a similar approach, but with different expectation. It would be a kind of screening test to be sure that my perception of the patient's state of consciousness is correct. . . .

For the truly unconscious patient, the nurse must "become" the patient's mind and nervous system, must anticipate bodily needs, including positioning and skin care, as though she felt for this patient with herself, much as a mother does for a newborn, or helplessly retarded, child. . . . (Schwartz)

Discussion

For a balanced and candid perspective on geriatric nursing, it should also be recorded that, at times, a puzzling interpretive problem presents itself. Subtle contrast in care requirements point to an existing paradox as though the thoughts and sentiments expressed on the subject originate from an underlying dilemma. While propounding the idea of no difference, these nurses cite or allude to differences in care that occurred or were suggested:

> Nursing care should be the same, differing only in areas of emphasis. . . . . The degree of responsibility assumed by the nurse for maintaining physical functions are intensified. . . . Nursing knowledge and skills are in greater demand in identifying patient needs and capacities in all areas, when caring for an unconscious patient.

And a nurse aide who would make no difference in care explained that she does all she can to make her patients comfortable; *but* the unconscious patient requires more physical care, and the person who is conscious, more emotional support. A charge nurse who quite firmly expressed her conviction that no difference is made in the care provided for her patients allowed, nevertheless, that it may take more time to care for a semi- or unconscious patient and that one's heart goes out a little more to the patient who is conscious and mentally alert, for he is apt to be anxious about his condition and in need of assurance.

What meaning is to be derived from this? Is there reflected a need on the part of nurses representing emergent quality in geriatric care to disassociate themselves and their views from the widespread criticism of the typically low quality of contemporary nursing? Or is there inherent in the dilemma an unresolved conflict between the traditional nursing concept of "equal care for all patients" and the newer concept of "comprehensive and individualized care for each person according to his need?" It is an issue worthy of further consideration.

Finally, it should be noted that some of these nurses felt that genuine personal and professional commitment to caring and care for aged comatose and dying patients can be anything but an easy assignment. They often find it difficult and frustrating to try to maintain a positive and constructive attitude toward, and to sustain an appreciative sense of dignity in and respect for, a more-or-less unfamiliar and completely unconscious patient "lying coldly in bed" day after day, totally and continuously out of contact, and frequently wetting and soiling himself. They imply how taxing it can become to be constantly changing linens and to keep on talking to the patient and treating him as though he were still there and in touch, somehow, with them and with what goes on around him. They testify to a sense of defeat that grows in them as they ever so often try to detect in the patient a flicker of response of the person that he once was and a sense of the personality that appears so completely gone or deeply buried.

Caring for seriously ill dying patients, particularly those who are unconscious, is perhaps one of the most stressful situations in which a nurse can find herself. It is also one for which most nurses have had little education or preparation.

SUMMARY

Statistical analyses of the data on the question of whether an aged patient's degree of consciousness or unconsciousness becomes a basis for making a difference in care reveals sharply contrasting viewpoints. Among the nurse practitioners, judgment is split almost down the middle. Slightly more than half of each of the three nursing ranks deny that a patient's state of consciousness makes any difference in the care provided for him, and somewhat less than half affirm that it does. In contrast, in the DRN rank this affirmation is supported by three times as many as deny it. These pros and cons are reflected in the following chart.

	NA's %	LPN's %	RN's %	DRN's %
There is no difference in nursing care	51.0	54.7	54.3	26.7
There is a difference in care	40.4	45.3	43.2	73.3

The general tone of the negative position can briefly be summed up in the words of one respondent who said that the same care is provided for conscious and unconscious patients—"You treat them all alike." Another commented that in the presence of an unconscious patient a nurse may tend to be less guarded in her overt behavior, such as facial expression, but that no difference is made in the care given. Others insisted, however, that a nurse should be as careful of her hands and voice with a patient who is semi- or unconscious as with one who is conscious and alert; for "who can say how much is taken in by the unconscious patient?" Still another respondent warned that if the nurse develops a negative attitude toward an unconscious patient, she is likely to express this in his presence in unpremeditated ways. But whether a nurse takes the negative or affirmative position on the question, in her discussion at times she wavers somewhat from one side to the other.

Among those nurses who claimed that a patient's state of consciousness does make a difference in the care provided, another dichotomy of opinion becomes evident. It is on the question of whether more nursing care goes, or should go, to a patient who is aware and conscious or to one who is semi- or unconscious. The LPN's were almost evenly divided on this issue; the RN's claimed, almost by 2 to 1, that more nursing care goes to those who are conscious; nearly 3 to 1 of the DRN's say that more care should go to the unconscious patient as compared to the one who is alert and conscious. The NA's side with the DRN's, but their ratio is much smaller. These positions appear in perspective on the following chart.

	NA's %	LPN's %	RN's %	DRN's %
More care for *conscious* patients	13.4	18.9	21.0	17.8
More care for *unconscious* patients	18.3	17.0	12.3	52.5
Differences not specified	8.7	9.4	9.9	3.0

Further diversity of nurse opinion became evident in *areas* of care differences. The three ranks of nursing practitioners ignore almost entirely possible needs of unconscious patients for extra psychological care, whereas the degree registered nurses favor this by more than 10 percent. And while only about 5 percent of the practitioner groups favor more physical *and* psychological care, the DRN's support this by more than 30 percent.

In broad overview, it appears that, while the concept of "no difference" in the nursing care of aged ill conscious and unconscious patients "dies hard," this may be due, in part, to the long-established ethical nursing standard or ideal of "sameness of care" for all patients which harks back to an earlier nursing epoch. At the present, especially in professional nursing, the trend is toward frank recognition of patient differences and needs. These are, in turn, linked to the contemporary ideal of comprehensive and individualized patient care. In historical perspective, perhaps the very divergencies of the nursing views expressed on this question indicate change and carry promise of a better future for nursing for the aged ill.

For tabulations used in this chapter see Appendix B, Table 6.

10 Relationship of Prognosis to Nursing Care

> *The last stages of life should not be seen as a defeat, but rather as life's fulfillment.*
>
> CICELY SAUNDERS

How does nursing care differ for an aged person who is expected soon to die in contrast to one who is expected to recover? Does the nurse take into consideration the possibilities in the outcome of a patient's ailment? Does she pay any heed to whether signs and symptoms point toward or away from a likely recovery? Do the portents of death, whether it be expected to occur within hours, days, weeks or months, significantly alter the care the nurse provides for her patient? Does the medical diagnosis, or the patient's awareness of it, or both, make any measurable difference in the nursing care that he may receive?

SOME IMPLICATIONS

Issues such as these are likely to have moral and ethical implications, for the concept one holds of life and death determines one's sentiments and influences one's behavior. In these matters, the unsophisticated heart can pull one way; the trained head, another. The commitment of physician and nurse to sustain life exerts pressure. Religious and philosophical beliefs are influencing factors, as are social and cultural norms.

Nurses occasionally hint at the dilemma in which they are caught. They find that philosophy of life and professional training are not always compatible. They may face situations in which it is difficult to reconcile what they believe in and what they have been taught for their nursing careers.

Optimum care implies that a nurse's practice be in harmony with

127

that of the attending physician. She is part of a team that ministers to, and administers on behalf of, the patient. By tradition, she conforms to the physician's attitude and practice, and many doctors refuse to admit to a fatally stricken patient that death is imminent.

Nurses in some geriatric facilities report a close and progressive working relationship between medical and nursing personnel, including cooperative planning for patient care; in other institutions there evidently is very little sharing, except of the most vital information, between doctor and nurse, and almost no cooperative planning for patient care. A dedicated and experienced nursing supervisor in a long-term care facility contends that nurses may actually be hampered by the physician in their efforts to provide comfort care for a dying patient, and illustrated this by the following account:

> The patient had been ill for some months, and for several weeks had been losing ground more rapidly than before. There seemed to be little hope of recovery. During the course of his illness, the patient had quite routinely undergone very stressful medical treatments designed to slow the progress of the disease and to give him relief from discomfort and pain. As time went on, the treatments were given more frequently, but with diminishing results and the patient was dreading them more and more. He continually begged nurses and doctors to leave him be and spare him the extra pain; but the physician paid little heed to his pleadings, except to assure him that the treatments were helping him.
>
> The efforts of the nursing staff to provide some comfort and to ease his mental anguish met with little success. They complied with the doctor's expressed wishes that they refrain from discussing any aspect of his illness with the patient, but no amount of diversionary conversation appeared to take his mind off his plight; no amount of rubbing his back, smoothing the bedlinens, or positioning him eased his obvious tension and discomfort.
>
> Then the nurse in charge asked the physician how essential he believed the treatments to be and would he consider stopping them in view of the patient's terminal condition and his feelings. The doctor responded along these lines, "The doctor's credo must always be to keep the patient alive with whatever means are at his command, regardless of the ultimate outcome; the public demands that the doctor do everything in his power to preserve life, and that is what I am doing; we must also protect ourselves—I don't want a lawsuit on my hands for alleged negligence."

The supervisor then added:

> I cannot help comparing this situation with a personal experience I had in another place of work. The particular patient exhibited similar symptoms and the medical diagnosis was the same. So were the medical treatments. But in this instance, the attending physician, the patient, and the nurses planned cooperatively for the patient's care. He

was given pain-killing medication, but not to the point of unawareness. Medical and nursing efforts were focused upon comfort care and
psychological support. He found attentive listeners in both doctor and
nurse, and on several occasions spoke freely about approaching death.
He had some time before put his house in order, but needed help in
accepting his increasing dependency upon others for "all the little
things I used to do for myself."

This patient also had found the medical treatments uncomfortable, and when they no longer seemed to help him, they were discontinued. As death came closer the pain seemed to diminish. His son
and daughter visited daily. He expressed relief that he no longer had
to endure the painful treatments. As much as circumstances permitted,
someone stayed with him; for he had expressed his fear of dying all
alone. He took comfort from the thought that those around him cared
for and respected him as a person of human worth. In various direct
and indirect comments, he expressed his appreciation that he still
mattered as a person.

It is conceivable that his life was shortened by several days because the treatments were discontinued, but he died as he had wanted
to die—at peace with himself and others and with dignity.

The foregoing examples suggest that, in addition to professional
ethics and morality, a physician's own philosophy of life and death is
a factor to be reckoned with in geriatric patient care. Indications also
are, that a nurse's practice may be enhanced or impeded, depending on
whether the attending physician esteems her as a professional colleague
or considers her his handmaiden. To be sure, an important consideration
in the physician-nurse relationship and its resultant influence upon the
care of the aged ill is whether the RN has the education and background
as well as the capability to practice geriatric nursing on a professional,
rather than a technical, level.

Excellence in nursing care also makes it imperative that nursing and
the general administration in the institution be of like mind in the major
areas of care provisions for patients. But in this area also one encounters
wide differences. It may be administrative policy, rather than medical authority, that exerts the stronger influence upon the practice of nursing. In
one facility the attending physician's philosophy and policy largely prevails, in another the director of nursing may have the freedom and the responsibility to develop the policy of the nursing department, and in a third
the administrator of the institution may make the rules for all departments,
including nursing. In some of these nursing homes, the medical director
may also be the administrator, or a nurse may have the dual role of director
of nursing and institutional administrator. In many proprietary nursing
homes, the administrator is also the owner or part owner. Since proprietary
institutions are business enterprises, the question may well be raised as to
whether the profit motive and the service principle are compatible. State
laws usually set minimum standards, and in most, if not all, states a nurs-

ing home administrator is not required to possess a medical or nursing background, and he most probably has no degree in health care administration.

That nursing home administrators, whether qualified or not, at times exert influence upon medical and nursing practice, is illustrated in the following incident:

> The RN was in the (lay) administrator's office when the telephone rang and was answered by the administrator. A physician was returning an earlier call made by the administrator. The following dialogue ensued:
> *Adm.* Oh, doctor, I was calling about Mrs. R.—the nurses are having a hard time managing her—can't you give her something to quiet her? *M.D.* What do you want me to do? *Adm.* Why don't you give her the same medicine you ordered for Mrs. X., it worked fine with her. *M.D.* That's all right. I'll call the drugstore and have some sent over—I'll be in one day next week to check on Mrs. R. *Adm.* Thanks, Doctor. The call completed, the administrator then dialed one of the nursing care units. He recognized the voice at the other end of the line as that of the RN in charge at the time; repeated to her the name, dosage, and frequency to be given of the medication; and told her that the physician had prescribed it for Mrs. R.

And in another geriatric facility, the administrator, who has since left the nursing home field, was heard to exclaim, "I can almost qualify for a medical license—but I wish these doctors would not leave so many medical decisions up to me."

Such practices may not be condoned in a court of law, but they are indicative of authority exercised by some administrators in the care provided for patients admitted to their facilities.

In some nursing homes, stringent regulations govern what the nursing staff may and may not tell their patients when one of them is dying or has died. Staff is admonished never to let on when a patient is terminally ill. Nurses are instructed to make no difference in the care they provide for a dying and a recovering patient. By implication, no patient is considered to be dying.

Not every nursing home has such strict rules. Particularly in some church-related institutions, no secret is made of death and dying. This does not mean, necessarily, that such a philosophy is accepted or adhered to by the care-giving personnel. Many nurses holding key positions in these facilities find it difficult to admit to their patients, much less discuss with them, that death may be close. Thus, the issue is further compounded.

And in some geriatric institutions, nurses categorically deny that they have any dying patients. In one such home, a supervisor commented that it is their policy to keep patients up and about for as long as possible. They rarely linger as bed patients. Some have fatal heart attacks even while up and about. Others go in their sleep. Also, when patients become critically ill, they are usually transferred to a nearby hospital where more life-sustaining apparatus is available. This practice is adhered to, even though a patient may wish to remain in his familiar surroundings instead of dying in a strange environment.

If the knowledge of impending death is not shared with the patient, can or should the prognosis be considered by the nurse when planning and implementing care for the patient? Some nurses admit to differences in care for a dying and a recovering patient *if the patient knows he is dying,* in which case they give more care, especially comfort-giving care. But what about the patient who is not aware of his impending death? Is he to be denied comfort-giving care? And who is to decide whether or not a dying patient is aware of his prognosis? There is considerable evidence that a fatally ill patient often "knows" that death is close, even though he has not explicitly been told. Indeed, dying persons are known to have predicted or to "choose" the exact time of death. Such intuitive awareness would seem to have enabled Miss E. to predict her approaching death—to the day:

> Miss E., a writer and former university professor, had undergone surgery for cancer three times in as many years. Having insisted from the beginning of her illness upon open and frank discussion of the nature of the disease, she was able to speak freely with her physician and a few close friends about her suffering and, later, about her approaching death. She appreciated having had sufficient time to become reconciled to death and to set her "house in order," which included plans for publication of her latest book and selecting the tombstone she wished to have placed on the grave and the inscription to be engraved on it.
>
> About three weeks before her death Miss E. phoned her closest friend and confidante of many years (who lived some 300 miles away) and asked her to visit and remain with her until her death. Though for months her condition had shown no dramatic change, Miss E. told her friend that she expected to die within the month. During the final week of her life, Miss E. telephoned a few friends and bade them good-bye, asking them at the same time not to visit any more, as she no longer felt up to such visits.
>
> The friend and confidante, who had promised to remain until the end, continued to visit Miss E. every day. The day before her death, Miss E. told her friend that this would be the last time they would see each other and she bade her a final good-bye. Then she telephoned her home to bid her housekeeper good-bye.
>
> The next morning her nurse gave Miss E. the usual routine care. Later in the morning Miss E. asked for paper and pencil, as she so often had done, to write verse. The nurse then left to have her lunch.

When she returned half an hour later, Miss E. had expired. The paper contained a poem, half finished. Those who had seen Miss E. during the final weeks of her life expressed surprise that death had come so soon.

Instances have been reported also of persons who lived beyond the time when others had expected that death would have come:

There was Mrs. F. who had been very ill for several months with a cardiac ailment. When the daughter with whom she made her home was unable to obtain nurses to help care for her mother, Mrs. F. expressed the desire to enter a nursing home. She realized that she would not live much longer, but she kept repeating to her daughter that she wanted very much to live until her granddaughter obtained her master's degree, which was to be some six weeks hence. No one expected her to live that long. But she did. When the granddaughter on her day of graduation showed Mrs. F. the diploma, she was visibly moved. Then she said, "Now I am ready to die." Two days later, she died.

Experiences such as these may not be very common occurrences, but they are indicative of differences in the manner in which dying persons view, and attempt to cope with, personal death.*

The suggestion has been made that the aged, more often than those who are younger, are aware of impending death when fatally ill; but the geriatric nursing personnel repeatedly contended that aged patients often do not realize when they are near death. Many elderly persons are senile and have lost touch with reality. Others, especially if very aged and spent, are overcome by a drowsiness which gradually deepens over a period of days, weeks, or even months before they enter their final sleep. One RN reported that more than half of their patients who die are confused or unaware months or years before they die. Among the aged who are mentally alert and conscious, also, differences are said to exist. One dying person may not realize that he is fatally ill; another may suspect but not be sure, and still another may "know" but not verbalize that he knows. A dying person's awareness or unawareness of impending death

* The famous British statesman, Sir Winston Churchill, is also reported to have died on the day he hoped he would. During a television interview (Channel 13, New York, November 26, 1968) a friend and associate of Churchill, Lord Mountbatten, related: "I was twelve when I first met Churchill. I knew him very well. He was tremendously, absolutely overpowering. When I was staying at Sandringham in January 1965, when he was so very ill, his private secretary told the duty private secretary, 'You don't need to worry. Sir Winston told me once he'd like to die on the anniversary of his father's death.' And he hung on for something like ten days and died at the same hour and on the same day that his father had died 70 years before. If that isn't a case of the power of mind over matter, I just don't know what is." (Channel 13 Program Guide, vol. VI, No. 5, March 1969)

may be an important factor for the nurse to consider when planning and implementing nursing care for a terminally ill patient.

Another important factor in the issue of care differences for aged dying and recovering patients is the nurse's attitude toward death. A great many nurses report going to great lengths to avoid "death talk" or otherwise becoming involved with the patient. Some nurses contend that, for their own protection and composure as well as that of the dying patient and the others involved in his care, it is essential not to admit to the truth, particularly since, during the period when there is "nothing more to do," the nurses often bear the major burden of caring for the patient—and, perhaps, the family. Other nurses expressed concern, lest the dying patient be isolated and neglected by staff, thus maybe bringing about an earlier death than nature intended. Still others contend that when an aged patient is not expected to live, his needs are not only greater, but also different, than those of the patient who is expected to live.

With the complexity of factors influencing the care that nurses would provide for aged patients, perhaps it comes as no surprise that considerable diversity is encountered on the issue of nurses coping with possible care differences for aged dying patients, as compared with the care for recovering patients.

No Differentiation in Nursing Care

The exploration of the issue of whether a terminal diagnosis is a justifiable basis for differentiation in geriatric nursing care revealed sharp differences that cut across all four ranks of nursing personnel. The three practitioner groups, who work in the various select geriatric facilities and are directly involved with the care of aged persons, are almost evenly divided on the issue of differences, with some 50 percent declaring that prognosis is no basis for making differences in care, and an almost equal number taking the opposite position—that prognosis does make a difference in the care they provide for their aged patients. Some degree nurses also supported the "equal care" concept, but by something less than one to two.*

Reasons put forth for providing equal care for all patients, regardless of prognosis, are many and varied. A common rationale is that God

---

* NA's, 51.8 percent; LPN's, 49.0 percent; RN's, 51.2 percent; DRN's, 29.4 percent. See Appendix B, Table 7, Items 1 to 4.

gives life and it is he who takes it; and since only God can know when a patient will die, it behooves nurses to make no distinction in the care they give to dying and recovering patients. An LPN spoke for a number of her co-workers when she declared:

> God determines when your time is up; but man has to help himself, and God expects us to give a helping hand to those who need it. So it is with very sick patients. You don't want any patient to feel that there is no hope. And if the doctor feels that patients can help and do things for themselves, they should, and you explain that it is good for them.

Similar sentiments were expressed by nursing personnel who justify equal care on the basis of an Omnipotent God.

Personal experiences were called upon to support this stand. An RN explained that one of their patients had some months back been seriously ill and though the doctor felt there was no hope for him, he recovered and is "still very much alive." Similarly:

> One of our patients, in his late eighties, was critically ill with pneumonia. He was not responding to treatment, and all who cared for him feared for his life. Then very unexpectedly he rallied and recovered.

Consideration of the emotional well-being of patients was also cited as justification for giving equal care to dying and recovering patients. Adherents to this idea stress the importance of continuance of familiar routine, so that the dying patient will not sense that death may be close. Besides, the other patients in the room or on the floor might become alarmed if differences were made and they realized that one of them was near death. Some patients might even become jealous if they see that more is being done for a dying patient:

> When one patient died, her 94-year-old neighbor said, "How peaceful she looks." Before this patient had died, she had been given more attention than her neighbors and the 94-year-old had complained a great deal that more was being done and that she herself had to do everything without help. She had also complained because a light was left on with the dying patient—but after a while she accepted it.

More often, however, the reason offered is that equal care is given because if "patients see you do more for one than for the others, they feel there is something wrong and so might get upset." The orientation is to the "here and now," and the prospect of pending death is to be denied. The assumption, often hinted at and at times clearly stated, is that we are all afraid to die and everyone wants to live as long as possible.

Equal care is further justified on the basis of moral commitment. The expected nursing role is to support and prolong life, and to alleviate pain and suffering. But there are times when the nurse has to abandon her goal of cure and let comfort for the patient take priority with its accompanying dilemma, as was illustrated by one RN:

> Only God knows who dies and who recovers—so the care must be the same. The whole concept of nursing is to help patients recover.
>
> One 94-year-old patient, who had been in the home about 15 years, had never developed any decubitus ulcers. Then some four weeks before she died her skin began to break down all over. No specific reason for the breakdown could be found, and it was attributed to her advanced age and her general condition. As a nurse, this was difficult to accept, but one must realize that if this patient had not lived this long, she would not have developed the sores.
>
> When our efforts to heal the sores were futile and meant additional suffering and pain for the patient, we changed our focus and considered her comfort first and foremost rather than healing the sores or trying to prevent further breakdown—her body had nothing left with which to fight the infection. But I still had guilt feelings.

Another RN recommended that both the dying and the recovering patient be treated similarly—as critically ill—on the basis that the aged are especially susceptible to pneumonias and other complications. All aged patients require intensive care, for the "general body structure" of elderly persons falls apart so quickly. An LPN stated that she never gives up because she is morally obliged to nurse those who are ill, and, "where there is life, there is hope." And a DRN maintained that nursing care should not differ in any respect, since only the *fact* of death can justify any differentiation. The nurse should not give in, or give up, to death psychologically, because attitudes are easily communicated, and a patient might lose his will to live if hopelessness is conveyed. In thought and in practice, these nurses expressed obligation to make *no distinction* in the care they provide for dying and recovering patients, and they emphasized that a nurse's commitment does not falter just because the critically ill patient is elderly.

Some of these nurses hold that while they cannot condone differentiation of care on the basis of a terminal prognosis, they admit to care differences on other grounds: specifically, that each individual patient in his situation is unique. One RN reflected the thinking of several of her co-workers when she said that "you give equal care on an individual basis." And another reported that "if personalized care is given as we practice it here, the care is the same for all, as we try to fit the nursing care to the individual patient's needs at the time."

The proponents of the equal care concept emphasized professional and ethical norms of equal care for all patients. They frequently expressed concern, lest aged patients be denied equal care and the charge be made that nurses have been known to provide less care for dying patients than for those expected to recover. A nurse in charge in one of the geriatric institutions commented that at times a staff member, by giving up too early, may actually add to a seriously ill patient's discomfort and pain; and she cited the following example:

> To avoid painful intravenous infusions or clyses, the concentration on getting nourishment, especially fluids, into the patient is vital and the nurse should not shirk this just because it requires patience. It is easy to leave a difficult feeder and turn to a patient who takes nourishment without effort on the nurse's part.

It is likely that a considerable number of nurses who believe in the equal care concept have, at one time or another, been witness to situations in which a dying patient was avoided by doctors and nurses alike, or even neglected. They want to make it known that they consider such behavior morally wrong, and that dying patients entrusted to their care would be treated the same as patients who are expected to recover. They strongly emphasize that a dying patient has the right to receive, and the nurse the obligation to provide, the same care as that given to a patient for whom there is hope of recovery.

Paradox or Matter of Interpretation

A fairly large number of nurses who subscribed to the equal care position alluded, nevertheless, to differences they actually do make, or believe should be made, in particular situations; and occasionally they voiced seemingly contradictory sentiments regarding nursing care for the two categories of aged patients. To illustrate:

> A nurse aide, whose assignment included two very aged patients, was giving A.M. care. One of these patients was recovering from injuries sustained when she had fallen some days before, the other had for several weeks been noticeably failing, and the staff did not expect her to live much longer.
> It was observed that the aide took special pains to make her patients comfortable, but she spent considerably more time with the patient who was not expected to live.
> When discussing her work with her later in the day, the aide emphasized that she makes no difference in the care she gives her patients, adding, however, that "your heart goes out more to the one who is dying," and that she takes special pains not to tax the waning

strength of the critically ill patient. She then went on to explain that she spends extra time with her dying patient, even though the time is not taken up with doing something for her physically, in order to convey to the dying person the feeling that she is not alone—that she still matters as a person and that here is someone who cares.

A registered nurse who stressed that prognosis is no basis for differentiation in patient care contended that the role of the nurse is to support life and ease suffering wherever she can, but that she should not deny to herself or to a dying patient that death is imminent. She added that the nurse has an obligation to allow the patient to die in his own way.

The implication is that, while the standard norm is "equal care for both," the dying patient is not, and should not, be denied special comfort-giving care. The paradox perhaps lies not so much in whether or not nurses admit to care differences, but in their interpretation of what constitutes nursing. That nursing encompasses both the physical and psychological realm is not a new concept, but the idea of patient care consisting mainly of technical procedures and the "laying on of hands" is more traditional and seemingly dies hard. Nursing may be said to have come "full circle"—for such early pioneers as Florence Nightingale and Pastor Fliedner were as much concerned with comforting the ill person as with the care of his bodily ills.

PROGNOSIS A BASIS FOR CARE DIFFERENTIATION

Nearly half of the nurse practitioners and slightly more than two thirds of the degree registered nurses affirmed that a terminal prognosis is a basis for differences in the care provided for aged patients.*

But a very few in all four nursing ranks who held that there are differences asserted that greater attention and care goes, or should go, to the patient who is expected to recover. This greater concern for aged patients expected to recover is based on the claim that it is better to invest in life than in death, that rehabilitative measures are time-consuming, and the recovering patient needs to be motivated and encouraged. A head nurse, stating that she "leans" more toward patients who are expected to live, said, "They need a boost, and you must let them know that you are there with them."

* NA's, 46.2 percent; LPN's, 49.0 percent; RN's, 47.6 percent; DRN's, 69.7 percent. See Appendix B, Table 7, Items 5 to 8.

However, the overwhelming majority of those who hold that a poor prognosis calls for differences in nursing care focused upon care and comfort of the patient whose life appears from a medical judgment to be drawing to a close. While the concern of this group leans toward the patient with a poor prognosis, considerable diversity is encountered in the particulars, as reflected in their responses. Some would provide more physical care for dying patients; others, more emotional support. The need for close cooperation among those involved in the care of the patient was emphasized. In addition, the idea was repeatedly stressed, particularly by the degree registered nurses, that each patient is an individual with needs and wants uniquely his own.

Physical Care and Comfort

A very small number of respondents, but which includes about one-tenth of the nurse aides, see differences largely in terms of extra physical care for the patient whose life is drawing to a close. This includes measures aimed at preventing complications, such as frequent turning and positioning, and intensive skin and mouth care, as well as special attention to those personal tasks which the patient is no longer able to do for himself, such as bathing, shaving, clipping and filing of nails, and the like.

The aged patient is apt to be weary to death during the final weeks or days of his life. Even a small effort such as wiping a brow may tax his strength. Moreover, dying patients, though conscious and mentally alert, may not always make their needs and wants known. This calls for anticipatory care on the part of staff, so that the bodily needs, including sufficient fluid intake and proper elimination, are met.

With the dying person, one provides for the moment. Comfort is all important. Procedures and treatments that are prescribed for future therapeutic value should no longer take priority. The dying person should not be taxed with procedures that have no immediate importance. Mrs. L. is a case where comfort was considered foremost:

> We did not force her out of bed, although we were concerned about her skin breaking down. To turn her caused her extreme pain. We held a staff conference to discuss her care and reached the decision that we would refrain from turning her because of the pain. She had a fondness for ice cream, so we made certain that there was some available on the floor at all times. All of us on the floor cooperated to provide the most complete care possible. We concentrated on seeing that she did not become dehydrated, for she would take fluids by teaspoon only. We spent a great deal of time with her. She was more important to us during her final days. I kept thinking about possible ways to ease her pain.

Nursing measures to ease the pain, to prevent complications, to provide comfort, are the overriding concerns of those who see care differences mainly in terms of physical well-being for the aged patient.

Emotional Support

A few nurses held that emotional support of dying patients is at least as essential as physical care, if not more so. They contend that most, if not all, dying persons are apt to manifest anxiety and express fear as death comes closer. Many individuals are said to be afraid to die alone—and many fatally ill patients will find solace and comfort in the nurse's presence. Having someone near to share with him his ultimate loneliness may be the dying person's uppermost need and want. A head nurse in a geriatric facility commented:

> We have one 80-year-old patient who is dying of cancer. She has a colostomy, and ever since her operation she has been very apprehensive. She is very alert. We try to alleviate her anxiety and try to have someone near her at all times. She has great fear to be left alone, fear of the unknown. She is a religious person, but she is still afraid to die.

Extra time must be provided. Extra attention is called for—beyond what the doctor ordered. And special consideration should be given to a dying person's personal whims and wishes. In brief, this extra care is directed largely toward personal comfort—mental ease and spiritual solace.

Physical and Psychosocial Ministrations

By far the largest group of nurses who believe in care differences based on prognosis considered these differences not in terms of *either* physical *or* psychological care, but in terms of physical *and* psychosocial considerations (22 percent to 48 percent). They indicated that a major difference in care hinges on patient-oriented goals of providing care and comfort instead of cure and hope for those deemed to be dying. Hence, nursing ministrations are determined on the grounds of comfort-care—physical, psychosocial and spiritual. When a patient reaches the helpless stage, he needs a kind and understanding nurse who will do things *for* him. But in attending to the patient's needs and wants, and in doing the little personal tasks he no longer is able to do for himself, care must be taken that these be done in such a way as not to rob him of his dignity. Timing must also be considered, for aged persons like to do things at their own pace and resent being hurried. Doing things slowly for a dying patient contributes to his comfort and peace of mind.

An experienced and dedicated nurse aide declared that she does more for dying patients because her conscience would bother her if she did not make them as comfortable as possible "in every way" during their last days or weeks on earth. A licensed practical nurse, in charge of a floor during the evening tour of duty, emphasized that staff must be more patient with those who are terminally ill, must do more for them, but must also allow them to do whatever they can and wish to do for themselves. She added that in every dying woman she cares for she "sees" her mother; in every dying man, her father—treating them as she would her mother and father, with respect, kindness, affection, understanding, and patience.

A registered nurse, who has devoted many years to the care of the aged ill, emphasized two significant factors in the care provided for dying patients: expenditure of extra time and consideration of the uniqueness of the individual patient. She feels that each situation has its own particular needs, and the nurse does what is called for. She takes her cue from the patient, attending him with kindness and gentleness. Her goal is to provide comfort for every remaining moment, unhurriedly and with deliberateness and understanding. The patient whose life is drawing to a close is, after all, "someone special."

The number of nurse practitioners who recognize and emphasize the comprehensive needs of the patient and support the idea of individualized patient care is considerably smaller than that of the degree registered nurses. Those who think in terms of a larger, more encompassing nursing role stressed the team concept, which implies collaboration and cooperation not only among nursing personnel, but also between nursing and the other disciplines involved in patient care and welfare: doctors, clergy, social workers. They emphasize as well the importance of working with the patient, to whatever extent he is able and wishes to participate and with the patient's family if he has any. Above all, they stressed that *each situation is unique* and must be evaluated in terms of the individual patient's past life and present needs.

Patient-oriented goals are seen as the major criteria upon which care is based. An aged patient for whom there is hope of recovery may be expected to forego some of the more immediate satisfactions and perhaps endure uncomfortable therapy and pain in order to realize more distant goals. Not so the dying patient whose goals appear more immediate, with comfort and peace of mind being most important, and including opportunities to have loved ones near him.

In the planning of nursing care, the expectations and concerns of the patient are seen as of prime importance and which, conceivably, may differ markedly from those of the nurse. If a person is aware of his impending death, he may wish for help in meeting death, personally and in terms of his family. If, on the other hand, a patient is not aware of his prognosis or seems unable to face the fact of death, it becomes difficult for nursing care to be different from that provided for a patient who is expected to live:

> Seventy-year-old Mr. D. was afflicted with Parkinson's disease. Though he was steadily and noticeably loosing ground, he continued to be full of hope of recovery. He had considerable speech difficulty as a result of his illness, and speech therapy was prescribed—for the sole purpose that *he felt it would help him.* The therapy did seem to improve his state of mind.
>
> He was not a religious person. When it was suggested to him and his wife that perhaps the priest, who routinely made visits in the home, could be of some solace, nothing came of it. The nurse in charge, a religious Sister, opened up the conversation about approaching death, but he never picked this up, though he was a very intelligent man.

Mr. D.'s unawareness of his prognosis, or his inability to face the fact of approaching death, was the major basis upon which his care was planned and implemented. The nurses acted upon the knowledge and insight gained about his attitude toward life; about his belief in himself and in Eternity; and about his hopes.

The way a patient feels about these things and the way the nurse feels about them will be reflected in the behavior of both. In order to relate with the patient in a positive way, it is essential that the nurse listen to, and understand, the patient's point of view. But first she must know her own. Moreover, she needs to know that too much anxiety in the presence of terminal illness and death may cause her to act in an inappropriate manner, such as avoiding the dying patient, being overly solicitous, or even treating the patient with levity. The responsibility of the nurse when caring for a dying patient is discussed by a DRN:

> The factor of death should alert the registered nurse to the understanding needed by the patient and his relatives of the approaching crisis in their lives. First, the nurse needs to resolve her own feelings about death. Regardless of her feelings and philosophy, she must provide and give emotional support and understanding to the patient's, and his family's, feelings and to their manner of meeting the impending crisis. In no way should the RN, LPN, or NA impose her own value judgment on the patient or his family. . . .
>
> The nurse's own resolution of her feelings will be sensed by the patient. Her acknowledgement of the gravity of the situation, her calm, and her skilled manner as she gives nursing care will certainly assist her to meet best the needs of the patient. She has the respon-

sibility of gaining understanding of the patient's, and the family's, awareness of the imminence of death, their spiritual and religious convictions, and their anxieties. Only in her sensitivity to the individual needs of the patient and his family can she reassure and share with them the impending crisis. . . .

She must also recognize the patient's need to maintain a sense of individuality and identity. . . . Concern and anticipation of methods whereby the nurse can provide the most skilled means to meet the patient's needs for comfort and emotional support is essential. (Quinlan)

In addition, the nurse needs to be sensitive to, and respectful of, a dying patient's feelings as to whether or not he desires to know that death is close and whether or not he wishes to reveal or discuss his feelings. But possible conflict in a terminally ill person's readiness to face death must also be recognized:

All people are alike in the sense that they have similar needs; and are different in that each individual is in some respects unique. . . .

Even when a patient's expectation of approaching death, and his philosophy, religious or otherwise, is one of considerable acceptance of the fact, his attitude is often one of "Not today, Death—come back a little later."

No one who has watched a terminally ill person continue to live day after day with a certain amount of effectiveness can doubt that a degree of conflict can exist between a philosophical readiness to die and a very practical unreadiness to "let go." (Schwartz)

The following account bears vivid witness to such a state of ambivalence:

Mr. A. had been a very independent and self-sufficient person. Autocratic in makeup, he had always been "master of the house," and his word was considered law by his wife and their four sons. He was born and raised in the Catholic faith, but for many years had not practiced his religion.

At the age of 91, Mr. A. became fatally ill and was admitted to the nursing home. The philosophy of this home is that a patient has the right to know when he is not expected to live much longer, and that opportunities be provided for preparing himself for death and Eternity. Shortly after his admission to the home, Mr. A. was persuaded to see the priest who regularly visited the patients.

Before long Mr. A. consented to have last rites. He was able to talk about death and dying and repeatedly indicated to the priest that he was ready to meet his Maker. But often, when awakening from sleep, his anguished cries would summon a staff member to his bedside, to whom he would cling with all his strength, while crying, "I don't want to die—help me, help me."

One might well ponder the ways in which those who cared for Mr. A. attempted to bring comfort and solace to him. Situations such as this give credence to the premise inherent in the above discourse and that can be summed up concisely in just two phrases: "Know thyself" and "Know thy patient" if optimum care is to be provided for aged dying persons.

Care for aged terminally ill patients, as it is practiced by few, but is seen as a goal toward which to strive by many of those who represent the thinking of nursing at a high level, is summed up by one DRN as follows:

> Nursing care for the aged patient who is expected to die soon should take into consideration that the person is facing an unknown task which he must complete alone; that is *death*. However, the process of dying is still part of living, and here social interaction and physical assistance can share each step of the way. Thus, the process of dying may be the person's principal nursing problem, depending on whether there is a family who is willing to share this final passage. Nursing the dying person, then, means a sharing of his life process—to its completion—as opposed to abandonment, which may easily occur if the patient is not given a kind of nursing that *shares*.
>
> Sharing his life process involves assisting the patient to cope with his own feelings regarding dying and (if he is ready for it) making a plan for the termination of his life. Since these personal feelings will vary from culture to culture, the patient must be (or become) known to the nurse. The nurse can operate efficiently only through the knowledge of, and trust from, the patient. She should accept the patient's behavior as he approaches this new and final act as she accepts the behavior of any person who is facing a new and threatening situation. She should try to read from it the cues that ask for assistance.
>
> Nursing care should be given by the fewest personnel in order to provide for continuity of nursing measures which prove effective for this particular patient and for adequate communication of those (personal) facts, the sharing of which may save effort for the patient.
>
> Nursing care for the aged dying patient should consider the characteristics and the values of his own family and include every possible opportunity to encourage the family's participation in his care. Support given a family member by the nurse may be one of the most important acts, which will in turn allow the family member to give support to the patient.
>
> Nursing care of the dying person, then, assumes the function of assisting the patient to prepare for death in so far as he indicates that he is ready to be assisted. It involves a nurse who is able to face this fact herself and who has committed her efforts to making death and dying a peaceful process which she can view without feeling defeat in lack of recovery. (Wolanin)

Issues and Trends

The issue of differences in the care provided for aged dying versus recovering patients, and as viewed by the four ranks of nursing personnel, is complex and not easily resolved. The type of inter- and intra-group differences in emphasis on certain aspects of nursing practice that emerged from the data warrants further inquiry.

A minor theme running through some of the findings is that a dying patient's awareness of his prognosis is a basis for differences in his care. Among all four groups of nursing personnel, differences in care are occasionally recognized on the basis of whether or not the patient knows that his death is close. If a dying patient is not aware of his prognosis, then the care provided for him may be the same as that of a patient for whom there is hope of recovery. If, on the other hand, he is aware that he is fatally ill, differences in care are suggested, and made, especially in the area of comfort-giving ministrations.

Opinions vary concerning a person's right to know that death may be close. There are those who feel strongly that a person needs to know that he may shortly be leaving this world in order to prepare for his exit mentally, spiritually, and perhaps in more mundane ways, such as tidying up his affairs and making provisions for his heirs. Others believe that all are afraid to die and that the dying person should be spared knowledge of the ordeal he is soon to face.

By far the most important concept inherent in the responses, especially in those of the nurse leadership (DRN group), is that of individualized and comprehensive care. Those who think in terms of this larger, more encompassing nursing role stress the team concept, not only among nursing personnel but also between the different disciplines involved in the patient's care and well-being. They emphasize as well the importance of working with the patient, to the extent that he is able and wishes to participate, and with the patient's family, if he has family. Above all, these nurses claim that each situation is somewhat unique and must be evaluated in terms of the individual patient's needs and wants.

If an aged patient is fatally stricken, his comfort is considered first and foremost, with relief from pain holding a high priority. If medication is prescribed, it is essential for the nurse, in cooperation with the physician, to find a safe mean between too little and too much. An important consideration here is that the patient not be under the influence of drugs to the point of excessive dullness. Though mental anguish and pain must be controlled, the nurse should try to understand and balance the degree of alertness against the liability of suffering.

It is also recognized that there is a real difference between a person who is dying of a lesion, such as cancer, and a patient who is dying of generalized deterioration or complications of old age. If a person is dying of a catastrophic illness and was, until stricken, very much involved with life's experiences, he may feel that the entire world is against him. If, on the other hand, the patient is advanced in age and, following a long life, is slowly wasting away, he may be more accepting of his fate. Moreover, it is conceivable that the very advanced ager, because of mental impairment and subsequent loss of touch with reality, is not aware of what is happening.

Often a dying patient finds solace in the mere presence of an empathetic person; but if there is evidence that he is looking for a listener, it may be well to remember that what he tells the listener, not what the listener tells him, is more important. Finding a sympathetic and supportive listener may well be more therapeutic and effective in relieving anxiety for the patient than the most potent medicine. The nurse, who spends much more time with patients than do other health professionals, cannot justifiably escape the supportive role as a good listener.

Isolation of the dying patient should be avoided as much as possible, as should the denial of opportunities for seeing and talking with fellow patients—especially if he has been in the habit of doing this and still desires to do so. On the other hand, the patient who craves to be alone should have his needs and wishes respected.

Above all, the nurse must have perceptivity and exercise judgment in order to ascertain the individual patient's needs and wants—physical, psychological, social, and spiritual. This implies that it behooves the nurse to become familiar with the patient's background and previous pattern of life, including religious practices, cultural and social values, personal interests, and likes and dislikes. Finally, sensitivity on the part of the nurse is essential so that she may be able to ascertain, and act upon, the dying person's wishes of the moment, whether expressed overtly or covertly.

A small number of respondents indicated, however, that a prognosis of probable recovery of an aged person implies a greater challenge for extra attention and individualized care, since the patient may have lost his zest for living and is dependent upon renewed motivation for his early recovery. They further pointed out that rehabilitative measures, which are often prescribed for such a patient, are time-consuming. The manifest implication made by these few nurses is that lavishing time and attention on the aged dying patient may actually be at the vital expense of recoverable patients who are in need of, and waiting for, additional care from the staff. This kind of choice, with which health personnel may be confronted, can create for the conscientious nurse a further complication of this already uncomfortable dilemma.

Recent studies in some general hospitals document extensively the practice by nursing staff of limiting, delaying, or even neglecting the nursing needs of dying patients under a rationale of implied prior obligation to patients diagnosed by physicians as having a chance of recovery. Doubtless, some of the motivations behind tendencies to neglect the dying are too illusive to be subjected to logical interpretations.

From the DRN's who supported differences and discriminating care of the dying, there were outspoken and abundant testimonials to the effect that the dying patient has extraordinary needs which should be recognized and included in the nursing care for him. They repeatedly emphasized that these needs are only partly obvious and call for keen perceptivity and sensitive judgments on the part of the caring person. They recommend that the nurse train and discipline herself to become acutely sensitive to the cues of needs of the patient, whether he is conscious of these indicators or not. They indicate that a nurse must be able to read the signs of urgent unmet needs and discern to what extent and in what ways the patient may wish for or welcome assistance in his terminal travail.

Another theme that runs through the data has to do with the recurrent issue of what is nursing; what are the essentials that make nursing unique; and what functions fit significantly into the emerging image of the professional nurse. Here one becomes aware once more of some of the dilemmas in nursing. On the one hand is the impelling pressure for the nurse to fit aptly into the organized system of health services, meshing like a cog into the institutionalized staff roles. On the other hand is the equally compelling notion that the individual needs of particular patients dictate a *special role* or function for the nurse. This major dilemma becomes more or less evident in all institutional situations and constitutes a contradictory value orientation for the nurse, creating tensions whenever she attempts to comply with the conflicting role prescription. Fortunate, indeed, is the nurse who is committed to individualized patient care and who also finds herself in a situation where the fulfillment of this professional goal meets with support and reinforcement within the immediate institutional context—and no less fortunate is her patient.

Another conflicting issue is the interpretation of nursing that stresses the care of the body in contrast to the psychologically oriented nursing that recognizes and takes into account the interrelationship of psyche and soma in the nursing to be provided. Still other views of nursing involve a myriad of elements that fuse and reinforce each other in the concept of giving care to the whole person—physically, psychologically, spiritually, and so on.

This progression from the technical, procedure-oriented, and functional pattern of nursing is not to be equated with any particular category of nursing personnel, nor does it arise solely with the training that nurses receive. The DRN's, though, tend to view the present issues more distinctly in terms of the larger and more professional perspective.

This more encompassing outlook for nursing is an outgrowth of the emerging image of the professional nurse as the provider of comprehensive, or psychologically perceptive, nursing care of the *whole* person within an individualized frame of reference. Apparently, a major key to ensuring this kind of nursing care for aged dying patients lies in the nurse's sharing and utilizing the knowledge of the medical prognosis in her relationships with her patient and in tempering and adapting her nursing procedures to his individual needs, perhaps more in terms of present realities than future uncertainties.

SUMMARY

In brief summary, the nurse practitioners of all three ranks were almost evenly divided on the issue of whether a terminal diagnosis is a justifiable basis for differentiation in nursing care, with slightly more than half of them claiming that awareness of such a prognosis makes no difference in the care they provide for their aged patients, while slightly less than half declare that, on the contrary, such awareness does result in differences in nursing care. The degree nurses supported the affirmative position by a ratio of more than 2 to 1:

	NA's %	LPN's %	RN's %	DRN's %
There is no difference in nursing care	51.8	49.0	51.2	29.4
There is a difference in care	46.2	49.0	47.6	69.7

Justification for the equal care concept touched upon three distinct areas: God, nurse, and patient. A small number of respondents reasoned that the life of man is in God's hands; hence the nurse must provide equal care irrespective of the projected outcome. A somewhat larger number of respondents stressed that the moral commitment of the nurse does not permit that distinctions be made on the basis of prognosis. Interestingly, this position is given the most support by the nurse aides and the least by the degree registered nurses. Still others declared that possible differences in care, if any, are related to factors other than a patient's prognosis. A considerable number of these nurses pointed out that each patient and his situation are somewhat unique and must be evaluated in order to determine a patient's nursing needs. This stand was most strongly supported by the DRN's and the least by the NA's. Still others took the negative position without further qualifying their stand. The exact figures on the "no difference" or negative position are as follows:

	NA's %	LPN's %	RN's %	DRN's %
No difference: God determines life and death	6.7	9.4	6.1	1.0
No difference: Nurses have moral commitment to help the living	16.3	11.3	8.5	5.9
No difference: general negative statements	24.0	9.4	22.0	0.0
Possible differences not related to prognosis	4.8	18.9	14.6	22.5

Respondents who took the positive position on the issue of differences in nursing care declared that the needs of dying versus recovering patients differ in some important aspects of care—physical or psychological or both. Additional physical care for the dying was stressed by the NA's, extra psychological care, by the LPN's. However, the idea that extra care for the dying encompasses more than either physical or psychological ministrations was attested to by the largest number of respondents who supported care differences based on prognosis.

Some of the respondents specified or implied that the psychological aspects of care for the dying person centers primarily on giving comfort and assistance to the patient in achieving a peaceful and, if possible, a dignified and appropriate conclusion to his life—a closure in accordance with the way he might have wished his life to end.

A very small number of nursing personnel affirmed, however, that a prognosis of probable recovery of an aged patient presents for them a greater challenge for extra attention and care. The exact figures on the affirmative position are:

	NA's %	LPN's %	RN's %	DRN's %
More physical care for the dying	11.5	0.0	4.9	3.9
More psychological care for the dying	8.7	22.6	7.3	15.7
More physical *and* psychosocial care	25.0	22.6	29.3	48.1
General positive statements, including those indicating more care for the recovering patient	1.0	3.8	6.1	2.0

Finally, some of the respondents who took the *equal care* position indicated, more or less directly, that they do, or would, make some differences in care, especially in the form of personalized attention to the needs and preferences of the dying person. In brief, they would prefer, if possible, to have their patients die in peace and comfort.

For tabulations used in this chapter, see Appendix B, Table 7.

11 Use of "Heroics" in Prolonging Life

> *There is a time to live and a time to die.*
> SIR WILLIAM OSLER

Health professionals are often confronted with the question of how far to push or carry a frail, flickering life into its extremities. Almost as critical is the issue of what available means may be justifiably used to keep an aged person alive as long as humanly possible; and, if the physician has initiated the use of artificial measures to prolong a life, when may he discontinue their use?

Decisions on these and similar issues are usually regarded as primarily the responsibility of physicians. But in nursing homes and other long-term care facilities, physicians are not usually in as constant attendance as in hospitals, and nurses frequently are confronted with such problems. A director of nursing, who has devoted many years to the care of the aged ill, stated that she often finds herself making decisions of a critical medical nature; and many geriatric nurses admittedly make or influence such judgments, probably more than do their counterparts in general hospitals.

Several RN's recalled incidents in which they had telephoned an attending physician and suggested to him that tube feedings or infusions be started on a particular patient. A registered nurse, in charge of a nursing unit in a geriatric facility, exemplified:

> I often ask myself why? The patient is often reduced to a mere vegetable, and still you have to give all sorts of vitamins and other medicines that prolong life. Our conscience tells us to do these things. . . .
> We now have a patient who is semiconscious. She sustained a brain hemorrage a few weeks ago and was transferred here last week. She is also an amputee. She is in her early eighties. This morning she refused to eat or to take any fluids, and I phoned the doctor about starting tube feedings and clyses. He agreed. . . . Here we do everything to keep them alive regardless.

149

Conversely, incidents were related in which RN's had questioned the decision of physicians to resort to life-sustaining measures when they felt that their judgment had been made on medical grounds only—to the exclusion of all human factors. To illustrate:

> We now have a patient who has been completely disoriented for a long time. Recently she became critically ill and is being kept alive with tube feedings, infusions, and the like. She is on vitamins as well as on antibiotics. All this is a great financial drain on the family. I have discussed it with the physician, but to no avail. . . . For my own parents I would not want this.

Another element was injected into the issue by an RN who indicated that there are times when the nurse can protect her aged patient from painful life-sustaining measures:

> When doctors and nurses work closely together, there is sometimes a great deal that the RN can do to save the patient unnecessary suffering. You subject persons to extra pain and discomfort whether you push a rubber tube up their nose or insert needles into their soft tissue or into a vein.
> The other day one of our doctors ordered that a clysis be started on a spent and weary octogenarian who was dying. When I told him that I would see to it that the patient would be given fluids every 15 minutes, he cancelled his order and the clysis was never started.

Some nurses implied that patients' relatives sometimes influence a doctor's decision. One RN spoke of the "selfishness" of the husband of a 73-year-old patient who was dying of cancer:

> The patient was obviously suffering. She was very obese and her body was breaking down all over. At times she was semiconscious. Her husband kept insisting that everything be done to keep her alive. She was given transfusions—everything was done to keep her heart beating. The husband came every day to stay with his wife. He watched her suffering for almost 3 weeks. Then he apparently could not take it any longer. When the physician visited one day, the husband told him, "No more of this—I want her left alone." The doctor went along with the husband's decision. All tubes and needles were removed from her body, and the transfusions were discontinued. The only medications continued were pain-killing drugs.

A different account involving relatives was recounted by an RN in another home:

> Several months ago we had a patient who had been unconscious for a couple of weeks. His physician prescribed all sorts of life-sustaining

procedures; besides having nourishment and fluids pumped into him, he was on oxygen therapy.

He had three children who visited regularly, a daughter, who was an M.D., and two sons, both priests. One day all three came at the same time, which was very unusual. They went into the father's room together, and after a while the daughter came into the hall and quietly informed the nurse in charge that she was taking full responsibility for her father's care and that she had just removed all life-sustaining equipment from the bedside. The three stayed with the patient until he died—some seven hours later. The daughter then telephoned her father's physician to inform him that their father had died.

The RN added that she keeps wondering what might have been the outcome if the daughter had not been a medical doctor and the family had asked the attending physician to discontinue all life-sustaining procedures and to let nature take its course.

A religious Sister confided that she prays to God that her parents, if they reach old age, be spared the kind of death where "everything" is done to prevent physiological death without considering any human factors. A nurse aide recalled the well-known phrase: "We have added years to their lives, but have we added life to their years?" And, Rousseau was quoted: "To live is not merely to breathe."

Another thought was injected into the issue as reflected by the poignant statement of a DRN:

> With the attitudes about the aged as they exist today on the part of most persons, even professional nursing and medical personnel, I think we need to be extremely cautious that we are not helping people to die before it is time to die. The attitude toward oldsters at this time may result in letting them die much too early due to the immature judgment and some projection of staff feelings and lack of knowledge and experience in dealing with old people, especially as related to their ability to rally and live small lives within limited life space; for it is their lives to be lived. We sometimes hear of an old person who is 109 and wants to be 110. I do not believe that we can reliably project that a person does not want to live because he is uncomfortable and his prognosis is poor. (Knowles)

Within the context of our contemporary culture and under the pressure of its stereotyped norms that emphasize supreme values for life and corresponding antipathies toward death, many dilemmas arise within the complex of age-illness-death. These cultural influences follow the elderly patient into the therapeutic setting and often plague or disrupt the supportive network of interpersonal relationships that surround him.

The critical opinions as well as the alternative objectives and means become counter-poised, such as, whether or not the terminal diagnosis is valid and, if so, whether to attempt to extend the dying process or to arrest it, ever so temporarily, and by any available extraordinary or heroic measures? Then, eventually, whether to shift from the all-out therapeutic goal of *cure* toward the more supportive *care* and *comfort* goals? And finally, somewhere along the patient's declining course, whether to shift major concern away from the patient and toward the needs of his close relatives and friends in the wake of their shock of bereavement? In time, indeed, the central issue may become whether to shift primary concern away from both the patient and his family and direct it back to the staff's own needs and interests, such as certain research potentials in the "case"; personal reconciliations or rationalizations for "failure to save a life"; or a transfer of attention and time to other urgently ill and possibly more recoverable patients? All these competing objectives are, of course, understandable and often justifiable.

Natural Life-Sustaining Measures

The nursing personnel leave little doubt that they consider it of great importance that so-called *natural* life-sustaining measures for aged and terminally diagnosed patients be continued as long as there is any sign of life left. They stressed again and again that there must be no let-up in meeting the patient's daily needs, and some of them asserted that with patience and time, a skillful nurse is able to accomplish wonders in maintaining the patient's nutritional needs and proper fluid balance and often his overall feelings of comfort. The geriatric nurse is urged, also, to encourage self-care activities for fulfilling the patient's sense of self-reliance and dignity—but not to the point of overtaxing his tolerance. Some of the nurses pointed out that when a patient's life is nearing its end, nursing takes on much of its original meaning. It then becomes a service of nourishing, protecting, and supporting the aged infirm person with all the attention and tenderness that the nurse can muster—somewhat as a good mother cares for her helpless infant, but within a very different context and social outlook.

There was less agreement among nurses, however, about the meaning of the terms "natural" and "artificial," or "ordinary" and "extraordinary" or "heroic." Some would rule out under natural any intrusive procedures such as tube feedings, clyses, or intravenous infusions. Others would include the more commonly used procedures such as infusions among the natural or ordinary means. Still others pointed out that time and place largely determine what is ordinary and what is extraordinary. For example, transfusions are fairly common medical procedures today, whereas some 50 or more years ago they constituted quite extraordinary procedures.

A religious Sister spoke of ordinary and extraordinary means as interpreted by her church. So did the chaplain in a geriatric institution administered by a Roman Catholic religious order. Each explained that any patient enters into a moral contract with an institution when he is admitted to it, a contract of justice which implies that whatever means are readily available in that particular institution must be used for sustaining his life. These are the ordinary means or "means of justice." Extraordinary means are "means of charity," as distinct from means of justice. Means of charity are not readily available. By their very definition, "someone will sacrifice" in order that the well-being of the afflicted person be fostered. In relating this concept to an individual who is aged and terminally ill, however, another religious Sister quoted Pope Pius, "A person has the right to live, but he also has the right to die." According to her also, Pope John, when on his deathbed, wanted no intravenous infusions.

A great many of the nursing personnel, however, interpreted as *natural* those means that are ordinarily practiced in a person's home under the supervision of a medical practitioner. These would include oral feedings, especially liquids, "as long as the patient can swallow," and indicated therapy to prevent complications from nonemptying of the bladder and rectum, and meticulous care of the body, including mouth hygiene for personal comfort and the prevention of complications such as pressure sores and chest involvement. In general, the following discourse is based upon this premise.

The question of purpose was also raised within the present context. Many of the nurses distinguished between life-sustaining procedures that are administered primarily for the comfort of the patient and those resorted to for prolongation of physiological existence—without consideration of the "quality of life" to be saved.

ARTIFICIAL OR EXTRAORDINARY LIFE-SUSTAINING MEASURES

In sharp contrast to the unanimity of opinion of nurses on the use of natural means to sustain a dwindling life, controversy and disparity prevailed concerning the possible use of artificial, extraordinary, or heroic life-extending measures. Some of the nurses took a clear-cut "yes or no" stand; others avoided the issue or rested their decisions on varied conditional factors.

Moreover, a difficulty arises again in the definition of the kind of heroic means for prolonging life. Some nurses believe in resorting to whatever medical discoveries have been made for prolonging life; others would limit life-sustaining means to the more traditional measures such as hypodermoclyses. Still others would not want to subject their patients to anything beyond a tube passed via nose or mouth into the stomach for nourishment. The question of expediency versus high quality nursing also was raised. Several nurses, including both LPN's and RN's, pointed out that it may take as much time and effort—and perhaps patience—to adequately manage equipment involved in the use of artificial measures as it does to use natural means to provide optimum nursing care for an aged terminally ill patient. For example: It requires time and patience, as well as skill and understanding, to feed a very spent and weary ager; but it may take as much time to regulate the equipment used when a patient is being given a hypodermoclysis, in order to prevent the pain associated with overdistention of the tissue or dislocation of the needles inserted. A very dedicated and experienced licensed practical nurse made the following observation:

> Life is up to God, but we should do everything in our power nursing-wise to help the dying patient. A while ago we had a patient here who was expected to live only a couple of days, but she lived for three months. The doctor told us that it was because of the loving care she received. An aged person who is very sick is apt to give up sooner if he knows there is no one who cares. When you try to give a patient some fluid and you talk "sweet talk" to him, he will take it, but if you just "shove it down" he often refuses. If he knows that someone cares, he fights harder—loving care is better than medicines—here we do not use any artificial measures to prolong life.

In nursing homes and similar long-term care institutions, artificial life-sustaining apparatus usually is limited to equipment for infusions and the like. The very advanced and sophisticated mechanical and electronic life-saving devices ordinarily are found only in modern hospitals and medical centers. But aged critically ill patients have been known to be transferred from nursing home to hospital to undergo artificial life-prolonging therapy.

AVOIDING THE ISSUE

From about one fifth to two fifths of the responding nursing personnel of varying ranks were unwilling to commit themselves when it came to accepting any responsibility for a decision on the use of artificial or heroic measures for prolonging the life of an aged, terminally diagnosed, patient.* The smallest proportion of this group skirted the issue on the grounds that the decisions are determined by the philosophy and policy of the institution, or that the question is resolved for the individual nurse by her professional standards and ethics. The largest proportion placed the responsibility entirely upon the physician.

A registered nurse reflected the views of some of her colleagues when she declared that it is up to the good nurse to carry out whatever orders the physician leaves for his patient, and that hers is not the responsibility to question his judgment about resorting to heroic means for sustaining a life. A degree registered nurse contended that while she recognizes that some nurses take the liberty to influence physicians in one way or another, she believes that "even today" the nurse is obliged to carry out his orders as these pertain to physical treatment regardless of her own philosophical or religious views. Another, who asserted that the question of artificial lifesaving therapy is not for the nurse to decide, nevertheless recognized that a nurse often gets caught up in the issue.

> I feel her (the nurse's) problem lies in the area of limiting artificial measures that the doctor orders and then leaves without realizing their full implications to the patient and the family. I have found that detaining the doctor in adjusting and manipulating all the equipment makes him see what is going on and then he often modifies his therapy. Once in a while, the direct approach of "Why are you doing these things," (artificial and extraordinary measures) brings about a mutual sharing of information about both patient and his family that either indicates that it is desirable therapy or that it is not so desirable and the plan of care is modified. (Kerrigan)

Other nurses claimed that it is a moral and religious issue and that the answers lie in the teachings of the church.

In brief, the issue of responsibility for a decision will not arise to plague the practice and the peace of mind of the nurse who tends to her nursing chores, relying upon and adhering to the standards, norms, and regulations of the nursing profession and the judgments of other responsible professionals and leaders in related fields.

OPPOSING THE USE OF HEROIC MEASURES

Other nursing respondents were quite outspoken in their opposition to the use of extraordinary or heroic measures for prolonging the lives of aged, terminally ill patients. Their theme seemed to be, "Let them die in

* NA's, 39.7 percent; LPN's, 28.3 percent; RN's, 17.1 percent; DRN's, 23.4 percent. See Appendix B, Table 8, Items 1 to 4.

peace and comfort and with dignity." This position received its strongest support from the registered nurse group.*

One nurse aide believes that with an aged and spent person there should be no artificial life-prolonging. She commented that there comes a time when "letting go" is best, and that it has been her experience that aged people usually do not want their life prolonged; most of them "beg to let them go peacefully. At that time, comfort and peace of mind is the most important consideration."

A registered nurse stated:

> We do not use life-prolonging measures such as venoclyses here. Our doctors do not go along with heroic measures—they believe that an aged dying person has the right to as peaceful and comfortable a death as we can make it. When you see them lonely and without family; when you see them confused; and when they are a total vegetable it seems almost criminal to prolong such a life. . . .
>
> It seems cruel when a patient is deteriorating—what is the sense of bringing them back for another week of suffering. We have a patient now who is dying of cancer. We do everything we can to make him comfortable. We coax him to eat, but we do not force him. This morning we made gruel for him—it was the only thing he wanted.

A director of nursing in one of the geriatric facilities pointed out that many of their patients are mentally impaired:

> The most tragic thing is to see these people who are physically remarkably well, but mentally so deteriorated that they can no longer help themselves. Some of these people have accomplished a great deal in their lives; some have left a rich heritage for those who come after them; and here you see them just bodies—no personality left. If one of them becomes critically ill, no one with any compassion would want to see their lives prolonged by means of medical heroics. The very best of nursing care, yes; but prolongation of their suffering by means of artificial procedures, no.
>
> We do everything we can to make our patients comfortable. But whatever you do, you want to make sure that you are not shortening their lives—by even the slightest neglect. Let them die in comfort and with dignity. Many of them have already endured social and psychological death—why prolong physiological death by use of mechanical means.

A degree registered nurse stated that, for the patient who is ill and aged and who has lost interest in life, heroic measures do not promote his welfare. Such a person should be able to die, when the time comes, in reasonable comfort "and as expeditiously as Fate allows, without being snatched from the brink by a lifesaving measure—lifesaving for what?"

* NA's, 13.6 percent; LPN's, 17.0 percent; RN's, 39.0 percent; DRN's, 10.2 percent. See Appendix B, Table 8, Item 5.

The tone of the nursing comments indicated that this position arises from strong convictions that the human qualities and characteristics in a life should be regarded as more valid and valued than are life's relatively brief extensions toward the very end—and at a heavy expense, perhaps, in suffering. This position seemed also to carry the implication that the way of dying, as a part of the way of living, may be cherished more by some individuals than a little more of a largely spent life. Nearly all respondents who supported this position appeared to recognize, at the same time, that no single, simple answer can resolve this issue for all nurses or other involved persons; but many of them did claim that their particular stand can provide a good anchor point for treating the patient, at long last, as a person of unique individuality and worth. It seems clear that these nurses would endorse the decision of the distinguished American surgeon who is reported to have insisted on being taken home to die in peace and quiet—without being surrounded by medical paraphernalia and tubes protruding from every orifice of his body.

These nurses held that generally, for the terminally diagnosed, critically ill, and aged patient, the dominant goal of nursing care moves away from priority for the extraordinary lifesaving measures and toward the priority for comfort-giving supports. They stressed that the time comes then, if ever, to concentrate upon personal reinforcements for the ailing and spent individual and to show concern for his immediate survivors. The task then becomes that of coping with the realities of dying as constructively as possible for the sake of the patient and his closely involved associates. From here on, the leading goal remains that of achieving some sense of creditable completion of a life valued as unique in its own individuality.

One DRN seemed to sum up for many of her colleagues the pertinent issues as she and others perceive them:

> If the philosophy of the nursing home is well understood by the medical and nursing staff as well as the patients themselves, I believe that the professional nurse can find freedom to operate within that frame of reference. She is the one who most often knows the patient, the family and friends, and the religious advisor, if there be one.
>
> I do not believe that dramatic lifesaving attempts should be made or begun when the condition of these patients with medically defined terminal illness becomes critical. They should have adequate medical attention and supervision; but I do not believe that they should be sent off to hospitals where extraordinary measures are used to continue their lives. Oxygen should be administered to relieve dyspnea, the trachea should be aspirated to ease breathing. Active and passive exercise should be continued if it increases comfort. Drugs such as are available in home situations should be given if indicated, but the very expensive antibiotics, the vasopressors, the

respirator-types of breathing apparatus have little or no place in the care of such a critically ill aged patient.

If this is the philosophy of the home for the aged, then I believe it is the nurse's responsibility to treat the illness with the ordinary nursing procedures and not the extraordinary. She should take those steps that are indicated for the patient's comfort and to prevent further injury or disease. She should notify the physician of the action that she has taken. If she does not create an emergency situation, the physician will not respond as if it were one and start a lot of lifesaving measures that neither he or anyone else will have the courage to stop at a later time. (Declan)

SUPPORTING THE USE OF HEROIC MEASURES

Justified Unto Death

A substantial proportion of all four nursing ranks supported, but on a variety of grounds, the use of extraordinary or heroic measures for prolonging the lives of aged terminally ill patients.* A considerable portion of this group unconditionally supported the extraordinary measures for keeping aged, critically ill patients alive "unto death." In other words, they emphasized no letup in life-sustaining attempts. Even if a patient seems weary of life and expresses a longing "to go," everything possible should be done. Incidents were related by nursing home staffs where patients have been kept alive for months. Some of these nurses held that doing anything less than everything possible can be regarded as supporting euthanasia, and that no one has the right to shorten the life of another.

Their justifications for this all-out supportive position vary and include the following reasons: in our society it is a matter of principle and law which must not be violated; God expects man to do everything to save life up to the very end; it is "wrong" for anyone to shorten the life of another either by commissive or omissive acts; it is never possible for human beings to know when one's time is up; miracles do happen in what appear to be impossible conditions; it is the safest course for humans to take because, should God not will it, He can disrupt the lifesaving plan and "take" the patient anytime He chooses to do so; the professional code of nursing demands the saving, not the ending, of lives; and, after all, it is human to want to live.

A nurse aide explained that God and science "work side by side" and

---

*. NA's, 30.8 percent; LPN's, 47.2 percent; RN's, 42.7 percent; DRN's, 61.2 percent. See Appendix B, Table 8, Items 6 to 8.

if He sees fit, He will take the person regardless of what is done to keep him alive. A registered nurse who supported this firm and positive stand on lifesaving measures unto death mused that a nurse can find herself in conflict when she is tempted to think that it might be better to let the patient go—"but you cannot do that."

Some of the degree registered nurses who hold the position of doing everything possible as long as there is any chance for life—until the patient is pronounced dead—expressed some reluctance about making such clear-cut commitments. One DRN reasoned that in our culture and under our legal system a nurse is obligated to urge natural *and* artificial life-sustaining measures until death actually occurs; and she reported experiences of conflict in certain critical situations when the patient or his relatives opposed an all-out course and produced in her such ambivalent feelings that she became inclined to side with them. But another nurse contended that some families feel an obligation to press for extraordinary measures. She recalled with some dismay how she had seen a woman literally eaten up with cancer, but who lingered on for weeks because her son felt guilty about any stoppage of intravenous therapy.

Other nurses referred to the fact that in our society there exists a widespread, publicly-shared expectation that physicians, nurses, and other health professionals are all committed to saving and prolonging life and will do everything in their power to do so; that many families tend to exert pressure to this end; and that the nurse is caught somewhere in the middle. This is elaborated upon by one respondent:

> The layman in our culture is afraid of death, and he will use many defense mechanisms to decrease his anxiety which is caused by his reluctance to accept an imminent certainty of the event. The loss of a patient often results in a feeling of failure among doctors and nurses. Our acquired feelings about death tend to promote the use of heroic measures to prolong life by those who work directly with dying patients. I think that closed chest cardiac massage plus the artificial methods, such as machines to breathe for the patient, are often resorted to because our cultural values emphasize the preservation of life at all costs. Many hospitals have teams of physicians and other personnel who rush to the bedside of every patient whose heart suddenly stops, or who shows signs of being near death. Every possible method of sustaining life is tried by those who respond to the emergency. The 85-year-old man whose heart stops will have just as much done as will the 25-year-old in similar circumstances. Once the heart is beating again, the patient will remain attached to the various machines which will keep his body alive, even in the face of the knowledge that irreparable brain damage has been suffered. The patient will live in this comalike state until someone makes the decision to shut off the machines. But who is to make the decision?
>
> Many patients, young and old alike, have been saved by these measures. The decision to shut off the machines is usually made by the

physician. The nurse usually does the actual removal of the machinery; so her voice should be heard whenever questions of how long to try are made. (Shumway)

Still other nurses claimed that it is neither the role of the physician nor the role of the nurse to sit in judgment on the value of human life. Society entrusts to them the task of promoting health, prolonging life, and alleviating pain and suffering. Only by supporting every possible life-saving measure can a nurse feel assured of having fulfilled her obligation to the patient and to society.

Intricate and scientific life-sustaining equipment, such as machines that breathe for the patient, is not usually available in nursing homes or other geriatric institutions, except in those specifically licensed as hospitals. In institutions established for long-term care of chronically ill and infirm persons, the question of life-prolonging measures most often revolves around procedures such as tube feedings when a patient is no longer able, or steadfastly refuses, to take nourishment by mouth and hypodermo- or venoclyses used to maintain proper fluid balance. To illustrate:

> The patient, a former professor, has been steadily going downhill since he came here a little more than two months ago. He is 85 years old and gives every indication that he does not want to go on living—he can no longer bear his infirmities and the physical and mental suffering. When he first came here, he still talked to some of us; but now he no longer speaks. All he wants is to be left alone and to sleep. He refuses to eat, even closing his lips tight when we try to give him some nourishment by mouth. He often pulls at the nasal tube we passed in order to get nourishment into him—and a private aide has been assigned to him. We also give him clyses regularly.

However, the question of *going all out*—of using the latest mechanical and electrical life-sustaining apparatus known to medicine—cannot be ignored. Being in a nursing home does not vouchsafe for an aged critically ill patient that he will remain there to die. If the doctor or the administration deems it advisable, he is transferred to the hospital, and in certain geriatric institutions this is done almost routinely. And, of course, many aged patients are admitted directly to a hospital from their home in the case of serious illness.

In the view of some nurses, the possibility of unexpected recovery should never be entirely overlooked by any responsible health personnel. Also, in some patients, it is assumed to be impossible for any mortal to determine precisely when the terminal phase in life begins, or when the cut-off point for potential recovery occurs. New lifesaving techniques have already brought back some of those once pronounced dead, and new discoveries are constantly made. Therefore, everything possible should be done to enable patients to live until they are dead, and even that point in time is becoming difficult to determine precisely.

Judgment Is Conditional To the Individual Situation

While siding with the position that a time comes for some patients when it seems wiser to limit extraordinary efforts in keeping aged terminally ill patients alive and to concentrate mainly on comfort-giving considerations, many of the nurses stipulated that such a shift should not result from routine commitment to a generalized rule. To the contrary, every decision should be reached on grounds of individual circumstances in which various contributing factors are considered.

These nurses suggested that the factors might well include any potential opportunities for the patient to enjoy the rest of whatever life is left to him; any degree of uncertainty about the diagnosis; any remaining mental capacity in the patient; the intensity and constancy of the pain suffered; the expressed wishes of the patient in any lucid moment; and some appraisal of the interests and capacities of the relatives or other responsible persons for prolongation of the patient's life. Moreover, some nurses urged that the reaching of a decision to resort to extraordinary measures, along with explanations of what is involved and can be expected, should be shared by the physician with the nursing staff; with members of the family, if possible; and with the patient, whenever feasible.

The thinking of this group, however, differs only in degree from that of their colleagues who *reject* the use of artificial lifesaving measures for aged patients with a terminal diagnosis. The nurses who unqualifiedly disapproved such measures appear to do so on the assumption that the terminal diagnosis *is* definite and that the promise of further meaningful living for the patient is almost nil. The nurses who would evaluate each situation, clearly do not presume this. If, upon consideration of many pertinent factors for a given patient, it appears that further extension of the patient's life by artificial means could mean no more than a kind of prolongation of death with no foreseeable good effect, these nurses join their colleagues in rejection of artificial lifesaving procedures.

But the individualized, conditional decisions are not at all easy to reach in a given situation:

> When an elderly patient is hopelessly ill, it would seem better not to begin the "heroic" means. Once begun, there is almost no morality to the decisions that follow; either to continue or to withhold them.
> Far better would be a plan made in advance in which the doctor and the family participate, and including the patient if he is aware and knowledgeable.

All things considered, what should be done? This question cuts deep into the finest contribution that a professional can make to any situation—the constructive use of his trained judgment. The goal of patient care is not the prevention of death, but the prevention of *untimely* death and of needless suffering. (Schwartz)

The DRN's frequently pointed out that a nurse must exercise professional judgment to guide her in particular situations. They left no doubt that she is morally obliged to use all *ordinary* means to promote and sustain life at any stage of illness. At times they also recognized the wisdom and expediency in the use of extraordinary procedures, but mainly when these fit constructively into the larger therapeutic situation, which is in the best interest of the patient and his family. In general, the use of heroics for aged terminally ill patients was considered ill advised when for the primary purpose of assuring someone that "everything is being done," or for any convenience of the hospital staff, especially when involving suffering for the patient or stress on his family.

If the chief aim is the comfort and welfare of the terminally ill patient as long as life lasts, then, these nurses seem to imply, all decisions to use special devices and heroic measures should be in accord with this principle. Prolongation of a life pronounced by medical diagnosis to be hopeless and that would be long-drawn-out and filled with suffering tends to be viewed by them as inhuman, torturous, and "wrong."

These nurses grant that it may be different with persons who are younger; but with many of the aged and infirm, a time comes when they are ready to accept, and even wish for death. When hope fades with the passing of time, nature should be permitted to take its course.

The following example reflects the tempered attitude and reasoning of a physician:

> A massive cerebral hemorrhage had left the 79-year-old patient in a comatose condition, and after a few days' hospitalization, he was transferred to a nearby nursing home where his physician, having attended the family for many years, continued to take responsibility for his medical care.
>
> Until he was stricken the patient had enjoyed fairly good health, and his wife found herself unable to accept that his condition was terminal; she implored the physician "to do something" so her husband would live. The doctor kept explaining to the wife that her husband's condition was grave and that in his judgment any medical heroics might prolong the process of dying, but could neither keep the patient alive for very long nor restore his health. When the wife continued to insist that extraordinary procedures be used to save her husband's life, the physician called a family conference to explain his position, during which he related an experience of his early medical practice which had weighed heavily upon him.
>
> As a young medical practitioner he had been called to attend a

patient who had suffered a severe cerebral hemorrhage. With the permission of the family, he had resorted to whatever medical science had put at his command to keep the patient alive. This patient continued to live for several months, completely dependent upon others, and suffering great mental and physical pain. The family also suffered, finding his care emotionally exhausting and financially a great burden.

Professional judgment and the physician's integrity prevailed. The patient died peacefully, without regaining consciousness, about a week after being transferred to the nursing home.

Some nursing support of the use of extraordinary lifesaving measures for aged dying patients was made conditional to assurances that the rights of the patient and his family be fully safeguarded. The importance of doing whatever is possible to recognize and insure these rights was stressed by relatively few practitioners, but by about a fifth of the DRN group. The steps to take seemingly could involve anything that clearly takes account of, and complies with these rights, such as getting permission from the patient, if it seems appropriate, or from responsible members of the family as well as preparing them for the measures to be taken and supporting them throughout the treatment procedures.

That the opposite may, and at times does, happen is illustrated in the following account, related by a DRN out of her personal experience in a modern medical center:

> The day before entering the hospital, my Aunt discussed with her widowed sister and me the possibility of not recovering from the contemplated surgery for cancer, and she begged us to let her die in peace should her condition become critical. She did not want all sorts of medical heroics used to keep her alive. She also made this known to the surgeon when he examined her prior to her hospitalization.
>
> My Aunt was 83. Despite arthritis which had stiffened her joints and made walking difficult and an occasional bout with diverticulitis, she led an active life. Some years before she had fallen, and the accident had left her with a completely ankylosed left elbow. She dreaded becoming an invalid and being dependent upon others for her basic daily needs. For many years she had made her home with a younger sister, a widow. She had a keen mind and loved life. She was a religious person and very active with church affairs.
>
> A radical mastectomy was performed, and the surgeon held out hope for complete recovery. For the first week her postoperative course was uneventful. Then she began complaining of tightness in her chest, and her temperature hovered between 101 and 104 degrees. She vomited whatever food was given her by mouth, and she also began having difficulty breathing. Following numerous laboratory tests, the doctor informed her and her family that she had a massive staphylococcus infestation. Various treatments were tried, but to no avail. Intravenous clyses were resumed, blood transfusions were given every few days, oxygen therapy was started, and she was placed on an oscillating bed. All medications were given by injection—and there were a

great many of them. Every day laboratory tests were done. Throughout all this, her mind remained remarkably keen.

Despite the complications and the painful and wearying treatments, she never lost hope of recovery and was waiting for the day that we would take her home. She never complained, not even when three days following her surgery two aides helped her to the toilet and forgot about her. She had no way of reaching the bell and her calls remained unheard. When the staff finally remembered, they found her semiconscious and shivering with cold and exhaustion. She did not complain when one Sunday afternoon she was placed in a wheelchair and taken for additional x-rays because of high temperature, and was left alone for well over an hour because there was no one available to take her back to her floor since it was Sunday. The pastor of her church had come to visit her that afternoon, had waited in her room for almost an hour, and then gone to the nurses' desk again to make inquiries about her whereabouts. A nurse telephoned the x-ray department and someone was sent to bring her back to her room. She seemed extremely exhausted, but begged the pastor not to report the incident.

Shortly thereafter, in the middle of the night she began "choking," and a tracheotomy was performed. Her condition worsened. It became exceedingly difficult to insert a needle into a vein when giving transfusions or venoclyses and her veins kept collapsing. Phlebitis set in in both legs. The mastectomy incision was breaking down. Her chest complaints continued. She began refusing nourishment.

Her hope of recovery had given way to despair. Whereas formerly she had always nodded her head and smiled when we encouraged her to "keep fighting" so she could go home soon, she now shook her head whenever reference was made to getting well. Her face looked drawn and thin, she seemed utterly exhausted, and she gave every indication that she was "giving up."

One day the patient's sister remonstrated with the doctor about discontinuing some of the extreme procedures. His answer was brief: "Do you want to play God?" He answered me similarly when a couple of days later I reminded him of my Aunt's attitude before her surgery and her wish to be permitted to die in peace and some comfort.

Four days after this the surgeon telephoned me at my place of work to inform me that my aunt had taken a sudden turn for the worse and asked that I come to the hospital at once. When I arrived there half an hour later, the nurse met me in the hall and told me that my aunt had died moments before.

The nurses who seemingly commit themselves to the "conditional" position spelled out the precautionary or conditioning factors in impressive details as reflected in the following reflective statement.

Urging the use of extraordinary lifesaving measures may be at times unjustifiable; health professionals often reject them when proposed for themselves as patients; they are less safe when a patient objects to them or is unconscious; and points are reached in patient tolerance when these procedures shorten life. There is danger of increased suffering and greater complications in the end; and once begun, it is very difficult to reach a decision to stop them. Extraordinary lifesaving measures become unrealistic when a patient is aged and slowly dying, but lingers on and on. Actually, though little is said about it, for years therapists have been reaching points in the use of such measures where, when practical prospects are exhausted, they let the patient go naturally.

The use of extraordinary measures can be justified on a practical basis *only* when the comfort of the aged patient is reasonably assured, his independence is not violated, and he is under constant care of a competent nursing staff. It is still better, to have the permission of the family and of the patient, if he is conscious and able to make a rational choice. As much as possible, the decision should be arrived at collectively through deliberations with such responsibility-sharing persons as consultant physician, nurse, social worker, clergy, and the like.

Generally, as far as nursing is involved, very heroic measures should be supported only when prospects for the patient's recovery look encouraging by medical judgment and when it is recognized that the aged patient still wants to live, has certain tasks or purposes that he wishes to fulfill, is willing to assume a modified existence, and is capable of making this kind of adaptation.

This point is illustrated by a statement from a DRN:

> Many of us who have worked together in nursing for years tell each other, "If they ever bring me in here in that shape, don't let them operate on me or use special lifesaving measures. Let me go in peace." Do we mean it?
>
> I have assisted with inward horror while a doctor attempted artificial respiration, injected adrenalin into the heart, and performed other similar procedures on an old man who had been ill and senile for years. Then again, I have seen another old and ill patient make a good recovery when his doctor persisted. . . .
>
> I definitely feel, however, that there is a time when a person should be permitted to die in peace rather than to be made to live. (Damon)

When justifying and qualifying their decisions on moral, religious, or philosophical grounds, the thinking of the nurses follows this way of reasoning: Granted that the full meaning of life is not known, it cannot be said of an aged person, even in pain and with wasted health, that his life is devoid of spiritual value. It is difficult to see, nevertheless, how the extraordinary measures will promote the welfare of a patient who is definitely ill beyond recovery and has lost interest in life. Such a person should be permitted to die, when his time is imminent, as comfortably and as expeditiously as Fate allows, without being snatched from the brink, perhaps again and again, by the drastic lifesaving devices. Morally, procedures which have the sole aim of keeping the organism breathing are difficult to justify. *The nurse's commitment should be to support and sustain dying when one's time has come as well as to promote and safeguard living until that time comes.* How can it be "right" for a nurse to urge the prolongation of the life of an elderly dying patient into a state of purely passive and negative existence? And how can it be "wrong" for her to suggest to the physician that to push any further for the continuation of such a life seems "out of place." Indeed, it may be the conscientious nurse's place to inform the physician in detail on her observations of the patient and to express her personal concern whether the push should go on, especially if her own philosophy and professional ethics recognizes the individual's right to die under certain circumstances as well as the right to live under others.

One DRN, who is also a religious Sister, expressed some of the same cautionary ideas in a rather pointed question:

> Until the full meaning of life is known, is it not as needful, or more so, to help the dying person over his death as to sustain a spark of life in a body that is "as good as dead?" (Hagen)

DISCUSSION

From the assembled information, it appears evident that whenever the nurse embraces some independent responsibility for sharing or influencing decision-making on the issue of resorting to extraordinary or heroic life-extending measures for medically diagnosed terminally ill patients and makes commitment to individualized conditional considerations, she is likely to face a complex and confusing situation. Many potential influencing factors may challenge her: she may find herself attempting to discriminate on definitions of terminal diagnosis and degrees of terminality implied; she may try to identify and weigh for a particular patient the potentials left to him for deriving further gains and satisfactions out of further small extensions of his life; she can become concerned about the effect upon both the patient and his family of prolonging the process of dying; or she may strive to perceive more clearly what is meant or implied in a situation by natural versus unnatural measures as they apply to a particular person, to cite but a few of the factors.

It seems obvious that a nurse, especially the RN and the DRN, who neither avoids nor subscribes to the position that "everything possible unto death" should be done for an aged terminally diagnosed patient tends to become involved in a situation of potential conflict. Conditions are probably optimum for this when the physician, on the one hand, prognosticates an early death but attempts to postpone it by extraordinary measures, while the nurse, on the other hand, comes to hope and even pray that the same patient—when his last days get tough and torturous—may obtain an early and peaceful release. Similarly, when a nurse receives orders from a physician to disconnect life-sustaining equipment from a patient whom he has earlier decided to keep alive as long as possible by heroic measures, the situation can become charged for her with emotional stress. Under such conditions, certain awkward and dilemma-laden relationships are very likely to arise, whether openly expressed or not. And when they do, they are not without price perhaps to all concerned, and especially to the patient or his family or both.

In a time of major medical advances—with cardiac pacemakers; more potent and effective drugs; linkups with mechanical substitutes for failing vital organs; and with implantations of vital body parts—there is likely to exist a middle knowledge between knowing when to use and when not to use these "extensions of life" and many competent professional persons of great integrity may lean too far either to one side or to the other.

Dr. M. F. A. Woodruff clearly brought the dilemma to the foreground when, in a British medical journal, he asked: "What degree of suffering should we be prepared to inflict on our patients in return for a faint hope of life?"*

SUMMARY

By a near consensus, the nursing respondents of all four ranks adamantly affirmed that so-called *natural* life-sustaining measures must be continued until the very end of an aged patient's life.

With respect to urging the use of *artificial* or extraordinary life-sustaining procedures, however, considerable diversity of opinion was encountered. Indeed, on issues such as this, one would anticipate the appearance of certain conflicts, paradoxes, and dilemmas.

The data relating to the use of extraordinary life-sustaining devices were separated into three major categories: 1) Avoidance of the issue; 2) rejection of resorting to such means for aged terminally ill patients; and, 3) Support of such measures.

* Quoted in an editorial, "Moments of Death: Interplay of Law, Ethics, and Science," published in *Medicine at Work*, October, 1965.

Of the respondents, about a fifth to two fifths, varying according to nursing ranks, appeared unwilling or at least very cautious to assume any responsibility for influencing decisions of this nature. They justified their stand by offering a variety of grounds which, essentially, amounted to an abdication of responsibility on their part for decision-making.

A very substantial number of the nursing respondents, however, made bold and took a firm stand in assuming some responsibility for influencing decisions on this issue. Those who unequivocally rejected the use of extraordinary lifesaving procedures for aged dying patients ranged from about 10 percent for the DRN's to a near 40 percent for the RN's. These nurses took the position that for aged and ailing persons with an early terminal diagnosis, the dominant goal of nursing should be shifted from lifesaving to comfort-giving measures and that major efforts should be concentrated on the personal support of the patient and his immediate family and friends in their attempts to come to terms with the pending realities of death with dignity, self-composure, and peace of mind. Some of the very devout respondents saw, of course, much richer fulfillments in prospect.

Nursing respondents who supported the use of extraordinary measures for sustaining life, on the other hand, ranged from a near third of the NA's to close to two thirds of the DRN's. Statistical details on the three major positions are as follows:

	NA's %	LPN's %	RN's %	DRN's %
Avoiding the issue	39.7	28.3	17.1	23.4
Opposing the use of heroic measures	13.6	17.0	39.0	10.2
Supporting heroic lifesaving devices	30.8	47.2	42.7	61.2

It should be noted, however, that the group endorsing the use of artificial life-sustaining means is divided on one important aspect: the issue of whether such measures should be used for all, or only some, aged, fatally ill individuals. Some declared unequivocally that everything possible should be done to save and prolong life in the terminally ill aged person; others tended strongly to qualify or condition the grounds upon which their opinions are formulated. The latter specified that each individual situation be examined and the factors inherent in it be carefully considered before a decision is made and a course of action determined. Important among such factors would be how definite the terminal diagnosis is and how promising is the life that the patient would be able to enjoy. Some of these nurses also made the point that special weight be accorded to the wishes of the patient, if he is capable of expressing them, and to those of the family. The following figures represent the supporting stance:

	NA's %	LPN's %	RN's %	DRN's %
Use heroic lifesaving measures "unto death"	20.5	21.5	24.5	14.3
Decision depends upon the individual situation	8.0	20.8	15.8	25.5
Respect the rights of patient and family	2.3	1.9	2.4	21.4

These figures reveal that the DRN's lead by a wide margin all three practitioner groups in supporting the heroic or extraordinary measures; but their representation for full and unqualified support is low as compared with the practitioner groups. Indeed, almost half of these DRN's give their support conditionally.

An interesting and quite relevant question to ponder is whether the fundamental or instrumental needs of aged patients are made more vulnerable by the differing positions which the several categories of nursing personnel support.

For full statistical details, see Appendix B, Table 8.

12 The Dying Patient

One cannot make rules about telling the patient about his illness, but must try and deal with each person individually.

CICELY SAUNDERS

The question of whether a patient should know that he is dying arouses controversy in our culture not only among professionals responsible for his care, but also among the patient's relatives and friends. Uncertainty about this issue—to know or not to know—may even exist in the mind of the patient himself. Those who would withhold from a patient the knowledge of the seriousness of his condition may do so for reasons such as: life is extraordinarily precious; nearly everyone wants to live as long as possible; and, in the face of the inevitable, a patient should be safeguarded from any unnecessary worry during his last days on earth. Some also hold that such knowledge tends to upset and disturb the patient to the point that he may give up the fight and thereby shorten his life.

Others, holding the opposite view, claim that a man or woman who has been diagnosed as terminally ill by competent physicians has a right to know it in time, if possible, to prepare for the eventuality. If he is able to do so, the patient may feel responsible, and desire opportunity, to make a final settlement of his affairs; to smoothe out any ruffled relationships with his fellows; to achieve a few possible "eleventh hour" objectives toward which his life has been directed; and, also, to prepare himself to meet the unknown. It is said that since human beings are probably the only creatures that can actually become aware of impending death and also possess some capacity to cope purposefully with it, they should have their chance to do so. The Shakespearean dilemma—to be or not to be—was put into the mouth of a young man; but how much more apt and timely would this be upon the lips of an old man?

Numerous variations on the above two divergent themes are encountered, and not without mental and emotional conflict for those involved.

170

Western tradition has invested the physician with the primary responsibility for deciding whether or not a patient is to be informed about the seriousness of his condition; and doctors are about as divided on the question as are other professionals. Many a nurse faces the issue at close range and, not infrequently, expresses relief at the thought that this decision is not hers to make. Some nurses, however, would welcome the freedom to discuss with the patient his thoughts, attitudes, and any anxieties with which he is preoccupied. Occasionally, a nurse may chide the physician who withholds from them such an opportunity and who keeps from the patient the graveness of his diagnosis.

There are nurses, also, who express the belief that an elderly person, much more often than one who is younger, realizes that he may be terminally ill and should be given ample opportunity to verbalize his concerns about dying, if and whenever he shows signs of his need and readiness to do so. A social atmosphere which allows free patient-staff communication on the subject can, and often does, contribute to the inner peace and well-being of the patient. However, not every aged patient has either the capacity or the desire to face the medical forecast on the nearness or manner of his death, and some individuals may be disinclined to admit anyone into the inner privacy of their fears and anxieties or of their individualized manner of coping with the terminal crisis in their lives. There is wide agreement among these nurses that such privacy, when really preferred by an elderly patient, should be both respected and safeguarded. "One must try and deal with each person individually."

PART 1. NURSES' PERCEPTION OF AGED PERSONS' VIEW OF DEATH

It was possible to gather some interesting interview data from staff nurses in the select geriatric facilities on the manner in which elderly patients view and react to their impending death. Nursing personnel generally focused their attention upon aged patients' attitude and behavior toward death and dying before dealing more specifically with their own beliefs and practices. The degree registered nurses, on the other hand, addressed themselves more directly to nursing philosophy and practices, and their responses contain few references to nurses' perceptions of the views elderly persons hold toward death.

It is natural to assume that a nurse takes into consideration her patients' views and reactions when coping with particular problems, and some of the nursing staff in the geriatric institutions evidently use their perceptions of patients' attitude and behavior as a basis for rationale in their own nursing practice. Others do not appear to make such useful linkage between their reflections and their practice.

PATIENTS SHOW NO CONCERN ABOUT DYING

Nearly a third of the respective groups of nurse practitioners reported that their aged patients rarely allude to death topics or appear to be overly concerned about the prospect of dying.* Their contention was that an aged person lives from day to day, from hour to hour, or even, in the latter phase of life, from moment to moment. He reminisces about the past—his own past; perhaps shows some interest in the present; and is quite unconcerned about, perhaps even oblivious to, his approaching death. With advancing age, man's senses become dulled to the point that he does not react as sensitively to the experiences of pending events as does a younger person. A very aged person's attention span is apt to be short, and senescence is said to be, in a sense, its own anesthesia. When death takes a fellow patient, the others do not appear overly upset and, before long, return to their more mundane preoccupations with immediate personal needs and wants. Having lived a long life and being spent and weary, the aged may be more accepting of their coming death than they might have been at an earlier age. A registered nurse reported:

> One of our patients died recently at the age of 89. During the years of her residency here she had always been cheerful. She remained mentally keen and alert until death. She never alluded to death or dying, but from time to time she would say, "It's time I went," or "It's time Saint Peter came for me." She was ill with pneumonia during her final illness. About half an hour before she died, she looked about the room and said, "Saint Peter is coming to get me." She did not appear anxious or fearful, and her death was peaceful from all that we could observe.

It was often implied or openly contended by these nurses that the aged ill, having come to terms with dying, are not disturbed about the prospect that death may be near, and their acceptance of death also eliminates for them the need to be vocal about it.

From a background of these and similar comments it comes as no

---

* NA's, 30.3 percent; LPN's, 28.3 percent; RN's, 32.0 percent. See Appendix B, Table 9, Items 1, 2. No figures on the issue are available for the DRN's.

surprise to hear a registered nurse declare that in her busy rounds of duty she rarely hears an elderly patient speak of death or dying. But within the same institution, other nurses voiced their concern that the institution's regulations and routines tend to impose a major degree of silence on the subject and that, in general, the social atmosphere is not conducive to free expression on death topics. They also alleged that, given a sympathetic nurse who knows how to listen, many of their aged patients would choose to voice their thoughts about this final event in their lives.

It is suspected, however, that more is needed than an officially permissive atmosphere; for many staff members voiced feelings of insecurity on their own part and find themselves ill prepared or incapable of positively and constructively handling the topic of individual, personal death. They feel on safer ground when they ignore the reality of the situation, and they often resort to false assurances when caring for dying patients. A registered nurse, who has devoted many years to the care of the aged ill, commented that "no matter how sick or how old the patient is, we tell them that they will feel better by tomorrow." Concerning this matter, it should be remembered that the nurses frequently are following the lead of the physician and the public in their pattern of behavior.

FEAR OF DEATH IS HUMAN NATURE

Other staff members took issue with those who hold that death and dying are not part of aged patients' serious concerns. These nurses claimed that fear is part of human nature, and they perceive this fear in their patients. Slightly more than one in five of the licensed practical, and the registered, nurses held this position, with about one in six of the nurse aides agreeing.* Irrespective of whether the patient is deeply religious or a professed agnostic; whether he is dying of a catastrophic illness or of a gradual and prolonged deterioration of the general body structure; whether he is a relatively young ager or an octogenarian; and whether he is highly intelligent and educated or a near-illiterate, these staff members conceive of fear of death being present in all of them. A licensed practical nurse said, "You know what you have now, but you do not know what you get afterwards"—an eloquently simple and profound remark. According to these respondents, facing an unknown, even if portrayed as the Kingdom of Heaven, produces anxiety, if not fear; and,

* NA's, 15.7 percent; LPN's, 22.7 percent; RN's, 20.5 percent. See Appendix B, Table 9, Items 3, 4.

while death may be a passage leading to a more glorious hereafter, it is nevertheless a point of uncertainty from which there is no return.

The experience of this group of nursing personnel was that while some of their aged patients articulate their fear, many others communicate their anxiety and apprehension in more covert fashion. Certain of these nurses distinguished between fear of death and fear of dying alone. Instances of seriously ill persons pleading with staff not to leave them were frequently related, but whether the distinction between fear of death and fear of being alone when facing death is a valid one seemed to some a moot question:

> Mr. M., 91 years old, was gradually getting weaker, and death did not seem far away. He realized that he was dying, but he kept pleading with whoever took care of him, "Don't leave me—don't let me die."

Wide agreement was encountered among the nurses, and quite unrelated to the particular position they took on the above issue, concerning the fact that aged dying patients usually do take comfort in having someone with them. Experiences were cited where patients, even though semiconscious and unable to communicate their needs and wants, seemed more relaxed when someone remained close by, apparently finding solace in the touch of a comforting hand or the tone of a familiar voice.

Some of the staff detected fear in their patients' eyes or in the way a dying patient would cling to them—not wanting them to leave the bedside. Requests of dying patients to have their door left open or a light left on all night also were interpreted as being prompted by fear of death. A few, however, saw little, if any, relationship between a patient's attitude toward death and his evident need to have another person share his final travail.

A PATIENT'S ATTITUDE TOWARD DEATH DEPENDS ON DIVERSE FACTORS

By far the largest number of the nursing staff took a less specific stand on the issue. About half proclaimed that the issue is complex and does not lend itself to generalizations, due to the number of diverse factors to be considered in the situation.* They stressed the individual differences rather than the common traits in their aged patients. These nurses held

---

* NA's, 54.0 percent; LPN's, 49.0 percent; RN's, 46.2 percent. See Appendix B, Table 9, Items 5 to 7.

that a person's background; his health, both mental and physical; and his religio-philosophical orientation all shape his attitude toward death and dying. The extent to which an aged person was involved with life's experiences before being fatally stricken and the degree to which a particular patient believes himself abandoned by his family also are considered to be important variables. A charge nurse in a nursing home contended that a sense of feeling abandoned very probably was a factor in the death of Mrs. E.:

> We never knew the reason why Mrs. E. was placed in the nursing home. She had been living with a married daughter and appeared to have been in relatively good health. She was in her late seventies. She must have been quite happy living in her daughter's home, for she often told about her lovely room, furnished with her own belongings which she had brought with her several years before when she was forced to give up her own home. She seemed to live for the day when she would be returning to her daughter's house.
>
> Shortly after entering the institution, Mrs. E. began to complain of abdominal discomfort and she expressed fear of having cancer. She was transferred to the hospital for diagnostic tests, which proved negative. When the patient's complaints increased, she was again taken to the hospital, where an exploratory operation was performed. It was negative. Several months later, it was discovered that the patient had diverticuli and surgery was performed. The doctors expected an uneventful recovery.
>
> During her most recent hospitalization, Mrs. E. was told by a friend who was visiting that her daughter had disposed of the furniture Mrs. E. had brought with her from her own home and had redecorated the room her mother had occupied. From that time on, Mrs. E. seemed even more depressed than she had been before. Her physical complaints also increased, even though the doctors said there was no physical reason for her "suffering." When she refused to eat, she was given artificial feedings and infusions. But she died because "we all knew that she did not want to live."

Some aged patients are said to welcome death, others are resigned to die, and still others manifest fear as death draws near. A religious Sister recalled:

> We had a 90-year-old patient, who had remained remarkably keen mentally and fully conscious until shortly before death. She suffered a great deal of pain during her final days, and she saw in death a release from suffering. Being a deeply religious person, she also looked forward to the promise of heaven. Her only fear appeared to be that of dying without someone being with her, and she implored us to remain with her until her last breath. Her wish was granted, of course. We always have someone stay with a person who is dying.

A registered nurse remembered:

> Mrs. P. was in her late eighties when she died. For some months she had been having a good deal of pain. She kept praying for death and for relief from suffering, though before her final illness this patient had often been heard to pray to God to spare her a little longer.
>
> God is good that way. The human body can stand pain and suffering for just so long—then the person is ready to go.

But instances of gradual and peaceful death, without pain, were cited much more frequently. A registered nurse spoke for many of her colleagues when she said that often aged patients, particularly when very old, just fade away, with the body slowly weakening and the mind becoming drowsy, until the person sinks into a final sleep. So it was with Miss T.:

> Ninety-year-old Miss T. is dying of old age. For several weeks now she has been sleeping most of the time. When she is awake, she seems calm and not at all apprehensive about the future. She is just old and weary.

The belief was also expressed that while physical pain and suffering may make a patient wish for death, mental deterioration may result in less awareness of the patient about what is happening to him. Patients with severe mental impairment are reported to exhibit little or no concern about death.

Some staff members distinguished between an attitude toward death manifested by a patient who, up to the time he was stricken, had been in relatively good health and engaged in a variety of endeavors and a person of advanced age who has lost all interest in, and purpose for, life—whose existence is quite devoid of meaningful activities. The person who is stricken at the time of active and zestful endeavors, irrespective of his chronological age, may lament and resent oncoming death; whereas the very weary and spent ager may welcome or at least be resigned to it. Certain staff members also saw a difference in the attitude of a patient whose death is the result of a sudden, brief illness, and one with a lingering ailment. A long-drawn-out sickbed allows the person to become somewhat reconciled to the idea of closure of his life.

Religion was often alluded to as an important variable in a patient's attitude toward death. It was often reiterated that a deeply devout person faces death more serenely than does one who is not very religious. A nurse aide said that she finds solace in the promise of Christ that the soul has eternal life and that she tries to convey this to her dying patients. Still others saw a variant in the aged person's background, his style of life. It was suggested that a person who has lived what he believes was a full and good life is more ready to go than one who has not.

Some nurses felt that patients may resort to allusions of death and dying as a sort of lament—as a means to express their unhappiness with their past or present lot in life. Their wish to die springs from a sense of bitterness or a feeling of having been abandoned by their loved ones. An LPN illustrated:

> Almost every day Mrs. C. would say, "Call my daughter. I am going to die." And I always gave her the same answer, "You're all right—you'll outlive me yet." And we would scold her a little for talking like that.
>
> But one morning I answered her wailing with, "All right, have it your way—tell me which dress do you want us to put on when you die?" She was startled, but then said, "The green one." Then we all laughed. For quite a while after that Mrs. C. did not mention death again.
>
> Basically, this patient resents being here. She wants to go home to her daughter. The older you get, the more you yearn for family, for being near loved ones. Many of our patients here feel rejected, but some cover it up more than others.

Staff contended that patients resort to this kind of behavior more often while still in comparatively good health than when death is close. Most times these patients do not mean it when they say, "I wish I could die" or "I am useless and a burden, why doesn't God take me."

Instances of patients' premonitions of approaching death were also repeatedly cited:

> Mr. Q., a 90-year-old and very alert patient who was in relatively good health and quite independent in his activities of daily living, one day told the nurse who brought him his medicine, "Spring is coming; I won't be here much longer." A week later he suffered a fatal heart attack.

> Mrs. B., in her eighties, said to the aide who was caring for her, "I won't see you when you come back in the morning." The patient was not considered close to death, but when the aide arrived on the floor the next day, she was told that Mrs. B. had died during the night.

An RN commented that such experiences are not uncommon. Some patients are said to have a sixth sense; they feel it in "their bones" when death is close, though observable signs and symptoms do not indicate this.

Some of the nurses and nurse aides related experiences to exemplify the different ways in which death comes to aged persons. An experienced and dedicated nurse aide, who claims "not to be afraid of death" and who is often assigned to stay with dying patients, reported that she cannot remember the number of dying patients whose final days and hours she has shared; but that each situation is different from any other. She indicated that about half of these patients had remained mentally alert and conscious until, or almost until, the end; the others lost consciousness hours, and sometimes days, before death took them. Some of them seemed apprehensive; others did not. But almost everyone of them had a quiet death—no suffering, no struggle.

A registered nurse commented upon the dignity in death of a patient whose final hours she had shared:

> Following a hip fracture, Mrs. G. had developed some complications and her condition quickly deteriorated. She "knew" that death was close and verbalized her feelings and concerns about the closure of her life quite freely. The previous evening, she bade her two nephews, the only surviving kin, farewell. Just before she died, the minister from her church visited and prayed with her. When, upon leaving the room, I spoke for a brief moment with the minister, he commented upon her serenity and upon a "beautiful expression" that had come over her face after the prayer. As I opened the door to Mrs. G.'s room, she was drawing her final breath, quietly, peacefully. She looked as though she was envisioning something beautiful, as though she had found fulfillment in death.

Nurses also contended that aged persons, who according to the law of averages are closer to death than those who are younger, rarely indulge in philosophical discussions of death. If they are concerned, their own death looms too close for them to be objective or detached about the topic; and when they do allude to death and dying, it is much more likely to be on a very personal and subjective basis.

Even a limited summarization of the nurses' perceptions of the experience and behavior of aged patients about death and dying brings out many contrasting ideas and interpretations:

> Some hold that the aged show little or no concern about death or dying; but others assert or assume that those who have the mental capacity and awareness are truly concerned.

> Some say that they have never seen an aged person fear his death; but others state that they have frequently witnessed fear in their aged patients.

> Some maintain that it is not fear of death, but the dread of dying *alone* that is feared; but others claim that the fear of death is a part of human nature which remains potentially present as long as there is any possible awareness.

> Some point out that prolonged suffering makes a patient welcome death; but others claim that no strong relationship appears to exist between suffering and an aged person's acceptance of death.

> Some affirm that the advanced ager is more receptive or resigned to death; but others say that age alone makes little difference.

Some hold that a deeply religious person faces death in old age calmly and without fear; but others doubt that religion always makes that much difference.

Some report that most aged persons lose consciousness days, or at least hours, before death comes; but others maintain that many aged patients, if not heavily drugged, remain alert and conscious until the moment of death.

More significant perhaps than the major contrasting positions held by geriatric nursing personnel concerning these issues is a concomitant phenomenon that clearly emerges. From the diversity of perceptions that they relate with their claims and counter claims, the idea of the uniqueness of the individual patient and the *differences* that exist among aged persons in experiencing dying is emphasized more than in any idea of a *common* pattern of coping with death among the aged. It appears that no two deaths are quite the same—that there is as much diversity in dying as there is in living. The nurses' perceptions leave open the axiomatic concept that "a man dies as he has lived."

PART 2. DISCUSSING DEATH AND DYING WITH AGED PATIENTS

It was noted earlier in this chapter that a discrepancy exists between the nurse practitioners' perceptions of patients' reaction to personal death and the influence that these perceptions exert upon their nursing practice. A few of these nurses seemed to use their reflected views as a basis for their practice, but a great many of them apparently did not. An RN seemed to speak for a large majority of the nurse practitioners when she contended that, while aged patients' attitudes and reactions to death and dying are very individualistic, she would not engage in any meaningful discussion on the topic with them—even if they asked for it.

The Question

The major portion of the data for the foregoing as well as for this section of the chapter was derived from responses to the question of whether certain facts about, or attitudes toward, death are influential elements in the nursing care of the aged ill. The question addressed to the nurse practitioners was: *How do certain facts about, or attitudes toward, death influence your care of an aged ill person? Does your care differ, depending on whether the patient seems ready to die, even wishing for death, or resists or fears death? If so, how?* On the questionnaire mailed to the selected degree registered nurses, it was worded: *How may certain facts about, or attitudes toward, death tend to help nurses and patients cope with this event? Under what conditions should a nurse discuss, or not discuss, the prospects of death with an aged person?*

The replies to this query proved to be anything but uniform, with the nurse practitioners and the degree registered nurses being at opposite extremes. The dominant position of those who care for the aged ill is that they do not engage in any death talk with their patients; that of the degree registered nurses, that the subject should be meaningfully discussed whenever opportunities present themselves. From the data on this issue, three major positions were identified: 1) the topic of death is taboo; 2) noncommittal comments are in order if a patient broaches the subject; and 3) discuss the topic meaningfully when opportunities arise.

THE TOPIC IS TABOO

Large numbers of the nurse practitioners in all three ranks held that they avoid or discourage any discussion of, or allusions to, death or dying, with a few of them taking the extreme position that the question never arises. In contrast, the DRN's who responded to the question supported the taboo position by a negligible two percent.*

A nurse aide, who had worked in three different geriatric facilities, commented that it is not right to let people know they are dying, and she illustrated her way of dealing with a situation when an aged dying patient speaks of death:

> We have one patient who is getting closer to death, and he cries a good deal. He cries because of the pain and the loneliness and the closeness of death; he wants someone with him whenever he is awake. He keeps saying, "Help me. I am going to die," but I keep telling him, "Oh no, you will be all right."

A licensed practical nurse contended that the best way to keep patients from dwelling on death is to avoid direct replies to their questions or comments on the topic. They "get the message" if they receive no direct answer to their pointed remarks about dying.

A registered nurse explained that when a patient is afraid of death

---

* NA's, 57.5 percent; LPN's, 43.4 percent; RN's, 40.5 percent; DRN's, 2.1 percent. See Appendix B, Table 10, Items 1, 2.

and dying and verbalizes this, she and other staff members ignore the issue or avoid him as much as possible—even leaving him alone. Then she added that she feels inadequate to comfort dying patients—that this is the responsibility of spiritual advisors. Another RN said that she would chide a patient for mentioning the subject with "That is no way of looking at things," or similar remarks. Still another RN with several years' experience in geriatrics told of an encounter with a "highly educated and intelligent patient in her nineties" who lately had had to curtail her activities because of general debilitation:

> Miss S. every once in a while remarks that she wished she would die, to which we always give such pat answers as, "Don't be silly, you'll live to be 100," or, "That's no way to talk; next week you will be feeling much better." One day recently Miss S. surprised the nurse who was bringing her her medicine by retorting, "Don't give me such nonsense—what do you know about it."

When nearly half of the selected nursing home staff who are entrusted with the care of the aged ill consider taboo any serious discussion of death with their patients, is it any wonder that many of their aged patients learn from these experiences that it is nonrewarding or even useless to keep referring to the topic?

SUFFERANCE OF ALLUSIONS TO DEATH

Another group of respondents concurred in principle with those who held that the topic of death is taboo; but they seemed less adamant in their stand and their number was somewhat smaller.* They claimed that they neither encourage nor discourage their patients when they speak of death or dying. They allow their patients free expression, but avoid entering into any meaningful discourse with them. A number of these nurses suggest that the use of light humor is helpful in such situations. Others explained that aged patients who allude to death and dying may do so out of a sense of insecurity, and they recommend answers that convey to their patients a feeling of love and of being wanted. A nurse aide who believes in kidding with her patients when they bring up the topic, exemplified:

> We have a 98-year-old patient who until recently kept up a lively correspondence with friends. He had all of his life been an avid reader.

---

* NA's, 40.6 percent; LPN's, 45.3 percent; RN's, 27.8 percent; DRN's, 24.2 percent. See Appendix B, Table 10, Items 3, 4.

Because of failing eyesight, he can now no longer indulge these cherished activities. Lately he has been despondent and often remarks to those of us who care for him that he wished he could die. When he said that to me the other day I told him, "Well, you were not supposed to be here a year ago, but here you are." He smiled when I said that.

A licensed practical nurse related:

One of our patients developed a sore in her mouth. When the physician recommended that she enter the hospital and have it removed, she countered with "Why bother; I am 80 years old, and it's time I died." But the surgery was done. Upon returning to the home she told the staff that it had been a waste of money.

From time to time she would say that she was prepared to die; she had lived her life and was ready for God to take her. When I was taking care of her the other day, she talked again about being ready to die. When I told her, "Oh, come now, Mrs. H., you wouldn't want to leave us yet," she replied, "I'll see you there."

Other nurses reported that they respond to patients' death talk with comments such as, "What would I do without you—you can't leave us yet" to give them a feeling that the staff cares about them. Keeping the conversation light, indulging in "small talk," or resorting to some kidding appeared to be their way of warding off any serious communication on death and dying their patients might seek. Of the degree registered nurses, nearly one fourth agreed with this stance—that if a patient initiates the topic, the nurse should respond, but without becoming deeply involved.

The difference between those who would avoid or at least discourage allusions to death on the part of their aged patients and those who would tolerate such mention, but refuse to be drawn into any meaningful discussion with their patients, seems to be a matter of degree. The significance appears to lie not so much in the extent of permissiveness on the topic, but in the evident fact that all of these nurse respondents consider the subject of death more or less taboo, or not to be used for therapeutic purposes. In the selected institutions, the number of the nursing personnel who adhered to these two positions add up to an impressively large proportion—almost 100 percent of the NA's, nearly 90 percent of the LPN's, and close to 70 percent of the RN's. Of the DRN's, about a quarter of the group held a similar position.*

One may wonder about the possible effects upon coping patterns of aged ill persons in dealing with problems of life's closure if they had received some competent and judicious communications when they were asking for them. The stance these nurses take on the subject appears to have little or no relevance to a patient's attitude toward death—whether

* See Appendix B, Table 10, total of Items 1 to 4.

he is fearful of death, resigned to die, or welcomes death—or even whether his attitude is a symptom of a more immediate need to cope with problems of living until he dies. The fact that imminent death is not frankly recognized in their communications with their aged patients places these nurses in a more defensible position for providing *the same kind of care* for all their patients, regardless of their prognoses.

Some of these nurses indicated that they believe they have little choice in the matter; others recognize that their own attitude toward the realities of dying get in the way—that they have little preparation for this aspect of nursing and have not come to terms with themselves about death.

Perhaps physicians feel somewhat the same way when an aged patient indicates a need to discuss the matter with them. In one geriatric facility, a physician commented during a group discussion on the subject that he would call in a psychiatrist if one of his patients exhibited such a morbid interest. The attending physician in another institution for the aged ill expressed the conviction that most dying persons really do not want to know anything specific about when and how they are likely to die, so he tries to keep such communications on the "light side." If a patient raises the issue, he tells them that their time has not come yet, or he will reassure a patient by saying that his heart is still good and to stop worrying. Another physician related how one of his elderly patients kept asking about his prognosis, only to be told each time that he was showing signs of improvement. After repeated dialogue of this kind on the topic, the patient retorted, "Doctor, when I have already one foot in the grave you will still be telling me that I am going to get well."

Some physicians would withhold information about a probable terminal diagnosis even from a seriously ill professional collegue. The following account, related by a DRN out of her own experience, tells about the illness and death of Dr. L. The medical colleagues who attended him attempted at various times to withhold important medical information from him; but Dr. L. not only insisted upon making his own diagnosis, but also prevailed upon these colleagues to desist from surgical intervention. From what is known, Dr. L. never openly discussed the prospect of his death, though he frequently alluded to it indirectly.

> Dr. L. was 73 when he gave up his medical practice. His work had been his life, but ill health had forced him to retire. The onset of his illness had been gradual and in the beginning had defied exact diagnosis according to the two physicians who attended him—both colleagues whom he had known for years.
>
> When the pain increased, Dr. L. entered the hospital for diagnostic tests. The question of a biopsy was raised, but he refused to have this done, believing that if he had cancer, it might spread more

rapidly following a biopsy. He demanded to see the x-ray plates and all laboratory findings and made a diagnosis of cancer. He ruled out surgical intervention which had been advised, but did consent to a series of treatments designed to relieve his pain.

He had always been a person who kept his own counsel and was not given to sharing his thoughts with others. For many years he had enjoyed good health, and the prospect of death had never before been close. When his condition worsened and the pain returned, he put his house in order. Since he was a religious person, this included detailed arrangements for his burial.

For many months before his death Dr. L. was in almost constant pain, and his nights were disturbed. His difficulty in walking increased; he ate little. He refused to take narcotics for his pain, but never explained his reason for this. Gradually his activities lessened, and he began to spend more and more time in his bedroom. One day he fell in the bathroom. He did not hurt himself, but after the fall he kept to his bed. He knew that his condition made him prone to fractures.

His wife, an RN, cared for him night and day. He seemed afraid of being alone and would call, often for some trivial thing, when no one was in the room with him.

For many years Dr. L. had been giving financial help to a brother who lived in a distant city, sending him a check on the first of each month. The last check had been sent, signed in his own hand, on the first of the month. Now it was the tenth. About midmorning he asked his wife about the date and when she told him, he remained silent for a moment and then said, "It'll be too late." When his wife asked what he meant, he shook his head and then asked her to write a letter for him and make out a check to his brother's order. In the letter he indicated that this would be the last time that the brother would hear from him and made mention of the fact that he was sending him his check some 3 weeks early—something Dr. L. had never done before. He apparently had a premonition that he would die before the first of the following month. He died on the seventeenth.

About a week before he died, he commented to a friend who was relieving his wife for a couple of hours, "The hardest thing about all of this is to have to ask for help with the little personal things I used to do for myself."

He kept his eyes closed much of the time, but responded quickly when spoken to and at times engaged in brief discussion. He seemed very restless, but refused to take any medication for this. He frequently asked for things to be done. Two days before his death, he looked up and noticed fresh flowers on a nearby table. He asked who had sent them, and upon being told said, "How thoughtful of them." For more than a week he had been taking only fluids, which he drank from a cup or a glass. He continued to keep count of his pulse rate, and had his temperature checked regularly, noting this in a little book. He spoke over the telephone until a few days before the end.

During the last 2 days his respiration rate increased rapidly, and on the morning of his death it varied between 50 and 60 breaths per minute. He dozed a good bit, and from time to time would speak, asking the time of day or about some recent event. He perspired a great deal, and his hands moved restlessly over the bedcovers. For about 2 hours before his death he no longer asked for anything, but would nod his head if asked whether he would like a drink. Half an hour before he died he took a sip of hot tea—drinking this out of a cup. He was propped up on several pillows, finding it easier to breathe. During the final half hour, his breaths came slower and slower, decreasing finally to ten, then to five a minute, until he drew his final breath very quietly, peacefully.

During the course of his illness, Dr. L. never mentioned the prospect of personal death directly, but in various indirect ways would allude to it. He repeatedly told his wife where she would find important papers in the event that anything should happen to him. From time to time he would allude to some details about his burial.

Following Dr. L.'s death, his wife found the papers exactly where he had said they would be. On top was a letter addressed to her. In it he told of their life together, how very much she had meant to him, and how he hated to leave her. According to the date on the letter, he had written it 11 months prior to his death—on his wife's birthday.

The account of Mrs. P.'s final illness and death tells a different story:

For several months Mrs. P. had been gradually losing weight. She was losing her appetite, and her strength was not what it had been. Prior to this she had always been healthy and felt well.

It was not until Mrs. P. felt a lump in her abdomen, which she believed to be a hernia, that she consulted her family physician. She was promptly hospitalized and underwent extensive diagnostic tests, followed by abdominal surgery. Two weeks after her surgery she was transferred to an extended care facility to recuperate.

When her condition did not improve, she was several times returned to the hospital for blood transfusions. She was given various medicines—some to help build her up and others to relieve her discomfort and pain—but she died seven weeks after her surgery. She had been bedridden for about a week before she died and had "slept almost constantly" for the final 24 hours.

When shortly after his wife's burial Mr. P. had occasion to visit the physician on his own behalf, the doctor told him that his wife had died of inoperable cancer. The surgery had consisted of "just opening and closing her up." When the surgeon had opened her up, he found that the cancer had spread too far for removal of the diseased part. Neither Mr. nor Mrs. P. had been told that Mrs. P. was terminally ill. The physician had shared this information with the parish minister who visited Mrs. P. a number of times, but he too, had not told them.

Several days later some friends visited Mr. P. and found him preoccupied with what the physician had told him. He found it difficult to become reconciled to the fact that the true facts had been kept from him and his wife, though he admittedly had not pressed the physician or the surgeon very much and had accepted at face value their pronouncements that surgery had been successful and that Mrs. P. would recover. He wondered why surgery had been attempted if the tests revealed extensive cancer, for he believed that present day medical facilities would have shown whether or not surgery was indicated. And he wondered, also, whether or not "the surgeon's knife" had shortened her life.

He said that he felt they should have been told the truth and also have been consulted and given explanations before surgery was attempted, and he said, "But as a lay person, I am at the mercy of the medical profession."

POSITIVE APPROACHES

A small minority of the geriatric nursing staff but an impressive majority of the degree registered nurses took a more positive approach to their patients' interest in death, whether their own or in the abstract.* They suggested that opportunities be provided for aged patients to freely express their apprehensions and anxieties about dying or their philosophical concerns about death, and that these expressions receive serious and pertinent responses from nursing staff. These nurses felt that a patient has the right to know when death is close, but they warned that not every aged person desires to have this knowledge.

Their thesis is that a social atmosphere conducive to frank expression about death and dying can and would be therapeutic in the sense that it provides opportunities to ease a patient's apprehensions concerning death. Talking out his concerns to a trusted and attentive listener may fulfill his need and be all that he really wants or expects. He may know as well as anybody else that not everyone finds completely satisfying answers on the ultimate. With nursing staff spending so much more time with patients than do representatives of related disciplines, such as medicine, social work, and clergy, nurses have special opportunities to be helpful and supportive to anxious and distressed patients. A psychosocial environment which ensures the aged person a sympathetic hearing on his concerns, whatever they may be, can result in mental and emotional catharsis with genuine therapeutic value. It is well known that a patient who is anxious and full of fear or resentment does not respond as readily to medications as does a person whose mind is more at ease. Moreover, care would be enhanced for patients who recover as well as for those who die; for in such an environment, nurses would find more incentive to prepare themselves for providing such care and would feel freer to respond to patients' queries instead of ignoring or denying such signs, as so often happens in institutions where the topic of death is taboo.

---

* NA's, 2.0 percent; LPN's, 11.3 percent; RN's, 24.1 percent; DRN's, 70.6 percent. See Appendix B, Table 10, Items 5 to 8.

Some patients seem to believe that being afraid of death constitutes a weakness, a human frailty that is somehow degrading, and this may dampen any voicing of their deeper concerns:

> A patient in her late seventies was dying of cancer. Visibly loosing ground, she nevertheless kept driving herself, getting out of bed and trying to gain strength by walking—often to the point of exhaustion. She kept trying to eat, despite nausea.
>
> One day she told the nurse, "I know I am going to die, and I am ready for it." Only then did she relate some of her fears and apprehensions—the isolation she felt because everyone around her kept assuring her that she was improving when in fact she was feeling sicker. She had come to accept the fact that "this thing" (cancer) was proving fatal. The nurse sensed that the patient was not looking for answers, but that she needed to talk to clarify her mind and dispel the false assurances regarding her prognosis which had built a wall around her and which inhibited communication.
>
> When the nurse told the patient's daughter of what had taken place the latter seemed horrified, but her physician expressed relief that he could now be honest with the patient about her plight and plan *with* her instead of *for* her about her future. The patient's wish to have attendants around the clock, because she was afraid of dying alone, was granted. With everyone involved in her care and *working together,* the patient stopped driving herself so mercilessly, but she was encouraged to do as much as her strength permitted. She kept expressing her relief that she could count on those around her for support and help in facing the inevitable—death.
>
> She died quietly less than three weeks after she had confided in the nurse, at peace with herself and with her God.

A nurse aide related the following:

> Mrs. S. had for several weeks been quite restless. One day she asked me if I had seen anyone die, to which I answered, "No, not really." Then she told me, "I am going to die—soon," and asked if I would be afraid if she died. I assured her that I would not be afraid. She was holding my hand and I stayed with her for some time—until I was asked to go to another floor to help out. When I returned to the room about an hour later, a nurse was with Mrs. S., who had just breathed her last. I do not know if Mrs. S. spoke to anyone else about being afraid to die.

Many nurses deplored situations which deny aged patients a sympathetic hearing when they voice their concerns about dying since these perhaps even deprive them of the right to die as they would wish to die:

> Mrs. R. said to the nurse who brought her medicine, "I just wish that I could go—I'm almost 90 and I am very tired," to which the nurse replied, "Now, you know you are talking nonsense."

An hour later the patient had a stroke which left her unconscious. She was given clyses and tube feedings to keep her alive. Antibiotics were administered to combat a congestion which had developed in her lungs. The patient's 70-year-old son kept saying to the nurses, "Do you think she has much pain—I wish she would not have to linger like this."

It was quite generally agreed, and often reemphasized, that a nurse should not discuss death or dying with a patient—even with a physician's permission—*unless* the patient has indicated that he wishes to have her do so. The contention was that a nurse, with sensitivity and special skill in interpersonal relations, will recognize clues, verbal and nonverbal, that can and should be pursued in order to render supportive care. Some of these nurses repeatedly stressed that perhaps most times aged patients are not interested in lengthy discussions or explanations, but rather are looking for the nurse's understanding—for her to try and see things as they do—or often just for quiet empathetic listening.

Some nurses, however, have been known to be overly zealous and not very perceptive to the needs and wants of critically ill patients, thereby adding to a dying patient's anxiety and stress instead of lessening it. This may well have happened in the following instance, related by a charge nurse in a geriatric facility whose policy was that a person has the right to know when he is critically ill:

> When one of our patients recently had a heart attack, he begged me not to call the doctor. When I telephoned the doctor to report the attack, I explained that the patient did not want him to know that he was feeling ill. Then I called the priest. When the priest came shortly thereafter, the patient almost shouted, "I don't want you—I am not going to die." He seemed petrified, and I stayed with him for a while. Then I told him, "It's up to God, but your condition is not good." He finally consented to have last rites. He died the third night after the attack.
>
> It is better to be honest with them. He appeared less frightened after he had received last rites.

Conversely, it was acknowledged as a common experience that elderly persons in permissive situations frequently indicate a desire to talk about impending death. There was the patient who was moved to grab her nurse's hand and exclaim, "Bless you for listening." A degree registered nurse reported that, in a study she had conducted, persons from 70 to 92 years of age were frequently candid, forthright, and open in talking about their impending death. (Schwartz) When we take into account the culturally imposed restraints and the fact that many of the nursing staff who provide care for the aged are relatively young persons, it may be that they, far more than their aged patients, are inhibited and ill-prepared to respond positively and appropriately to topics of death.

But these nurses also recognize that dangers lie either in relying upon simple evasive tactics or in being too forward and forthright in such a delicate and sensitive area of human crises. To quote a few cautions:

> Often when patients who want to know are not told about their diagnosis or prognosis, they try to trap the nurse into admission of the fact that their physician has held back this information. Then the nurse is placed in the position of appearing to lie to the patient; and any relationship of trust that has been built up between the patient and herself tends to be weakened or even destroyed at the very time when it should be strongest. (Dithridge)

> If the nurse perceives that the patient has need to discuss the prospects of death, she usually should provide the opportunity; but she should not encourage such discussion if she has only a minute and a half to devote to it. People are slow in expressing ideas that are associated with deep anxiety and that are intensely personal. There may be other persons available better prepared than herself. It is her responsibility to provide the opportunity, but not necessarily to perform the service without help. (Macquinn)

> The nurse generally does well in waiting for genuine leads from the patient, and whatever she does about the matter should be with the approval and cooperation of the doctor and the family and the possible support of the spiritual advisor and friends of the patient. It is easy for variance and potential conflicts about the patient to spring up between these persons—conflicts that could be avoided by an astute and careful nurse. (Wald)

SUMMARY

It is obvious from the foregoing discourse and the statistical summary below that the geriatric nursing personnel differ considerably in the opinions they hold on the concerns of their aged patients toward impending death and, also, in their attitudes, judgments, and practices in coping with these problems. An example of the variance may be seen in the percentage of nurse practitioners who perceive that patients' attitudes toward death are highly individualistic, as contrasted with the percentage who state that they would be willing to discuss the subject meaningfully with a patient when opportunities present themselves:

	NA's %	LPN's %	RN's %
Patients' attitudes depend on diverse factors*	54.0	49.0	46.2
Discuss topic meaningfully if opportune†	2.0	11.3	24.1

* See Appendix B, Table 9, Items 5 to 7, subtotal
† See Appendix B, Table 10, Items 5 to 8, subtotal

It is to be expected, perhaps, that of the NA's, only a negligible number would discuss death meaningfully with an aged patient; but more significant are the respective figures for the LPN's, and especially for the RN's; only about one-quarter of the RN's would be ready and willing to discuss the topic with them, if an opportunity to do so arose.

It is surprising, also, that among the nurse practitioners almost a third in each of the ranks does not recognize that any problem exists in the minds of their patients with respect to pending death. Approximately a fifth hold that concerns over dying are natural and should be expected; and the remaining almost a half of the practitioners believe that whether or not an aged patient worries about dying depends upon diverse factors, such as their state of health, religio-philosophical beliefs, and the like. The exact figures are:*

	NA's %	LPN's %	RN's %
Presents no problem; patients are not concerned	30.3	28.3	32.0
Fear of death is a normal experience	15.7	22.7	20.5
Patients' attitude depends upon diverse factors	54.0	49.0	46.2

* See Appendix B, Table 9, subtotals.

When all four categories of nursing personnel were asked whether or not aged patients are or should be told about a possible pending terminal prognosis, or whether they would engage in serious discussion about death with them, an impressively large number of the nurse practitioners considered any death talk taboo or merely tolerated it, whereas an overwhelming majority of the degree registered nurses took the opposite stand, holding that the subject should be meaningfully discussed whenever opportunities arise to do so. These are the figures:†

	NA's %	LPN's %	RN's %	DRN's %
Negative approach: topic is taboo	57.5	43.4	40.5	2.1
Neutral position: death talk is tolerated	40.6	45.3	27.8	24.2
Positive approach: discuss meaningfully	2.0	11.3	24.1	70.6

† See Appendix B, Table 10, subtotals.

It seems reasonable to interpret these statistical data as indicating that within these institutions the chances are slim that an elderly patient with a terminal diagnosis will have an opportunity to learn from these nurses the truth about his medical prognosis or engage in frank talk with one of them about his worries over death and dying.

The situation is viewed more favorably by the degree registered nurses, with only 2 percent of them proposing a negative approach; about one fourth of the group tolerating inquiry and talk, though responding with neutral comments; and nearly three fourths of them subscribing to the positive approach of preparing for, and encouraging patients to talk about the subject if they so desire.

From available data, it would appear, also, that if an aged patient is fortunate enough to be in a geriatric institution of high repute *and* which is under the auspices of a voluntary, nonprofit, religious or church-related organization, his chances of being provided with opportunities to talk freely and frankly with his nurse about the subject will be greatly enhanced. Whether his nurse will be adequately prepared to help him cope effectively with his problem is another matter.

It is well known that physicians are divided on the issue of revealing to a patient his terminal diagnosis. In a recent publication of the Group for the Advancement of Psychiatry, Dr. Alvin Goldfarb who headed a committee to explore the issue, concluded his statement as follows.

> We appear to agree that the fact he may die should be part of the awareness of the patient faced by death as well as in the awareness of those who want to help him. Awareness on the part of the patient that he is dying may be psychologically helpful rather than harmful if it is part of—or leads to what are believed to be—constructive efforts to prevent death or to deal with its problems.*

* Group for the Advancement of Psychiatry. Death and Dying: Attitudes of Patient and Doctor. Symposium No. 11. New York, Group for the Advancement of Psychiatry, 1965, p. 655.

For figures used in this chapter, see Appendix B, Tables 9 and 10.

13 Death of a Fellow Patient

For each, when gyves are fretting,
A different balm must be.
Some find it in forgetting,
And some in memory.

MARGARET ROOT GARVIN

Whenever and however death comes, shock and strain on human reserves generally accompany the event. This is especially true for those within the immediate situation who identify closely with the person who is dying or deceased. Rarely are such persons fully prepared for the exigencies that arise or for the sense of ultimate reality that is conveyed to them—be they fellow patients, close relatives and friends, or involved staff members.

Since few human beings are ever completely prepared for the impact of death, many interdependencies arise within the group closely allied with the dying person. For these "in-groupers," recurrent needs prompt giving something supportive to the situation and gaining some reciprocal reinforcements within it. Often in such a crisis context, individuals with unexpected resources rise to the occasion. Not infrequently the dying person himself becomes an extraordinarily adaptive and supportive influence within the "inner circle." Many physicians and nurses can recall a patient who was able to meet death in a manner reinforcing for all concerned and who contributed significantly to transforming what could have become a defeating experience into something positive and memorable.

But whenever breakdowns occur in these mutually supportive relationships, the in-group resources are threatened and individual self-protective responses arise to cripple the group potentials.

When a person dies within the institutional context of a nursing home or similar facility, the two variables that largely determine whatever support is rendered to the bereaved, whether they be fellow patients or others, are the policy of the particular institution and the behaviors of the attending staff in the face of death. It is fallacious, however, to assume that a particular institutional policy is routinely adhered to by all the staff or that each member works to reinforce efforts of the others in the crisis situations involving death. Moreover, institutional policies shift from time to time and vary greatly between institutions.

But in a few of the facilities included in the present study, death is confronted openly, and the philosophy of the administration permeates all departments and tends to be strongly reflected in the attitudes and practices of the responsible personnel. In these institutions death is treated as a natural part of life. The dying person is kept in his own room, if at all possible, and a staff member remains in almost constant attendance. The gravity of the patient's condition is shared with other patients who may come and visit if they are able and wish to do so, especially if the patient formerly enjoyed being with people and still seems to benefit from such visits. These other patients are encouraged to pray with the patient at his bedside and go to the chapel to pray for him. This is done for the possible benefit of the dying person and, also, in order that fellow patients may observe the care that is provided for him so that they may see just how peaceful death can be. The experience may become a shared source of comfort, encouraging the patients to anticipate a peaceful death for themselves and to feel assured that when their time comes they will not be left alone.

When a patient dies, notices are posted so that all may know what has occurred. An announcement is made before chapel service, and the deceased is remembered in the service. If burial services are held in the chapel on the grounds or within reasonable distance, the fellow residents are encouraged to attend, with transportation provided if necessary.

Every attempt is made to accentuate the positive aspects of death as a natural and inevitable passage in life. It is viewed as the completion of this life and, in accordance with many religions, it is seen as the beginning of a new and fuller life. No attempt is made to hide or disguise death.

In many of the facilities included in the study, however, dying and death are tabooed topics. This is especially so in the various proprietary nursing homes. In accordance with institutional policy, the dying patient is apt to be moved to another bed or room in order that the seriousness of his condition be kept from his fellow patients. Depending upon the particular situation, the dying patient may even be moved to a nearby hospital. Half-truths or "little white lies" are resorted to by staff to keep the facts from the other patients. The cloak of secrecy extends over the removal of the body. In some communities, the undertaker uses a converted, or specially outfitted, station wagon to remove the corpse in an attempt to hide the death. The nursing director of a geriatric institution explained:

When one of our patients enters the critical phase, we move him to a room nearer to the nurses' station where the nurses can watch him more closely. Another reason for the move is to keep the seriousness of the situation from the other patients. The door is kept closed, or a screen placed in front of it so that passersby cannot observe what goes on in the room. If they inquire, they are told that the particular patient needs special treatment and is getting along all right. Our staff is trained never to rush or in any other way reveal that there is any urgency about the situation. This again is to convey to the others that there is no emergency and that nothing unusual is happening.

When the patient has died and the postmortem care is completed, the body is taken on a stretcher to the linen room which is at the end of the hall. The undertaker conveys the body through another door which leads to the service elevator, so that the patients cannot observe the body's removal. When they ask about the missing patient, they are told that he was taken to the hospital.

Sooner or later they may find out what happened, but by that time everything is back to normal. Aged persons often sense when someone has died. Also, notices are placed on the bulletin board downstairs, and at the next chapel service the deceased is given special remembrance in the service. When residents from the other floors come to the nursing unit to visit they are apt to tell the others.

The patients all take it calmly when someone has died, but I think it best to keep the knowledge of dying and death from them when it is happening—why expose them? They are old and sick, their own time may be running out fast, and no one wants to be reminded that one's death may be near.

PART 1. NURSES' PERCEPTION OF PATIENTS' REACTIONS

Detailed information is scanty for understanding the reactions of elderly patients in extended-care institutions when death is taking one of them. Whether the often feeble attempts to hide a death from other patients results in less or more stress on the other patients remains an unsettled issue. However, constructive and positive effects have been reported from patients when openly expressed awareness of a pending death is shared appropriately with them.

Concerning the question of rendering support to fellow patients in the event of death of one of them, a great many nurse practitioners focused upon *their perception of patients' reactions* to a death in their midst before they would comment on particular practices they follow in such crisis situations.* This response pattern was similar to that of the

* Data on nurses' perceptions of aged patients' reactions to the death of a fellow patient were not gathered from the degree registered nurses.

issue of whether a dying patient should know the seriousness of his condition, discussed in Chapter 11. Therefore identical code guides were used.

No Problem Exists

By far the largest number of nurse practitioners contended that their aged patients exhibit no stress and show no conscious concern when one of them is critically ill or deceased.* According to these nurses, old people are more philosophical than those who are younger; old age dulls one's senses; and many aged persons are senile and not keenly aware of what goes on around them. They related many memorable instances to support their contention. An NA reported:

> One of our patients asked me to wash a blouse for her which she said had belonged to Mrs. B. who had died. She had visited her when she was critically ill, at which time Mrs. B. had told her to take of her belongings what she liked—and she had chosen the blouse. Then she said to me, "Every time I wear the blouse I keep thinking what a nice person Mrs. B. was."

An RN recalled several incidents in which a surviving patient had asked for some item that had belonged to a deceased person, or even to occupy the bed of one who had died:

> Two weeks ago in a multiple-bed room a patient died. As soon as the deceased had been removed, her 91-year-old neighbor asked if she could have that bed, as it was closer to the window than her own and she would be able to look out and watch the birds and flowers and shrubs in bloom.
> This 91-year-old had always been a very quiet person, but since we moved her to the location she had asked for she "has been coming out of her shell—all of us have noticed this change in her but we don't know why she is so much more lively than before."

Other staff members claim the problem is nonexistent for the reason that the policy of the institution does not permit any death talk and the patients are quick to learn this. According to several nurses, the patients also come to know that some staff members avoid the topic. As one RN explained, nurses are too busy and therefore patients do not make their feelings known—"No one wants to be known as a pain in the neck."

* NA's, 57.7 percent; LPN's, 43.4 percent; RN's, 54.5 percent. See Appendix B, Table 11, Items 1, 2.

FEAR OF DEATH IS UNIVERSAL

Other nurses, however, believe that aged patients do become upset and grieve because all of us fear death. The death of a fellow patient reminds them that their own death may not be far off.* An NA related the following example:

> A few weeks ago a patient who was old and had been sick for some months died. Another patient on the floor became so upset that she insisted upon leaving the nursing home. She kept crying out that she did not want to die there. Finally, against the doctor's advice, her family came to take her home.

In another home, an NA reported that one of their patients, the widow of a physician, "gets very panicky" whenever anyone on the floor dies. The patients in this particular institution are not told when one of them is dying or has died; but according to the staff, the patients find out "through the grapevine" what has happened.

An LPN who believes that fear of death is part of human nature reflected the views of several of her co-workers when she said aged patients show their stress and grief in various ways when someone dies in their midst: Some become very restless at such times and may even ask, "Will I be next?" Others lose their appetite or complain all of a sudden of a headache, though ordinarily headaches are not one of their complaints. Still others have the urge to go to the bathroom "twice as often" as usual.

PATIENTS' ATTITUDES DEPEND ON DIVERSE FACTORS

Other practitioners voiced the opinion that many factors need to be examined in order to determine to what extent aged institutionalized patients experience stress when death takes one of them—factors such as the person's religio-philosophical orientation, his particular state of health, whether the death was sudden or expected, whether or not a close bond existed between the deceased and a particular fellow patient, or any combination of these and similar circumstances.†

An NA recounted a recent incident:

* NA's, 11.3 percent; LPN's, 18.9 percent; RN's, 8.9 percent. See Appendix B, Table 11, Items 3, 4.
† NA's, 27.8 percent; LPN's, 33.9 percent; RN's, 33.0 percent. See Appendix B, Table 11, Items 5 to 7.

We have a patient whose roommate had died. They had shared the room for years and had become friends. The surviving patient became so upset that the nurse had to give her something to quiet her. She wept and moaned and kept repeating how much she missed her dead roommate.

An LPN related a similar experience:

The other day the head nurse asked me to check on a patient whose roommate had died. When I went in to see her the patient was sitting at her bedside, breakfast tray in front of her, the food untouched. She began to cry when she saw me and said she could not eat—she missed her roommate and felt too lonely to do anything.

An RN used the following example:

Older people don't often make new friends, but we had a man and a woman on this floor who enjoyed a fine friendship. They shared many interests including reading and discussion of books. The woman's eye sight was very poor and the man read to her by the hour.

Then he became ill and died. She grieved so much that it affected her mentally and physically. She began to eat very sparsely and became noticeably withdrawn. Other patients tried to cheer her up and several residents began reading to her—but it was not the same as before. Ever since the death of her friend this patient has steadily been deteriorating, mentally and physically.

Several staff members distinguished between the difference in stress experienced by relatively young agers and that by those of more advanced years. Others emphasized the personality of the deceased as a factor related to grief experienced by the fellow patients:

Not long ago one of our patients died of an embolism. It was a sudden and very unexpected death. The deceased had been well and active in the many social affairs on the floor. Always interested in people, he had been solicitous of the welfare of others. He was in his mid-seventies when he died.

His death was felt by almost everyone on the floor and he was sorely missed. We could sense the grief his fellow patients were experiencing, and for quite a while they were very subdued. They were upset and showed this in various ways: few had heart to play games in which he had always participated; others complained of loss of appetite or insomnia. Comments were heard such as: "He was still so young"; "What a dreadful way to die"; and "He still had so much to give."

The illustrative experiences related by staff members tended to be varied in a variety of ways. The influencing elements inherent in them added up to a myriad of interwoven and complex factors that defy simple explanation. Briefly, they pointed once again to the uniqueness of the individual patient and the particular situation in which he finds himself at the time. Concerning grief and grieving, it seemed necessary to examine the complexity of the life of the departed as well as the lives of the survivors in order to ascertain the manner and degree to which the death of a person affects his fellow patients.

No matter what the nurses' individual perception of aged patients' reactions to a death in their midst, inherent in their responses was the idea that man grieves more often for himself than for the departed. We mourn our *own* loss when someone dies. Hence, in ascertaining some of the needs of aged patients when death takes one of them, it is imperative to look at the position of the departed as seen by his fellow patients. How close was he to them? How much difference, if any, will the loss make in their daily lives? What are the prospects of their own deaths and how do they view death for themselves?

In addition, one needs to examine the kind of congregate living in the particular institution. It is said that man dies a sociological, psychological, and biological death, and in that order. Have some of these patients already sustained social or psychological "death" or both? There is also considerable staff conviction that aged persons are apt to be more accepting of the death of an associate than those who are younger. Whatever the commonalities of old age, however, individual differences cannot be ignored without deficits in understanding of the behavior of elderly patients.

PART 2. COPING WITH PATIENTS' STRESSES WHEN DEATH TAKES ONE OF THEM

When death occurs on the geriatric ward or floor, an arresting issue arises with respect to nursing perceptions as these affect nursing practice in planning and caring for survivors. From the testimony of nurse practitioners in the selected nursing homes, the assumption that the staff's perceptions of the stress and grief of the fellow patients determine in any large measure the nursing care that they receive, appears tenuous or even dubious. Indeed the reverse may be suggested—that the staff's prescribed practices influence their perceptions of what is going on in the minds of these fellow patients. In certain instances, to be sure, a direct relationship does appear between a nurse's perception of the plight of a disturbed and bereaved patient and the course of nursing care that she initiates; but more often such a connection is difficult to see. For example, one RN strongly voiced her convictions that aged patients are not upset and do not grieve when one of them dies, and she went on to say that she had found it "almost incredible" how well the elderly accept death. She made a strong point, nevertheless, of insisting that it is best for the staff to make every effort to keep death and dying hidden from the other patients, even by resorting to subterfuges, if necessary. In another geriatric facility a nurse stated that she avoids any and all "references" to the subject of dying; but if a fellow patient asks a direct question, she usually does admit the condition. Another declared, "I never tell, and we may lie a little." A third nurse commented that her standard response is, "We don't talk about that," and then explained, "Our patients quickly catch on and don't ask questions."

With respect to institutionalized geriatric care, it should be borne in mind that certain differences in reporting occur by virtue of varying staff ranks and positions. Also, very similar nursing practices can be described as fulfilling quite different purposes according to the perception of the respondents. A good example of this is the moving of a critically ill patient to another room on the ward or within the institution. A patient may be moved for other purposes than keeping his prognosis a top secret. His bed may be brought closer to the nurses' station to enable the staff to provide more intensive care for him. Or the family may request that the patient be placed in a single room so that more time can be spent in private with him. Conversely, when a patient is left in an accustomed place among other patients, this may not mean that they freely share awareness of dying—every effort may be made by the staff to avoid this. Even with these and other differences, however, there was sufficient consistency in the nursing responses—from nursing aide to director of a nursing unit—for overall policy and general practice in a given unit to become apparent.

Topic Is Taboo

In analysis of the data on dealing with death and dying in geriatric settings, the nursing responses tended to cluster about three distinctive positions: 1) the topic of death is taboo; 2) death talk from patients is tolerated, but nurse replies are guarded; and 3) a positive approach is made toward sharing information and discussing death and dying with concerned fellow patients. It may be recalled that this is similar to the pattern encountered in the issue of whether a patient should know his own prognosis.

A relatively large number of the geriatric nursing personnel declared that they avoid and discourage any talk about a fellow patient's death, but of the degree registered nurses only seven percent held this position.*

The nurse practitioners who take the "taboo" position, told of various ruses being used to keep awareness of dying and death from the other patients. Those inquiring may be told that the dying patient is doing all right or has been transferred to a hospital. Visits by fellow patients are not permitted. After death, halls may be cleared by telling patients that it is cleaning time; so that the deceased may be removed without being observed. Or the corpse is put onto a stretcher and the covers arranged to make it appear that a living person is being transported. If a death occurs close to a mealtime or rest period, the staff may wait until the meal is being served or the patients are in bed resting before the body is taken away. If a patient finds out about a death and demands to know why they were not told about it, he may be informed that the patient died sooner than anticipated; or the staff may admit the death but refuse to be drawn into a discussion. An LPN who works in a proprietary nursing home where death is kept a secret commented:

> We try not to let the patients know and are successful most times in keeping it from them; I don't like to tell the others when one of them has died, but neither do I like to tell a lie. I evade the question and have gotten to the place where they don't ask me. I don't want them to feel sad, and we don't want this place to be known as one where people come to die.

That the issue of telling or not telling patients when someone is dying or a death has occurred is not an easy one to resolve is implied by another LPN, a charge nurse on the evening tour of duty in another home where the staff is not permitted to divulge such information to patients:

> I let it slide when patients ask me; I don't believe in lying. I cannot see anyone dying alone and whenever I can, I go in and often recite the 23rd Psalm. Sometimes when I do this I catch myself and stop— and often a dying patient will say, "Don't stop." . . . . I am upset by the whole affair and get angry—and I get to thinking, "Is this the way I would want my mother treated?"

An RN explained:

> We never discuss a patient's illness or death with other patients. If a patient asks, "Who died last night?" I say, "Did someone die?" If I am sure they know, I will say, "It's too bad," or "He's better off now," or "He is happier now." I hedge with them and they learn not to ask.

---

* NA's, 58.4 percent; LPN's, 41.5 percent; RN's, 34.2 percent; DRN's, 7.5 percent. See Appendix B, Table 12, Items 1, 2.

A director of nursing admitted that often she hears patients talk among themselves about a person who has died but that she never enters into the conversation. According to her, no one is resigned to die; everyone wants to live as long as possible; and everyone is a little afraid of death—"It's a blessing when they go into a coma before they die."

Several nurses commented that they had never been asked by the patients about another who was dying or had died. And a charge nurse contended that saying a patient was transferred to the hospital, when in truth he died, "is the only lie you can get by with." A DRN who would try to keep the other patients from knowing when one of them is dying or has died recommended that the dying patient be removed from the others before the situation becomes distressing but felt that questions should be answered truthfully, "falling back on platitudes if necessary."

TOPIC IS TOLERATED

A more neutral stand is taken by other nurses.* They support the position that death talk be permitted, but not encouraged and that patients be told the truth, not lied to, when a death occurs. One nurse made the observation that it is not always what we tell patients, but how well we tell it, that is important—and in telling the truth, one need not necessarily tell "the whole truth." Often a patient may only wish to know that another is dying or has died and not want to have a detailed description of the situation.

In one nursing unit the NA may be permitted to give brief truthful answers to an inquiring patient when another is dying; in another facility the policy may be to "send them to the nurse" who will then discuss the event briefly with the patient and assure him that everything is being done or that the deceased "did not suffer." An LPN explained that the other patients find out sooner or later when one of them dies, and that there is apt to be a more trusting relationship between patients and staff if the truth is told. An RN would not withhold the truth from patients, "but I don't know how the other nurses handle this—we have no set rule about this."

Some nurses expressed the belief that tolerating death talk and entering upon cursory discourse about death and dying with patients who initiate such talk is helpful to aged patients rather than upsetting to them.

* NA's, 25.7 percent; LPN's, 34.0 percent; RN's, 18.3 percent; DRN's, 29.1 percent. See Appendix B, Table 12, Items 3, 4.

Most are apt to take it in their stride when a death occurs in their midst, and for some of them it is like any other item of conversation—even gossip. But other nurses who would enter into such discussions briefly and on a superficial basis declared that patients *are* upset when one of them dies; but after the first shock, they recover quickly and go about their usual routines.

To support their contention that aged patients in general accept death without severe or lasting stress, several of these nurses cited patients' comments when told of the death of another: "He was not well anyway"; "She lived a full life"; "It's good to know his suffering is ended"; "She had a peaceful death"; "They did everything possible for her"; and the like. Other patients are said to reflect more upon their own condition or situation when a death has occurred. They compare their own state of health with that of the deceased, or their own age with that of the person who is critically ill or has died, or express satisfaction that they are still able to do things for themselves. One elderly lady was heard to exclaim, "Oh, she was an old lady like me—it's what we all have to look forward to sooner or later—when we leave this place, it's feet first."

POSITIVE APPROACHES

Other nursing respondents, which included a majority of the degree registered nurses, took a more positive approach to the problem.* They decry the practice of nurses who treat death with discomfiture before other patients. Several of them expressed the belief that hiding a death is apt to be frightening to those who watch, and one of them asked, "Have we lost all sense of the uniqueness of the individual—of the dignity of man?"

These nurses believe in being honest and gentle with patients who are witnessing the dying of another, and they emphasize that specific responses to individual patients be geared to what the nurse believes to be the survivor's real concern. Is the surviving patient fearful that his own condition is comparable to that of the dying patient; is he anxious and concerned because he cannot approve of the kind of care provided for the critically ill person; or does he mourn the loss of a deceased patient because of a close emotional bond between them? Indications are that among the elderly, and especially in institutional living, few new relationships are formed. When

---

* NA's 13.9 percent; LPN's, 13.2 percent; RN's, 32.9 percent; DRN's 59.1 percent. See Appendix B, Table 12, Items 5 to 8.

a friendship develops into more than a casual relationship it is of inestimable value. The sensitive and perceptive nurse will recognize and meet the needs of fellow patients when death takes one of them; but first of all she must accept the fact that different patients will have different needs in such death crises.

Protecting the dying person's right to privacy is also considered important. When a fellow patient inquires about the condition of a critically ill person, it is deemed important that the nurse be truthful in her answer but not elaborate on details. One DRN gave the following example: If a fellow patient asked how Mr. J. was, I would answer, "Not so well this morning," without going into detail that Mr. J. had another heart attack. A few nurses asserted that it is unethical for a nurse to discuss with patients the dying or death of a fellow patient in anything but very general terms. Thus, focusing upon the acceptance of the death of a fatally ill patient and the comfort care provided for him without divulging any details of a personal or medical nature will serve not only to protect the departing person, but also to convey to the survivors that when their time comes, their very private world will be also respected.

Several RN's who believe in a positive approach in death crises related some illustrative experiences:

> Mr. E. had been a resident in the [church-related] home for more than a decade and a patient in the infirmary of the home for 6 months. He had no close relatives.
>
> An outgoing person with a keen sense of humor and a cheerful disposition, he had made many friends in the institution. He was a "helpful" person, always doing little favors for those who seemed helped by them and making himself useful by attending to some non-nursing needs of other patients, such as reading to a patient, fetching a newspaper, and the like. He was well liked by staff and residents alike; doctors and nurses considered him a "morale booster."
>
> His health steadily declined. He lost weight; the pain became worse. Instead of helping and doing for others, it became now his turn to be helped—to have someone sit at his bedside to read to him, engage in conversation with him, or provide a closeness, conveying affection and caring by just sitting quietly near his bed. As he grew sicker he became quieter, but he never ceased to be interested in people and enjoyed the company of others.
>
> Four weeks before he died, the physician requested that he be moved to a single room where he would have privacy and be protected from others and the others would be protected from the travail through which he was passing. The nurse in charge, sensing how closely Mr. E. related to his fellow patients and they to him, discussed the contemplated move with him. He indicated that he would prefer to remain where he was—in the eight-bed ward—among his friends and neighbors, not alone—unless the others in the room would have it otherwise. They indicated that they would not. He died as he had wished, with friends and a caring staff close by.

In the ensuing weeks the manner of his death was a fairly frequent topic of discussion among the patients. Several of those who had shared his last weeks with him commented that they would wish for themselves the same kind of death.

The director of nursing in another church-affiliated home recalled two recent occasions when a patient had died in a four-bed room:

The patient had been steadily getting weaker and the other patients knew that she was rapidly failing. They had also observed that the staff had been spending more time with her.

It was mealtime the day she was obviously dying and there were two nurses with her. The curtain had been drawn because of the need for suctioning. When death came, three of us were with her and stayed to pray for a few minutes; then we just lowered the head of the bed and left her body. Then I talked with the other patients in the room who were still not aware that she had died.

After lunch, when all the arrangements were ready and the undertaker came for the body, only one patient was still in the room. I went over to her bed and explained, "God just called her home—I want you to say a special prayer for her." The patient just looked at me and said, "He did?" and started to pray with her beads. Then I said, "I am going to pull your curtains for a few minutes—they are going to take——."

The patient did not get upset, but told me how she would pray for her late roommate.

The second death occurred in the same room a few weeks later. I went in to pass the four o'clock medications, and as I talked with one of the patients I noted that the patient sitting in a chair across the room looked dead—in fact I was sure she was, but there was nothing I could do for the moment for her. Rather than getting the patient with whom I had been talking upset, I continued to talk with her; and when an aide came into the room a few minutes later, I turned to her and said, "I'll help you put Mrs. C. back into bed" and just walked over and pulled the curtain. Only then did the aide realize what had happened, and we put Mrs. C. into her bed and left the curtain drawn. Since it was almost time for supper trays to be passed, we made the necessary arrangements and requested that the body not be called for until after supper. After the other patients had eaten, we took two of them out of the room. Then I went over to the other patient, who was really the only one who might become upset, and asked her to say a special prayer for Mrs. C. because God had called her home. She looked at me strangely and said, "How do you know it's going to be tonight?" Then I explained again that God had already called Mrs. C. home. Then I realized fully that this patient had not been aware of anything at all, though it had happened within 10 feet of her bed. She was very surprised when she understood that Mrs. C. had died, but she did not seem greatly upset. When I left her, she was praying for Mrs. C.

It may be pertinent to ask what the special needs of aged patients who suffer stress at the death of an elderly fellow patient might be. It becomes difficult to define these needs specifically and to identify patterns of reactions under which they arise and are resolved. However, a few general statements or principles can be derived from the nursing comments. They may serve as tentative guidelines until more adequate concepts are available.

1. It is highly probable that such needs of aged persons differ greatly from those of much younger fellow patients. It is also very likely that individual differences vary widely among the aged themselves. This idea of age group and individual differences is recurrent in the nursing observations.

2. While the experiences and reactions of aged fellow patients to a death among them tend to become individualized, the person who is conscious and "in contact" generally identifies more easily with the dying person who is regarded as a friend, and, thereby, undergoes greater anxiety.

3. It is also generally held that the mental or emotional stress that fails to find open and direct outlet tends to be expressed in disguised or masked form and often with devious symptoms requiring extra attention and care. It is held by many nurses that open expression and direct coping with the "death stresses" make for better patient adjustment, while suppressive tendencies create handicapping barriers for both the patient and the nurse.

4. Wherever administrative and medical rules permit some freedom for the nurse, it is generally the better course for her to meet the inquiries of aged patients about another patient who has been placed on the "danger list" or who has died with brief, simple, and truthful statements—tempering the truth by her perception of the concerns of the patient and his capacity to deal with the particular problem. Revealing any medical details or personal confidences are to be avoided, and generally no more information is indicated than that for which the patients asks.

When the sharing of information is prohibited, it is proposed that the nurse, with due respect for the inquiring patient, state simply that she is presently not permitted to discuss the situation, but that she will remember his request, should permission be granted later. There usually seems to be no necessity to explain by whom the permission is withheld, whether by administrator, physician, or others.

An overriding principle stressed in such a situation is that every effort be made by the nurse to maintain in the eyes of the concerned patients her integrity and genuine interest in them, her willingness to give attention to what they have to communicate, and her interest in responding to their needs as circumstances permit. Probably, more by what she is and does, than by what she can say, the nurse is able to imply and convey that what is happening "has to be" and that she is doing everything in her power to "make it right."

A foremost need of a fellow patient who is alert and under stress because of the death of another seems to be his inclination to do something or to find some means of expressing a supportive act or relationship with the dying person—and almost any opportunity for a meaningful activity or gesture helps to satisfy this need. Closely associated with this is the need to be kept informed of how things are going with the friend or associate, and often without being exposed to the situation. Here bits of generalized information at suitable intervals—little assurances such as "resting comfortably"; "unconscious of any suffering"; "dying peacefully"; or "It is all over now"—can fill a void that lack of information will leave open and stressful.

A very personal need may arise for assurances that this particular event brings the fellow patient's death no nearer either by some special coincidence or some possible medical or nursing neglect due to the extra care going to the dying patient.

Another keenly felt need is for some form of rational and positive orientation to, and interpretation of, death when it comes. The fellow patient may be groping for a view point or perspective on the threat that will make it appear reasonable and acceptable within a natural, hopeful, or at least tolerable, order of things as they are or have to be—a perspective that permits and supports a commendable confrontation for those who would try for it.

A philosophical or religious interpretation will meet the need well when it fits into the background of the person's life. Perhaps a rationale that presents the death as more to be welcomed than any other realistic alternative may be acceptable and helpful. Possibly the essence of coping effectively with inevitable death, whether for another or for oneself, is in coming to acceptable terms with it.

Nursing testimonies are replete with commendations for elderly persons of varied backgrounds who confront and adapt remarkably well to the death of a fellow patient. One DRN appraised the situation and what to do about it in this way:

> When a person lies dying, a fellow patient feels helpless and distressed. His nurse can be of help by encouraging him to express his feelings rather than keeping them sealed up inside. For to say, "You must not think of it now," becomes a falsely supportive statement

that only compounds his anxieties. The personal talk should come as soon as possible or at the time that he finds out about the death. After the discussion, the subject should be dropped and the emphasis placed back on events and experiences of daily living.

If the fellow patient is near the dying person, he may raise his problems directly with the nurse. She must take care regarding everything that she communicates to him, for he may be appraising the entire experience vicariously. Her values and attitudes will be perceived by him, often even though she tries to hide them. Her respect for the dignity of man, her attitude toward death, and her beliefs about what nurses should accomplish are all communicated. She should avoid betraying the privacy of the dying person or the confidences of the family. She should try to be honest without causing anguish to the inquirer. She may have to simply say, "He is as comfortable as possible—we just don't know."

She should try to communicate the conviction that all patients are important and that she has time to care for those who rely on her. If, indeed, this proves false during a lengthy emergency, it is her responsibility to call her supervisor for extra help. (Nagy)

Another DRN stated:

It has been my experience that some aged patients are jubilant when a fellow patient dies. It seems as though they are happy that they have been able to overcome death which is their close partner day by day. Others are very discouraged and identify so closely with the one who has died that a great deal of nursing and patient conversation on a 1 to 1 basis is needed in order to explore what the death means to each of them. (Knowles)

These suggestive guidelines for geriatric nursing care gain their pertinence primarily when viewed in the broad perspective of nursing experience with what is generally done about dying in American institutions. In a typical situation in hospitals in the United States, death is considered a dreadful event: all too often the patient is isolated and his personal needs ignored. "Everyone around him knows what is happening, but no one is free to talk or cry about it."

SUMMARY

The interview data on the question of coping with grieving patients when death takes one of them revealed so many references to *nurses' perception of aged patients' reaction* to a death in their midst to warrant tabulation of this information. Similar data were not obtained from degree registered nurse responses on this issue.

A majority of the nurse aides and registered nurses, and more than two fifths of the licensed practical nurses, reported that the situation presents no problem to them; their aged patients either show no special concern about the death of another patient or the environmental tone in the nursing unit is not conducive to death talk.

A small minority, roughly one in ten, declared that fear of death is normal in human beings. A more substantial minority, approximately a third, reported that aged patients often are concerned and disturbed by the death of one of them, but that the prevalence and degree of their interest and distress is determined by individual differences and variable circumstances.

Since the nurse practitioners expressed their views not only on aged patients' reaction to the death of a fellow patient, but also on the possible stresses experienced by them concerning their own death (which was discussed in the previous chapter) it may be of interest to juxtapose the figures that reflect their perceptions of these two aspects of death:

Nurses' perceptions of patients' reaction to the death of a fellow patient:

	NA's %	LPN's %	RN's %
Presents no problem; patients are not concerned	57.7	43.4	54.5
Fear of death is part of human nature	11.3	18.9	8.9
Patients' attitude depends on diverse factors	27.8	33.9	33.0

Nurses' perceptions of patients' reaction to prospects of own death:

	NA's %	LPN's %	RN's %
Presents no problem; patients are not concerned	30.3	28.3	32.0
Fear of death is part of human nature	15.7	22.7	20.5
Patients' attitude depends on diverse factors	54.0	49.0	46.2

Further exploration of this issue is needed for any valid or meaningful interpretation of these figures, but the considerable discrepancies in the support of the different positions on the issues, as reflected by these figures, once more raises the question as to whether the nurses' comments reflect their own attitudes and reactions toward personal death and to that of another person, rather than the attitude and reactions of their aged patients. It should be noted, however, that certain of these nurses did show great sensitivity to, and understanding of, their patient's reactions in time of such stress.

To the question of what coping patterns are utilized or available to nurses in their care of aged patients who might become concerned or disturbed by the death of one of them, responses were obtained from all four categories of nursing personnel.

A negative approach was reflected by at least two out of five of the nurse practitioners but less than one out of ten of the degree registered nurses. According to these respondents, discussion of death of a fellow patient was either avoided and discouraged, or attempts were made to keep information on the event from the patients.

A neutral position was taken by about a fifth to a third of the respondents. They indicated that any discussion of the subject was merely tolerated, with noncommittal or guarded remarks being made by them when patients raise the issue.

A minority of the nurse practitioners, amounting to slightly more than a tenth for the NA's and LPN's and a near third for the RN's, but a majority of the DRN's expressed a positive approach to the issue. The statistical details are as follows:

	NA's %	LPN's %	RN's %	DRN's %
Negative approach: subject is taboo	58.4	41.5	34.2	7.5
Neutral stand: topic is tolerated	25.7	34.0	18.3	29.1
Positive approach	13.9	13.2	32.9	59.1

For those respondents subscribing to the more positive approach toward helping aged patients cope with their concern or distress over the death of a fellow patient, the dominant proposal is to have ready a plan and policy of insuring and encouraging easy opportunities for such patients, or groups of them, to discuss with staff whatever their concerns may be, and to have provisions, whenever indicated, for the most competent staff member to take the lead. Modifications of this proposal were the suggestions that staff members keep themselves ready and prepared to enter into such discussions with concerned patients whenever the occasion arises. (Table 12, Items 5 to 8)

For full statistical details, see Appendix B, Tables 11 and 12.

14 Bereaved Relatives and the Nurse

> Each hath his drug for Sorrow
> (Or else the pain would slay!)
> For one it is "Tomorrow"
> For one, 'tis "Yesterday."
>
> MARGARET ROOT GARVIN

It is generally assumed that bereavement at the death of a family member is commonly, and, indeed, almost universally, experienced. In anthropological perspective, it tends to occur in some form and degree almost everywhere in spite of sharply contrasting social and cultural differences in time and place.*

It is reasonable to assume, also, that in our society the nurse tends to occupy a unique position in the frequent expression of grief in its varied forms and degrees. The geriatric nurse may be frequently confronted with opportunities and responsibilities for sharing the grief and in lending support to the bereaved—at least as long as they linger about the bedside of the dying or deceased. Indeed, it would appear difficult for her to avoid this.

Concerning this issue, an interview question directed to the nurse practitioners in the selected geriatric institutions was: What part, if any, do you have in aiding and supporting the bereaved? In correspondence with the selected sample of degree registered nurses, the question was: In what ways may the nurse render aid and support to the bereaved?

The coded responses were somewhat surprising. The replies of the three practitioner groups split into three distinct factions. These were: 1) The aged dying patients they have known and cared for appeared to have no relatives or their relatives seemed not to care about the death of an aged kinsman—hence, no problem existed; 2) Aiding and comforting bereaved relatives is the responsibility of persons other than nurses;

---

* Simmons, Leo W. *The Role of the Aged in Primitive Society.* New Haven, Yale University Press, 1945, Chap. 8.

and 3) Nurses have a responsibility of aiding and comforting bereaved persons. Of the degree registered nurses nearly 100 percent took the positive position, declaring that, indeed, nurses have such a responsibility.

Furthermore, during the interviews many of the practitioners expressed definite opinions about the behavior and reactions of relatives of patients before defining their own position on the issue of helping bereaved relatives. Even a very cursory summary of the nurses' perceptions about relatives of aged dying patients attests to a diversity inherent in their statements:

> Some nurses say that their aged patients have no relatives; but others claim they do.
>
> Some nurses assert that an aged person's death is not upsetting; but others maintain that it is.
>
> Some nurses declare that most aged patients' relatives seem indifferent and even callous; but others see them as devoted and solicitous.
>
> Some nurses contend that for many relatives an aged kinsman's death cannot come soon enough; but others claim that relatives often insist that "everything" be done to prolong his life.
>
> Some nurses allege that when an aged patient is dying the relatives are apt to stay away even more than before; others say the contrary is true.
>
> Some nurses maintain that, when a patient is dying, relatives do not wish to assist in any way with his care; others point to help that has been rendered.
>
> Some nurses relate that relatives do not grieve about the death of an aged kinsman; others insist that relatives are often greatly upset and heartbroken when he dies.
>
> Some nurses indicate that relatives are friendly toward the staff; others that they are often indifferent to the staff, at times to the point of ignoring them.
>
> Some nurses say that they never see the relative again after a patient's death; but others insist that often relatives make a point of thanking them, often writing notes of appreciation—and that an occasional relative returns to visit other patients on the floor or to become a regular volunteer worker.

To what extent these perceptions reflect the nurses' own attitude and behavior would be difficult to ascertain, but the views of a small group of involved relatives may be relevant to the situation.

During a preliminary phase of this study some twenty-odd relatives of elderly patients who had died in nursing homes were interviewed. Only two of these spoke warmly and appreciatively of the caring attitude of the staff and of the helping hand extended to them by the nurse both before and after the death of their kinsman. A few others indicated that the nurses' major responsibility is the physical care of patients; hence they did not expect to be shown any special consideration by the staff. The majority of these relatives, on the other hand, voiced dissatisfaction with the treatment they had received during such a stressful time, mostly related to the apparent indifference of the nurses toward them. The daughter of one of the patients who had recently died related her experience:

> My 86-year-old mother had been critically ill for 10 days, during which I spent the greater part of each day at her bedside. I had a clear understanding with the administrator, who was also the nursing director, that I would be notified at once if my mother's condition should worsen at a time that I was not with her.
>
> On the day my mother died the phone rang at about 8:30 A.M. It was the nursing home administrator who informed me that my mother had passed away a few hours earlier, and that they had waited until now to notify me since they did not wish to disturb me earlier. When I said that I would come right over, she informed me that the undertaker had already been there, but that I should feel free at any time to fetch my mother's belongings. I was upset and angry that I had not been called at the time of my mother's death.
>
> I went to the funeral home to verify arrangements that had been made when my mother had entered the nursing home nearly 2 years before. From there I drove to the nursing home to call for the few personal belongings my mother had treasured and kept with her: a small bedside clock, her wristwatch, two small photos, and a few other keepsakes.
>
> At the nurses' desk I was told that my mother's room had been cleaned and the bed remade and that her personal belongings had been sent to the front office. At the office no one seemed to know what had become of them, but after some searching a nurse aide found the bundle, in which my mother's few treasures had been tied, in a corner near the stairwell.
>
> I shall never forget how lonely I felt when I took the bundle and walked out of the place which had been my mother's home for the last 2 years of her life.

NO BEREAVEMENT PROBLEM

Let us consider now the group of nurse practitioners who asserted that they encounter no problem with grieving relatives when one of their aged patients dies, either because the patient has no relatives, relatives seem not to care about his death, or senescent death is not upsetting.*

* NA's, 21.8 percent; LPN's, 28.9 percent; RN's, 38.2 percent; DRN's, 0.0 percent. See Appendix B, Table 13, Items 1 and 2.

A nurse aide stated that during the 7 years she had worked in the home she had not seen one relative visit a dying patient. In another home an NA recalled three or four instances when a relative had come to visit a very critically ill patient during her 8 years of employment there. Still another NA declared that some relatives "couldn't care less" and illustrated this:

> The niece of one of my patients got hold of my home telephone number and kept calling from time to time about her aunt who was critically ill. When she called not long ago and I told her that her aunt was beginning to talk and walk again, the niece exclaimed, "Oh my God—I hope she does not get well enough to come home." She had been expecting her aunt to die—and she seemed to be saying, "Aunt Alice, please die, so I can have your money."

A licensed practical nurse echoed the sentiment expressed by some of her colleagues when she said:

> Relatives don't get disturbed. They often see death as a release; often they don't care. Not long ago we had a patient who became critical and was expected to die shortly. We notified the family and it took them a whole week before anyone came to visit the dying patient— it is different in a hospital where people are younger.

Another LPN injected an attitude of "Do unto others as they do unto you" when she spoke of having been to a wake once because she knew the family of the deceased patient well, and she added that generally she has no contact with patients' relatives. "It depends on how well you know them—in any case, if a family gives, they get back more."

A foreign born and educated registered nurse who had been working in a nursing home for about 8 years commented:

> Most times the relatives don't come. And sometimes when they do come, a patient will refuse to speak with them though he will speak with me. Resentment may be part of this. In my country the families are closer—we do not put old people in homes as you do here. . . . If a patient has money, the relatives sometimes cannot wait for death to come—they say, "He is just a vegetable." Families don't want to be bothered. I don't see much of them at any time.

Several practitioners expressed bitterness at the apparent callousness of relatives. An RN gave this example:

> An 86-year-old patient was brought in here. She was semiconscious and appeared to be very ill. She had been living alone and no one seemed to know what had happened to her. Soon after being admitted, she had a severe convulsion and lapsed into a deep coma. The

doctors held little hope for her recovery and so informed the family.

Her son, who visited almost daily, seemed most solicitous and implored the doctors and nurses to do everything possible for his mother, insisting that "nothing but the best" would do for her.

The patient responded to treatment. She regained consciousness. After a few weeks she knew where she was and began to eat; and after a few months, she was well enough to be out of bed.

That was 6 months ago. Of late the son has been visiting very rarely, and when he does he ignores the nursing staff and refuses to discuss his mother's condition with the physician.

In sentiment and in practice these nurses convey the idea that most of their aged patients have no relatives and have outlived their peers or that in general relatives view senescent death as a release or, at least, a timely occurrence. This feeling, and the frequently voiced assertion by staff that for the institutionalized aged patients *they*—the staff—represent "family," may be the reason why in a number of the selected homes some staff members go to a patient's wake or attend funeral services.

Not a Nursing Responsibility

While a considerable number of the three ranks of practitioners insisted that the death of an aged patient presents no bereavement problem for them, many of their co-workers and colleagues acknowledged the problem but disavowed any responsibility on their part concerning it. This group of practitioners asserted that any aid and comfort to be provided for bereaved relatives is the responsibility of others, not the nursing personnel. One degree registered nurse concurred in this.*

In the few institutions where there are social service departments the task of aiding and comforting the bereaved relatives is often considered to be the responsibility of the social worker; in others, it may be the administrator of the institution or his assistant who assumes this role. In two of the participating institutions, social workers suggested that since they get to know the patients and their families more intimately than do the nurses and also are better equipped than nurses to cope with stressful situations such as bereavement, it is their job to aid and comfort the bereaved relatives.

In another home, the assistant administrator serves as a liaison between the nursing department and the family. It is the responsibility of her office to contact the family when there is a change in a patient's

---

* NA's, 61.4 percent; LPN's, 40.4 percent; RN's, 22.2 percent; DRN's, 1.1 percent. See Appendix B, Table 13, Item 3.

condition or if a patient has died. According to some of the nursing personnel in this institution, the assistant administrator works very closely with the relatives at all times; this was corroborated by her. She indicated that she knows the families better than any of the nurses and works closely with the nursing department to keep informed about any untoward change in a patient's condition. She emphasized, also, that often relatives stop by and ask her about a patient before going to visit with the patient. In some other institutions, practicality supersedes personal consideration, and the aid and support rendered to bereaved relatives may be limited to verification of burial arrangements and the like.

A nurse aide who declared that it is not her responsibility to comfort bereaved relatives stated that it is better not to become involved with families: they might ask questions the NA's are not permitted to answer, and becoming involved with relatives takes away from the time that should be spent with patients. Inquiring relatives in this home are referred to the head nurse or the front office.

A licensed practical nurse, in charge of a nursing unit during the afternoon tour of duty, refers relatives to the social worker or, if it is after 5 P.M., to the nursing supervisor. She contends that most relatives "do not bother" with the nursing staff and that she does not get to know them.

Some nurses indicated, also, that they discourage relatives from visiting dying patients. If the relatives insist on visiting, they may be asked to spend no more than a few moments at a time with the patient. The reason given for such practices is that the patient's comfort and welfare have to be considered first or that a relative at the bedside hinders the staff in giving care to the patient.

Several of the RN's hinted or frankly acknowledged that there may be a difference between a *given* and a *real* reason for taking the position that it is not a nurse's responsibility to aid and comfort bereaved relatives, and that the real reason may be that nurses feel ill prepared to cope with bereavement. A director of nursing reflected the attitude of a number of others in this group when she said:

> We usually see the family during the acute phase when the patient is critically ill, though we discourage them from visiting as much as we can. My own feelings enter into this—I don't want to face them with their suffering. Besides, we have to consider the other patients. Some relatives have guilt feelings about placing the patient here in the first place, and they often "carry on," which is upsetting for everyone. The present generation has not fully accepted institutional care for the aged.
>
> Our first responsibility is to our patients; we try not to become involved with families. Besides, they have relatives and friends to comfort them.

The proportion of nurse practitioners who disavowed any responsibility in aiding and supporting bereaved relatives together with those who deny the existence of such a need add up to an impressive total. About 80 percent of the nurse aides, 70 percent of the licensed practical nurses, and 60 percent of the registered nurses seem to assert, on one ground or another, that they have no occasion for feeling responsible for providing aid and support to bereaved relatives when their aged kin dies. One degree registered nurse took a similar position.

AID AND COMFORT TO BEREAVED RELATIVES

A third faction of the nurse practitioners and all but one of the degree registered nurse group took issue with the two positions discussed in the foregoing pages. They declared that nursing has a responsibility to bereaved relatives when an aged kinsman is dying or has died. Some of this group would aid and comfort any bereaved relative who seeks help or appears to need it; others would offer such help. Also, a small percentage of the practitioners indicate that they follow a planned policy of attempting to aid and support bereaved relatives. Almost all of the degree registered nurses would do likewise.*

This group considers it as important for the nurse to know the family as it is for her to know the patient and that a first principle is to make the family feel welcome and wanted. Many of them reiterated, also, that in order to be of constructive help, it is essential that the nurse accept and respect individual as well as group differences.

Many diverse variables in an aged patient-family relationship that need to be analyzed were suggested, such as: whether the terminal illness is the result of a catastrophic disease or the outcome of a long-term debilitating condition; whether the patient knows of and is accepting of his impending death or has hopes of recovery; whether the patient has retained his mental alertness or sustained mental impairment so that he has more or less lost touch with reality; whether the family members are an emotionally demonstrative group or stoical in expressing their emotions; whether the patient is a relatively young ager or is very advanced in years; whether the blood relationship is a close one, such as mate or child, or more remote, such as a grandniece, perhaps, or a distant cousin; and, finally, whether the patient entered the institution of his own volition or was placed there by his family.

If the dying patient was placed in the institution without being con-

* NA's, 10.9 percent; LPN's, 21.2 percent; RN's, 30.9 percent; DRN's, 98.9 percent. See Appendix B, Table 13, items 4, 5.

sulted or much against his will, a strained relationship may have resulted between the patient and certain family members. Instances were related by staff members when a patient would refuse to speak with visiting relatives—perhaps carrying his resentment to his grave. Relatives, on the one hand, may be seeking either a reconciliation or a relief from guilt feelings during the terminal phase of the aged kinsman's life or, on the other hand, may hesitate to visit for fear of arousing additional stress in themselves or the patient.

Furthermore, some persons may feel uncomfortable or even frightened in the face of death, while others may have a real need to be doing something for, or on behalf of, the dying patient. An RN explained:

> Some relatives don't want to be at the bedside, particularly when the patient is in a coma. Some stay for long hours, others are more content to come and stay for short periods with the patient. I try to talk with the family to find out how they feel—it helps me to bring them into the situation. The nurse should be right in there, so she can be of help to the family and, if necessary, to bring others, such as a doctor, social worker, minister, priest, or rabbi, into the situation.
>
> A relative may wish a quiet chat away from the patient; another appreciates a hot cup of coffee or tea; some relish a humorous or endearing comment the nurse remembers the patient to have made during his healthier days. If relatives are with the patient at the time of death, the nurse must not be too hasty to attend to practical things such as cleaning up the room, but should allow the family time to be with the deceased if they wish.

These nurses also hold, that many relatives do care and cited instances to support this assertion. A licensed practical nurse spoke of a loving daughter who for many weeks had come day after day to be with her dying mother, even assisting the staff with care. A registered nurse spoke of a devoted son:

> When Mr. M. became critically ill, we wired his son, who lived on the West Coast. He flew East as soon as he heard about his father's condition and remained with his father until he died—even sleeping in the same room.
>
> The patient's 84-year-old sister, who lived closer by, had visited Mr. M. quite regularly during the time he had been in the home. She was with him when Mr. M. died. Standing at his bedside and looking at the deceased for some moments, she remarked: "He seems to be laughing at me that he got there first." She then explained that by all odds she should have been the one to die first.

A nurse aide related:

> When Mrs. S. was dying, her daughter came daily. I thought that the patient would eat a little better if the daughter fed her—so the daugh-

ter came every day to do so. This was strictly between me and the daughter. But when the patient died, the daughter seemed relieved.

Some of these nurses were critical of certain of their co-workers and colleagues who seemed indifferent, avoided getting to know the relatives, or even discouraged family members from visiting a dying patient. Instances of such indifference, even situations causing suffering, were related. A licensed practical nurse spoke of a "most shocking" experience she had in her former place of employment:

> It had been a very trying afternoon and evening. Two or three patients needed intensive care, and we were short of staff. One aged patient was dying. She had been in the home for many months and had always been a very demanding patient. For more than a week—ever since her condition became critical—her son had been visiting her every evening, coming directly from his place of work. Often the patient sent her son to the nurses' desk to ask for something she wanted: a sip of hot tea, medicine for her pain, and the like. This particular evening the patient had been especially demanding, and when the son came to the desk and told the nurse in charge that his mother thought her medicine was overdue, the nurse answered sharply along these lines: "Can't she wait a little—what difference can it make—She's old and she is dying."

A contrasting experience was related in another facility:

> Mr. B. died suddenly one Sunday morning. He had been in the nursing home about 2 months, having been transferred from a nearby hospital. At the time of transfer, the hospital doctors had told the family that this was being done so Mr. B. would recuperate more quickly; but in truth they did not expect him to recover.
>
> Mr. B.'s wife, who had a cardiac condition, visited her husband regularly while he was in the home. Two children were married and lived in nearby villages. On Sundays the wife would attend church services, have dinner at home, and then spend the rest of the day with her husband.
>
> Death occurred without much warning while Mrs. B. was in church. When the assistant nursing administrator, who was in charge of the service that particular weekend, telephoned Mr. B.'s son to tell him what had happened, they discussed how best to break the news to Mrs. B. They decided that the assistant administrator would meet the son at his mother's home to await her return from church, at which time they would tell her about her husband's death. As had been anticipated, Mrs. B. asked if she might see her husband once more—before the undertaker would call for his body. Her request was granted, for instruction had been left that Mr. B.'s body be left untouched until the assistant administrator returned to the home. Son and daughter then accompanied their mother to Mr. B.'s room to bid him a final good-bye.

Predeath Bereavement

Nurses who would give aid and comfort to a bereaved family may profit considerably by their awareness of the stage of mourning and grief through which relatives are passing. Mourning ordinarily starts well before actual death occurs, especially when the patient is afflicted with a long-term illness or debilitating condition. In fact, the sorrowful period may have begun the moment the patient was institutionalized. Furthermore, it is conceivable that some relatives grieved more when the patient was admitted to the institution than at the time of death of their kinsman. For nursing personnel who attempt to aid and support relatives in their predeath bereavement, the following guidelines, derived from nursing comments, may prove useful. They are drawn primarily from the contributions of degree registered nurses.

1. By accepting the relatives' predeath bereavement behavior as normal, lending her approval and support to its expression, fitting it into the plan of care for the patient, and suggesting appropriate ways for its manifestations, the nurse may be able to make of it a mutually constructive experience for both the bereaved relative and the dying patient.

2. It usually is helpful for the nurse to find in the family a key member who appears especially concerned, relatively stable, and responsible and who obviously exercises some influence in the family group. It can become distinctly advantageous to the nurse to direct special attention to preparing this person to serve as an intermediary between herself and the family in coping with the approaching crisis.

3. A plan of action could involve being especially available to this relative, listening for his reports of family expressions of anxiety, grief, or guilt, correcting any false or unfounded alarms, and, through this person, keeping the family posted with truthful and appropriate information on the progress and the expectations for the patient. Part of the useful service here lies, also, in safeguarding the family from building up false hopes on the one hand or facing sudden shock on the other. A central idea appears to be pacing the progress of predeath grief work of the concerned relatives with the approaching death of the patient in order that both the patient and his loved ones may be, to some degree, reconciled and prepared when death comes.

4. Many nurses encourage sharing with the bereaved, through the selected family representative, current information on what is taking place with the patient during the periods of their absence. Although subject to any specific restraints on giving out information, the nurse can almost always find some truthful, well-chosen, and supportive details to relate about the patient, such as, having spent an exceptionally good night or day, if true; sleeping without the usual sedation; showing pleasure at some particular incident or expressing appreciation for some thoughtful service from family or staff; manifesting some personal characteristic known to and cherished by the bereaved; inquiring about particular family members; demonstrating a gamy spirit or even some occasional touches of humor about amusing or awkward situations; or almost anything else reflecting warm, human responses. Any such bits of personal information stand a chance of being welcomed by the bereaved and interpreted by them as evidence of genuine staff interest and attention or even as memorable bits of family solace.

5. It is further proposed by nursing testimony that opportunities be arranged for the bereaved to participate actively in some of the care of the patient both by their presence beside the bed and by some simple and safe services suited to their desires and capabilities as well as the desires of the patient. Some nurses would also include the presence and limited participation of young persons, such as grandchildren, where it appears appropriate and welcome by the patient. A caution is expressed, however, that no participation of bereaved relatives be permitted to reach the point of replacing the responsibilities of the staff.

With approaching death, the nurse's role carries double duty, for in addition to her concern for, and responsibility to, her aged patient, she has a responsibility to the family, to whom she may need to render aid and comfort in various ways. Her contact with, and knowledge of, the patient and his family enables her to anticipate certain of their special needs. They may appreciate some privacy, some opportunity to talk about their pending loss, and, perhaps, some nourishment.

If the relatives are asked to leave the room of a dying patient, the nurse should explain the reasons for this and make provisions for their privacy and comfort while they wait. She should respect the family's wishes about being notified in the event of a major change in the patient's condition or of any sudden signs of actual dying. She should also anticipate and prepare herself in advance for guiding and assisting the relatives in the routine details to be handled when death has come, for her responsibility to the family does not end with the death of the patient. Rather, it may take precedence over her other work responsibilities at that time.

Bereavement following Death

According to much nursing testimony, our culture encourages all of us at the time of death to give aid and solace to the bereaved family, and it is in the role of nurses, both as professionals and human beings, to offer aid and comfort to those who suffer great grief. As often affirmed by respondents, a last office of a nurse in the care of her dying patient is sustaining his loved ones in their sorrow. Even though the deceased may have been completely senile over a long period of time, the sense of loss to surviving members of his family may still be great, the feelings of grief and guilt very real, and the loneliness something that will take weeks or months to heal. In addition to insuring privacy for the outflow of grief and certain conveniences and comforts for the sense of shock suffered, the nurse's very concern for, acceptance of, and encouragement of the free manifestations of mourning may be the most significant thing that she can do for these relatives. When she can show genuine concern on a warm, human basis and not be ashamed of her own tears when she feels them, almost any simple and sincere act of caring and assisting is likely to be noted and appreciated. The bereaved rarely demand and may not expect or want more than this. Just being *with* them—not too busy with current nursing details and conveying by silences and occasional touches something that words are inadequate to express—often proves to be the exceptional and long remembered nursing contribution.

The nursing counsel is to avoid such platitudes as, "it is better this way." Let the bereaved reach a conclusion for himself from his own beliefs and experience and what he may recall about those of the patient. Try not to provide ready-made solutions to the problems and the mystery, but reflect and support the hopeful and realistic approaches that the bereaved takes toward resolution of his own loss. (Baziak, Declan, Matthews, Reiter, Wilkinson, Wolanin)

If the illness has been a long and stressful one and if the family is really relieved by the passing "in peace" of the patient, why shouldn't the nurse accept this expression, too, and without building up their feelings of guilt by her attitude.

Should the nurse become a target of accusation that the patient was neglected or mishandled, the nursing consensus seems to be that it must be remembered that such behavior on the part of the bereaved may reflect no more than current feelings of guilt about his own relationship to the deceased and that it is likely soon to pass. Above all, the nurse should avoid being drawn into any argument on the subject.

The request to see the dying or deceased should not be denied the family member—to take leave by touch, kiss, or some other endearment may be of special meaning and lasting significance to the bereaved.

It is recommended that the nurse and her staff prepare the body and the room for a family visit, but it is considered better for her to forestall any extensive handling of the body until the relatives are no longer in the vicinity.

While the family is with the deceased, the nurse should be ready to remain with them or step aside, but staying within reach, and, in no case, should leave the family entirely alone during the period immediately following death. She should give to the family any personal items of the patient which will not accompany the body and should assist the family with special respect in the packing of them, at least to the degree that this is welcomed and desired by the family members. This help should be unhurried and with attention to anything that they may wish to say. (Malipaard, Schwartz, Shumway)

Several nurses suggested ways of using the life of the patient for comfort to the bereaved. This involves learning enough about the patient to comment intelligently on the achievements in his life that redound to the good of his family or community or reciting some heroics of his last illness that can be commended by all. A discerning nurse will find many possibilities in this area. Talking about the dead person will help the bereaved acquire a deep sense of reality that the death has actually occurred.

It is emphasized over and over again by nurses that a quiet and private place, with telephone, refreshments, and other suitable conveniences, is indispensable for the nurse in providing her best aid and support. And, lastly, as one nurse put it, "I do feel that at the time of the family's departure, the nurse should escort the party to the hospital door. For me there is nothing colder than seeing an obviously grief-stricken family trying to find its way out of the building and without any support from the attending staff."

Other nurses conclude that the rules of courtesy that apply in one's home apply here: sitting with the bereaved, speaking of the deceased as freely as the occasion prompts, and supporting a comforting relationship for facing the reality. Under such circumstances the requirements transcend any purely professional and technical roles or responsibilities. This is a time when the right nurse can render a very special service to the bereaved by her concern, permissiveness, and warmth and by giving personal attention to *any* details that the grieved one feels unable to cope with. (Jayne, Kerrigan, Lanigan, Muir, Nagy, Wolanin)

Lest the above discourse give the impression that the needs of bereaved relatives can be met by following a fairly standardized set of procedures, a caution is in order. The situation calls for very discerning and personalized consideration on the part of the nurse. Variables to be considered in accommodating nursing supports to the needs of bereaved relatives when an aged, institutionalized kinsman dies include:

1. When the deceased has become elderly and decrepit instead of being relatively youthful and still active, the difference may be substantial in the reassurances required by the bereaved. .

2. The number of family members at the time of death creates differences in the course the nurse may take. If only the spouse is there, the nurse has a much different responsibility than if five family members are present.

3. The position in the family of the closest and the most involved survivor makes a difference. If it is the spouse, the loss may be very great, especially when two elderly people have shared their long lives. If sons and daughters are the closest of kin, they may take some comfort in thoughts that their parents are together again.

4. The value of religion for both the deceased and the bereaved can alter the impact of the situation. The strength and reconciliation that comes with faith helps the bereaved to maintain composure and also overcomes some of the emotional pain of the loneliness and loss.

5. The length of time that has elapsed between the first death crisis and the final passing may make an important difference. If the time was short, the loss may seem more unreal and the bereaved may suffer greater feelings of guilt because the time was too brief "to try everything." But the bereaved in this situation are likely to be more physically rested, not having been subjected to a lengthy emotional strain. If the time has been long, the bereaved are more likely to be worn down, somewhat ready to accept the loss as real, and may even have prayed for the end to come without further suffering. In a sense, they are more receptive to whatever aid and comfort the nurse can give.

6. The attitude the deceased held toward his impending death may influence the feelings and responses of the bereaved. With approaching signs of death, some patients show far more fear and

stress than do others who often manifest genuine feelings of peace. This difference can profoundly affect the feelings and behavior of the bereaved and what the nurse finds possible to do for them.

7. The amount of time available to the nurse for aiding and supporting the bereaved may make a major difference. And if she has developed a warm and trusting relationship with the family prior to the death, the bereaved will be more inclined to linger afterwards with the nurse for the comfort and help that she can give.

8. The social organization of the institution and the working relationships among members of the different departments may make a difference. If certain details related to a death are the prerogatives of another department, such as social service or administration, the nurse's responsibility toward the family may largely be limited to predeath bereavement and one of her final actions of supporting the bereaved may consist of escorting the bereaved to whoever "takes over" from there.

9. Finally, one of the most important variables in rendering aid and support to bereaved relatives when an aged patient dies in a geriatric institution is the philosophy of the director or administrator of the department of nursing and the philosophy and policy of the institution.

Perhaps the full and detailed statement of a degree registered nurse will reflect more effectively the spirit and service of a sensitive and competent nurse in her relationship with the bereaved:

> One way that we can provide help and support to the bereaved is to let them know that we as nurses are human beings, too. I always try to get on the same physical level with them. If they are sitting, I sit. If they are standing, I stand. I try to give them some kind of food, since food often means, "I love you" or "I care for you." It can become a kind of evidence of a nurturing function. Nearly everyone will say that a cup of coffee would be welcomed, whether one drinks it or not, and it helps to start conversation.
>
> I nearly always touch the relative to let him or her know I understand. I explore at least three feelings that are seen to be fairly prevalent: 1) guilt: no one ever believes that he has done enough. There are many more things that one can think of having done; 2) anger: very often it comes out that the relative feels anger that the deceased has left him, literally walked out on him; 3) I try to find out what images the deceased had of those who survive and grieve—what would he want them to be doing. In nearly every case, strengthening ideas are derived from these approaches.

It does not surprise me that people cry one moment when they think of the sad things that have happened in their lives, laugh another moment at the thoughts of the good things that have happened, and cry again when they think of the sad things. After sessions of this kind, people certainly appear drained emotionally; but I have the feeling that if I have reached people at all, they in some way thank me: they sigh, take a deep breath, or look a little more relieved. If the signals I get are correctly interpreted, they seem to be saying, "Well, it is pretty awful, but I have got to go through with it, and I can." (Knowles)

Postfuneral Bereavement

There is, also, a third well-defined and very important phase in bereavement—the grief work that needs to be completed before the saddened relative can return to normal relationships and feelings of normal well-being to his readjusting family and to his community. In the present survey it was exceptionally rare for the nurse of any rank to take note of this phase or to offer any reports or firm proposals on what nurses can do about it.

DISCUSSION

There is pathos in the realization that for many aged Americans the nursing homes are places "where they go to die." Allusions to this were fairly common in the nursing responses. Nursing home staff at times qualified pertinent statements with phrases such as "Our patients realize that they will be here for the rest of their lives." Not long ago a very elderly gentleman who had been confined to a nursing home for more than a year commented, "This is the waiting room for death." Another nursing home resident, who expressed bitterness and resentment about being placed there by her children, said, "I wonder if they realize just what they are doing to me—maybe they will find out when they reach my age and *their* children put them in a place such as this to live out their lives." And the administrator and co-owner of a suburban nursing home lamented that when attending social functions or shopping, she is at times introduced with such "complimentary" statements as, "She owns the place where So-and-so died."

Since an aged person frequently is expected to remain in the geriatric facility until death, it may be expected that at the time of admission the question of burial arrangements is raised, so that in the event of death there need be no waiting for such plans from relatives or other responsible persons. Besides, unlike hospitals, nursing homes or similar long-term care facilities rarely have morgues where the body of a deceased person may be kept to await funeral arrangements including the selection of an undertaker. Under prevailing practices the undertaker can be notified as soon as death occurs and the body removed from the geriatric institution without delay. There is evidence that this at times is done without a physician having certified the death of the patient and even before the family is notified of the death.

Certain differences between nonprofit and profit-making institutions that may have a bearing on the procedures and routines in the event of death of a patient should be noted here. Nonprofit facilities such as homes for the aged have as their primary purpose the fulfilling of multiple needs—social, psychological, spiritual, and health and medical wants. Most of their residents enter of their own volition and apply for admission in the hope of finding a "home"—a substitute "family." If in need of skilled nursing care, it is provided for in the infirmary or nursing unit of the institution. A death among the residents is considered much the same as a death in one's own family. Fellow residents are notified of the death and a memorial or burial service may be conducted in the chapel belonging to the home. In some of these institutions, the residents have the privilege to be buried in the burial plot belonging to the home if they so desire and have no cemetery plot of their own.

Proprietary nursing homes on the other hand, are business enterprises which are concerned with patients whose primary need is seen to be nursing therapy or "custodial" care. Most of these patients come from homes of their own or of a relative, often after an accident or illness that required hospitalization prior to being admitted to the long-term care facility. Usually they have no other choice; they may enter because they are no longer capable of independent living or their relatives feel they are no longer able to provide the care that is required.

There is evidence that these institutional differences affect staff-patient as well as staff-relative relationships, and, as has been stated, they may also affect the relationship between patient and relative. At times, staff members as well as patients expressed resentment when it was believed that the patient had been placed in the institution because the children found it inconvenient to have the parent at home.*

The particular system, its philosophy, and its policy, may also affect the position that nurses take on the issue of responsibility toward the

---

* Particularly relevant to what is said here is a chapter by Jules Henry, "Personality and Aging—With Special Reference to Hospitals for the Aged Poor," in McKinney, John C. and de Vyver, Frank T. Aging and Social Policy. New York, Appleton-Century-Crofts, 1966, Chap. 10.

bereaved in the event of a patient's death. Nurses who do not wish to become involved are often aided and abetted by the system within which they work. If the administration frowns upon any death talk, it quite naturally follows that stressful situations related to death and dying can easily be averted. One way to accomplish this, of course, is to discourage visits by relatives when an aged kinsman is dying or has died.

If the physical facilities in a nursing home are such that it is well-nigh impossible to find the privacy needed for quiet talk, a warming cup of coffee, or a good cry, it becomes difficult for the nurse to establish an atmosphere conducive to aiding and supporting an overwrought relative.

If the working relationship among the different departments, such as nursing and social service, or nursing and administration, is not very close or harmonious or does not encompass all facets of patient care and support of surviving relatives, this tends to work to the advantage of the nurse who shies away from becoming involved with the family.

If within the department of nursing there is no real teamwork, or if the philosophy differs among those who occupy leadership positions in the department or among the different nursing ranks, it is not difficult for individual staff members to disavow any responsibility in aiding and supporting bereaved relatives.

It thus requires professional skill and knowledge on the part of the responsible registered nurses who occupy positions of leadership in geriatric institutions—and an understanding heart—to adequately provide for the needs and wants relatives may have when an aged kinsman is dying or has died in the institution.

SUMMARY

A very sharp contrast exists between the concepts and attitudes of the geriatric nurse practitioners and the degree registered nurse respondents on the needs and issues of providing support for the relatives of dying aged persons.

Almost a third of the practitioners take a predominantly negative approach toward the issue, maintaining that they encounter no bereavement problem. A somewhat larger proportion recognizes such a problem, but disclaims any responsibility for providing aid and comfort to any grieving relatives when an aged kinsman dies.

All of the ninety DRN's who responded to this question recognize a bereavement problem, and only one of them would shift the responsibility for comforting and supporting the bereaved to others.

However, one tenth to three tenths of the practitioner ranks and ninety-nine percent of the degree registered nurses take a strong positive approach, subscribing to nursing concern for, and sustaining support of, the bereaved relatives of the dying aged, and providing plans and policies for insuring nursing attention and service. The statistical details are as follows:

	NA's %	LPN's %	RN's %	DRN's %
Negative approach; problem does not exist	21.8	28.9	38.2	0.0
Aiding the bereaved is the responsibility of others	61.4	40.4	22.2	1.1
Positive approach; nurses have such responsibility	10.9	21.2	30.9	98.9

For full statistical details, see Appendix B, Table 13.

15 Nurses' Likes and Dislikes about Geriatrics

In order that people may be happy in their work, these three things are needed: They must be fit for their work; they must not do too much of it; and they must gain a sense of success from it.

JOHN RUSKIN

It is no secret that geriatric nursing has little appeal as a career to young and promising persons, committed though they may be to nursing as a profession. Any attraction geriatrics has is far from commensurate to the existing need. Registered nurses who work in gerontological nursing often commented upon the low status of this specialty and the difficulties they often encountered when attempting to recruit other RN's for work in this area. Some nursing directors justified not having registered nurses in charge positions on such grounds. For some other RN's, however, the very lack of prestige of geriatric nursing was allegedly an added factor for entering the field. They felt challenged by the possibilities of care to be provided for the aged ill; of raising standards for geriatric nursing practice; and of changing attitudes in order that geriatrics would be considered a more prestigious specialty.

Some nurses suggested that the demeaning attitude so many Americans hold toward the elderly may well be related to the low status with which health professionals so often view geriatrics. They indicated that in medicine, also, geriatrics seemingly holds little attraction for physicians; often medical doctors are not interested in providing care for the aged. A few nurses were full of praise and admiration of the physicians with whom they were working. They spoke glowingly of their doctors' compassion for, and rapport with, their patients; the harmonious and ongoing nurse-doctor relationship; their teamwork toward the common goal of providing the best possible care for their patients. Many other nurses, however, related very negative experiences with physicians, tell-

229

ing of poor and inadequate medical care; of doctors' perfunctory visits to the institution; and of prescribing by phone—often without having seen the patient for a week or more. A licensed practical nurse who was critical of some nursing and medical procedures when she assumed charge of a nursing unit exemplified this:

> When I came here most patients were wearing diapers and rubber pants. I got rid of them and we now "time" our patients for toileting. It works. The patients are more comfortable and the smell of stale urine has disappeared. The aides are happier that they no longer have to change diapers. This practice has the added benefit that the patients get more exercise by being walked to toilet at regular intervals.
>
> When I came here the patients, also, were much more inactive than they are now. Most of them were heavily sedated—the doctors kept ordering tranquilizers on a p.r.n. basis. I used my own judgment in this, and now most of our patients are off tranquilizers and they no longer behave like so many zombies. I think at least twice a year all medications should be discontinued and then have the doctors reorder them on *the basis of need.*

A well-qualified and dedicated director of nursing in a geriatric facility commented:

> There is a tremendous need to raise work standards in this field and to attract well qualified nurses. Gerontological nursing is not for the more technically oriented nurse or for one who looks for dramatic recoveries such as one often sees in hospitals following surgery or some medical therapy. The challenge here is to help elderly and ill individuals find some further fulfillments in life and, when the time comes, to assist them to whatever extent they wish to find some comfort and dignity in death. The typical hospital patient expects to return to the larger community in better health than he had before entering, whereas most of our patients here have little to look forward to—and most of them are here until they die.
>
> The RN who works with the aged ill needs—in addition to basic, and including psychiatric, nursing skills—to be well grounded in the social and biological sciences. And, in addition to being knowledgeable in the biological, psychological, and social areas of aging, she must have sincerity of purpose and have achieved within herself a religiophilosophical orientation toward life and death. Such a nurse could be tremendously challenged by the work in this area.

And a degree registered nurse contended that:

> Geriatric nursing needs to have something very special to offer. At present, students rate it fairly low on their list of interests—yet the need grows rapidly. (Conn)

Because of the recognition of general lack of prestige for geriatric nursing in the profession, the widespread shortage of qualified nurses in the field, and the relatively poor preparation of those employed in most of the nursing homes in this country, special consideration was given in this study to the compensations and the discouragements that nursing practitioners experience in the daily fulfillment of their functions. By interview, the three categories of nursing practitioners were asked about the two or three things or conditions that they liked "best" about their work with the aged ill, on the one hand, and the two or three that they liked "least" on the other hand. A question somewhat related to the possible satisfactions of nursing personnel in the field of geriatrics was asked of the degree registered nurses: What would be the potential effects of granting greater freedom to the professional nurse for independent action in the care of aged terminally ill patients? Would you recommend this, and if so, under what circumstances? The responses to this question are analyzed and discussed later in this chapter.

BEST LIKED THINGS OR CONDITIONS

The practitioners' responses to the open-ended questions on best and least liked things or conditions were coded in eight categories on the basis of some preliminary experience with the data. In the resultant tabulation of responses from all three ranks of nursing practitioners, the most "like-able" aspect of geriatric nursing turned out to be the satisfactions derived from the staff-patient relationships. With a third or more in the three ranks considering this their biggest reward, the significance of this recompence appears outstanding.* When we recall and consider the "bargaining at the bedside" concept (see Chap. 1), the finding can be interpreted as a way of saying that whatever the aged ill have to give—perhaps in intangibles—for the nursing care that they receive, this element constitutes for nurse practitioners a major compensating component, and largely irrespective of their nursing rank.

A nurse aide commented:

> I like old people. I feel very close to them. Some have helped me with my personal problems. Some say funny things. I like to know about their history. Many of them have lived interesting lives and I learn from them. The aged seem to have affection for me. Perhaps

---

* NA's, 36.3 percent; LPN's, 40.4 percent; RN's, 33.3 percent. See Appendix B, Table 14, Item 5.

it is because I took care of my grandmother when she was sick. She died in our house and I dressed her after she died. These people are like my own relatives—they need me.

And another:

They are all so nice—they are like my grandparents. My grandparents were nice. Older people are affectionate. You do little things for them and they throw an arm around you and kiss you—they are so grateful, it just makes you feel good inside. They will say, "Tina, you are my friend—I love you." You try to ease their heartache and they repay you a thousand-fold.

A licensed practical nurse in charge of a unit declared:

The elderly are marvelous to work with. They appreciate so much what you do for them. Men as well as women are adorable and I love to see them happy. They are part of my life. A human being needs to give love as well as receive love—otherwise you just die.

Some of our people here have accomplished so much in their lives and now they are old and forgotten. They deserve more respect than people generally give them. You want for these people what you want for yourself in later years—you run a bank for your old age.

An RN, a director of nursing, said:

I appreciate the friendship that comes with their being able to trust me and, by so doing, perhaps they live their last days with a little more joy and comfort. I love them and enjoy them for what they once were and for what they are now. They can be interesting, help- ful, noble, humorous, grateful, angry, proud, loving—in short, they are no different from any other segment of the population, only older and perhaps wiser.

The consensus of this group of practitioners appears to be that their elderly patients are quite remarkable and in many ways a joy to be with. The smallest thing pleases them and they are grateful for all the little things one does for them. They can be fun to be with and interesting to talk to. One can learn from them, for some of them are very wise.

They admit that some patients are moody at times or difficult to care for; some are withdrawn and not easy "to reach" and they often try your patience—but you realize that they are old and ill and that this is the end of the road for them. An RN reflected the sentiment expressed by many of these nurses when she stated, "The 'what I don't like' is eclipsed so much by 'what I do like.' "

The next highest ranking compensation, identified again by all three ranks of practitioners, contributed an illuminating concept that seems closely related to the former idea. It consists of nursing satisfactions relevant to the fulfillment of altruistic sentiments and purposes, including religious, moral, and philosophical inclinations. Approximately a fourth of each of the three nursing groups made this choice.*

Some of these practitioners expressed an inner need to feel useful, to be of help to others, to do something worthwhile. Some indicated that they felt impelled to care for the aged ill because they are the "forgotten people" in our society. So often their families don't want them. They put an aged parent into a home where they can forget about them. A nurse aide elaborated:

> We get so many here who are all alone or whose families have left them here to die. Sometimes a mother can give up the best years of her life to bring up her children, but often the children feel no responsibility to take care of the mother. This is wrong.
>
> When you get them to walk a step or to dress themselves, they give you a smile and it makes your entire day all right. They are grateful for even the smallest thing you do for them. It gives you satisfaction because these people really need you; you grow to know them and to love them; we miss them when they die.

An RN related:

> We try to rebuild in them a sense of dignity and to alleviate their loneliness. One of our patients is the widow of a former ambassador. She has lost everyone and everything and has no one close. Loneliness and not being wanted is suffering. Another patient keeps telling us that he is here because his son could not both take care of him *and* educate his children. In his son's home this patient had for 2 years been kept in his room without going out. He was kept like that—a prisoner.
>
> Still another patient had been on public welfare. She had lived alone, very isolated, and she came here because her case worker felt that she could no longer manage on her own. For many years her children had seen very little of their mother. Their parents had separated many years before, and the children left home, one by one as soon as they left school. When she came here she was so withdrawn that no one was able to get a response from her. She would just sit wherever we put her and stare into space. We contacted her children, but when they visited she would not talk to them. Then came Christmas and the staff gave her a doll. She almost fiercely grabbed it and she has held onto it ever since. Before long she began to talk to this doll, and since then, in a low monologue, keeps confiding to the doll much of the pent-up feelings of bitterness and hostility that were part of her life. Of late she has begun to respond when the staff talk to her.

* NA's, 27.5 percent; LPN's, 28.8 percent; RN's, 21.0 percent. See Appendix B, Table 14, Item 7.

A director of nursing stated that she first entered the field because of her need to make someone comfortable and give personalized care which she had not been able to do in the hospital in which she had worked. Then, when her peers criticized her for working in a nursing home and kept telling her that as a nurse she was lowering herself, it became a challenge. "I was hurt by their attitude and half in anger I set about improving patient care and raising work standards."

A few practitioners indicated that "in order to be a whole person, you have to give to others and be interested in something beyond yourself." Others who believed in doing a good deed, such as caring for the aged ill, said that recompense will not be wanting and God will bless them for helping a fellow human being.

A dedicated and experienced male nurse, who evidently enjoys taking care of geriatric patients, said:

> People should respect the elderly more than they do. In China, old people are considered wise. When old folks come here, I like to make them feel like the Chinese—the wise ones.

An LPN added another dimension to patient care:

> I fill a need. They look for you in the morning, and when you have been off for a weekend they tell you how much they have missed you. They want to know how you are and ask about your children.
> I have brought my children here many times. Just now my children are practicing carols they want to sing here. The children enjoy coming here, but they ask, "Why do they make such a fuss over us?"

Some of these practitioners entered the field because of altruism; others had ulterior motives for working in a geriatric facility and stayed on because they found a great deal of satisfaction in their work. This is illustrated by an RN:

> I live close by. When my children no longer needed me I looked for work, but did not want to work in a hospital because of the pressures there and, also, because I had been out of nursing for many years. So I decided to apply here.
> At first I saw only the hideous side. Old people are not pretty—and the work can be very frustrating. But soon you get to know them as individuals; you begin to see the inner person and you grow to love them. I have the same feeling toward them as I have toward my children—they are my children now and they need me. It is also "but for the grace of God, there go I."

The third priority is somewhat less definable than the above two concepts. About a tenth of both the NA and LPN groups, and a fifth of the RN's, expressed their priority compensations in nonspecific terms, but which do not seem unrelated to the above two ideas. Their preferences were couched in more general phrases such as having a sincere liking for geriatrics or enjoying taking care of old people.*

The two top "job satisfactions" of geriatric nursing personnel, when combined, constitute a majority of chosen best things in spite of the fact that eight categories of "best things" were available for coding of the responses.

When we add to these two the third highest priority in best things —the general positive statements—the results show very impressive majorities of best liked things or conditions identified by all three ranks of geriatric nursing staff, accounting for more than three fourths in each of these ranks. (Table 14, total of Items 5, 7, and 8.)

It should be noted, also, that the very lowest or most neglected code category was the staff-relatives' relationship including society's general attitude toward the aged. Not a single respondent named this as a best liked aspect of her or his experience in geriatric nursing.

LEAST LIKED THINGS OR CONDITIONS

Responses to the corresponding question, the naming of two or three things or conditions liked the very "least," lent themselves to coding under an identical eight-category plan. There was less agreement on what geriatric nursing personnel consider the most disliked thing or condition in their work situation, but their choices tended to confirm the former selection of best things.

Approximately a fifth of both the LPN's and the RN groups and a third of the NA's considered personnel policies the most unrewarding single item in their work situation.† Among the RN's, however, this category vied with that of frustrating interstaff relationships for top priority in dissatisfactions.

Inadequacies or unfairness in tangible or material compensations included wages and fringe benefits, such as hospital insurance or retirement plans; policies concerning time schedules, sick and vacation leaves, and the

---

* NA's, 11.8 percent; LPN's, 13.5 percent; RN's, 21.0 percent. See Appendix B, Table 14, Item 8.
† NA's, 33.3 percent; LPN's, 20.0 percent; RN's, 22.2 percent. See Appendix B, Table 15, Item 2.

number of holidays allowed per annum. Among the nurse aides, particularly, wages often were considered to be far from adequate, and some expressed the belief that low wages was a major reason for the perennial staff turnover in their particular institutions. Others found fault with time schedules. Several NA's said that they would appreciate having more weekends off—"the nurses seem to manage more than a weekend a month off." Others found it a hardship to be required to work so many Sundays— "I hardly ever have a Sunday off; if it were not for the patients I would have left here long ago." In another institution the criticism dealt with having no set policy on increments and with salary increases being made more on the basis of favoritism than on ability. Said one nurse, "We are told not to tell anyone how much money we get." An occasional nurse suggested that a dietitian be employed to supervise patients' diets or at least a cook or chef who is knowledgeable in dietetics. Others suggested that in geriatric institutions there is need for social workers.

Some staff members considered poor pay a major reason for staff shortages, but others blamed administration policy for setting unreasonable limits on the number and ratio of the different categories of staff to be employed for X number of patients. The implication was that lack of time does not permit staff to provide adequate patient care or that there is insufficient time, beyond that required for physical care, for meeting some social needs of their patients. It was repeatedly stressed, also, that elderly persons become quickly upset and agitated when there is insufficient time for meeting their needs.

Some of the RN's who were critical of administration policy stated that if they knew more about their patients' backgrounds they would be able to do more for them and with them. In some institutions, the personal histories of patients evidently are kept in the social service department or in the administrator's office and generally are not available to nurses. Indications are, also, that some institutions show little concern for a patient's background beyond medical and economic factors.

Fewer RN's found their salaries inadequate than did the NA's. In fact, a nursing director named her high salary as the number one incentive for remaining in her position, while in the same institution ancillary staff voiced dissatisfaction with monetary and other material compensations.

For the second and the third top priority for least liked things or conditions, two areas vied with one another: frustrations in interstaff relations and staff-patient relationships. The NA's considered staff-patient relationships the more frustrating of the two, with 21 percent of them indicating this category, and only 6 percent named interstaff relations. The opposite is seen in the figures for the RN's, of whom 22 percent named interstaff relations and only 6 percent pointed to staff-patient relationships as being very frustrating or unsatisfactory. The licensed practical nurses are more evenly divided between these two categories.*

The following are some representative responses concerning least liked aspects in interstaff and in staff-patient relationships:

Nurse Aides:

> I'd like to replace some aides; some are mean when talking with patients—even slapping them—or they don't bathe them properly—but they are careful *when* they do it; one aide here is lazy and it irks the rest of us.

> When I have to go to a floor and am given assignments and no one explains to me about the patients. You should know something about a patient before you take care of him—he may get upset.

> Unfairness in assigning patients—the nurse in charge thinks the aides are below her.

> Demanding patients: you do your best and they still say hurtful things. Some patients are ungrateful, some are selfish—I don't like it when a patient treats me like a maid.

> When I can't get patients to do things—when they bicker—you must sometimes be firm with them to get them to do things.

> Incontinent patients and the very disoriented—the real psychos —that's hard.

> Caring for very senile patients—it brings death closer—working here gives you food for thought—you realize there are different stages in dying.

> When they die—but I try not to be emotional—when someone dies, the girls all get upset.

> When a patient is upset—I may have approached him the wrong way. . . .

Licensed practical nurses:

> Supervising the aides; you have to keep your eyes and ears open; you cannot have aides who say one thing and then do another—we have a shortage of competent aides.

* Frustrating personnel relationships: NA's, 6.7 percent; LPN's, 16.0 percent; RN's, 22.2 percent. Frustrating staff-patient relations: NA's, 21.1 percent; LPN's, 12.0 percent; RN's, 6.9 percent. See Appendix B, Table 15, Items 4 and 5.

What I don't like is not being able to do bedside nursing—I am happier when the aide is off and I get to do bedside care.

I wish I could do something about the help—too many don't give a dollars' worth of work. When you do something a little extra for a sick patient the other nurses call you names.

I don't like to be accused of stealing—and when a patient has an accident—but you can't really be angry with them.

I wish I could do something about incontinency besides diapering them. I can't fathom the idea of putting old people into homes.

When a patient is admitted and has been neglected mentally and physically—some have been permitted to lose contact with the world—a patient comes here sometimes debilitated mentally and physically—in hospitals you are concerned with the living, but here you are concerned with the dying.

When patients make themselves sicker than they really are; when they complain without reason—the chronic complainers.

The fact that this is the end road for them; you live in old age before you reach your own old age—you face old age daily; you cannot forget about it.

When patients are sloppy—senility and poor vision is the reason for this—it's hard to keep some of them clean. Its depressing sometimes—so many helpless people without hope.

Registered nurses:

Disappointment in my peers; aides who are petty and uncooperative —I hate firing people. How I wish I could imbue some of my coworkers with my ideals and interest, having them see patients as whole persons.

There should be more cooperation between the different tours of duty. In theory the A.M. nurse is in charge 24 hours, but it does not work because for 16 hours you are not here, and the nurses on the different shifts do what they want to do.

Nurses who are cruel; aides who are uncooperative; and when a patient wishes to die, the staff not being ready to let him go.

The nursing supervisor who says, "Do as I say, not as I do. Friction between RN's and LPN's.

When a patient develops decubitus ulcers—we often get them like that from the hospital. It's hard to see people you grow to love decline so rapidly before your eyes.

When they get particularly stubborn and difficult to reason with I feel frustrated and impatient, and disturbed patients you cannot help—too many tranquilizers sometimes. When you become attached to people and they are transferred to mental hospitals—you feel it more than death—not being able to do more for them.

It is conceivable that respective positions in the nursing hierarchy with their differing functions and responsibilities largely account for the reversal of NA and RN figures for least liked aspects in interpersonal relationships discussed above. Nurse aides generally are closer to the bedside and spend much more time with patients than do the registered nurses. According to one nursing supervisor, aides give 99 percent of the care provided for their patients. The RN usually is further away from the bedside, but it is she who is responsible for making staff assignments and planning for overall staff coverage, depending on whether hers is a head nurse, supervising or director position. This situational element may account for the fact that more nurse aides reported frustrating staff-patient situations, whereas the registered nurse finds interpersonnel relations the more aggravating of these two social factors.

Reference should be made to another possible variable which was shown by the data to strongly influence the practitioners when they responded to the questions on the best and the least liked aspects of their work with aged patients. This variable is the individualized social structure within which a respondent finds himself or herself.

The variant here is not the type of administration, whether non-profit, profit-making, or public; nor the particular admissions policy, whether open or restrictive. Rather, it is the social milieu—factors such as organizational pattern, policies dealing with patient care and with personnel, communication, degree of permissiveness—which appeared to influence nursing respondents when they identified certain best and least liked aspects of the work situation.

Following are some of the organizational differences reflected by the data:

Some institutions have a well-defined goal or purpose toward which to strive; others have not;

In some facilities the democratic principle prevails; in others the organization follows a more or less authoritarian pattern;

In some places well qualified and dedicated professionals occupy key positions; in others this may not be so;

In some institutions one finds dynamic in-service programs; in others there are none;

In some nursing departments the staff is encouraged to make suggestions and express ideas about possible improvements in patient care or welfare of staff; in others staff is discouraged from expressing such opinions;

In some organizations every staff member is respected no matter how "lowly" the job and is made to feel an essential and worthwhile part of the larger group; in others this may not be true;

In some institutions the profit motive is of uppermost concern; in others the service principle prevails—service for the aged ill who are dependent on others for help.

In certain geriatric facilities staff orientation and in-service education are geared to help the staff understand about the human aging processes, including some of the why's of untoward patient behavior. Clarification of the why's of various patient behaviors, for example seeing overt acts of hostility as being symptomatic of stresses the patient experiences, is said by staff to make them more accepting of such conduct. A nurse aide explained, "You cannot really be angry with a patient who accuses you of stealing when you know he is ill and would not do that if he were well. We are told about those things in staff conferences." Concomitantly, such on-going education may reinforce an individual staff member's feelings of doing an essential job and being an important and respected member of the nursing team. Such programs may also serve as incentives for improving one's work performance.

The three top choices of best liked things or conditions did not seem sensitive to the individual milieu; but from a negative perspective, they evidently were, particularly as these concerned the second or third choice: institutional policy and interpersonnel relationships, and, to a lesser extent, staff-patient relationships.

In all fairness it should be stated that some practitioners, though their number was small, lauded interpersonnel staff relationships. They stressed the value of conferences and pointed to harmonious working relations and teamwork. Nurse aides praised the understanding and fairness as well as helpfulness of RN's in various positions, and registered nurses spoke of competent and cooperating aides.

Finally, it should be noted that the positive and the negative statements were not always mutually exclusive. In fact, on occasion a disliked, frustrating, or negative element identified by a respondent might serve to reinforce a positive aspect within the work situation. Thus, a nurse might select as a least liked item the indifferent or demanding attitude exhibited by certain co-workers toward her patients, while at the same time, choosing as a best liked item the harmonious staff-patient relationship, or an altruistic aspect, such as the opportunity to serve those who are neglected in our society. Perhaps, paradoxes such as these augur well for the future of geriatric nursing.

GREATER FREEDOM FOR THE PROFESSIONAL NURSE IN GERIATRICS

Reference was made earlier in this chapter to a question addressed to the degree registered nurses on granting greater freedom for independent action to the professional nurse in geriatrics—an issue somewhat related to the possible work satisfactions discussed in the foregoing pages (see p. 231).

The question met with very considerable response by the DRN group. While some reticence and caution were shown, for the most part, the replies were ample for the purpose, well thought out, and stated with pertinent qualifications.

Categories for coding the responses were first divided into negative and positive decisions on the critical issue: "Would you recommend this?" These were then subdivided into the qualifying grounds indicated for reaching either decision.

The tabulations revealed that slightly more than a third of those responding made clearly negative statements; affirmative responses added up to slightly more than half. About ten percent of those responding made statements which did not lend themselves for coding as either opposing or supporting the critical issue of greater freedom for professional nurses in geriatric services.

Present day practices in this area vary widely. In some geriatric facilities, physicians' standing orders cover a wide variety of treatments such as enemata, laxatives, cough syrups, and the like, while medications such as tranquilizers are frequently prescribed on a p.r.n. basis. In some other facilities, however, the nurse is much more dependent upon the physician for specific treatments when a patient exhibits untoward symptoms of one kind or another. It is suggested by some nurses that often doctors do not leave adequate orders for the needs of aged patients; on the other hand, one of the DRN's pointed out that, "Nurses must not practice medicine." Various studies have shown, and it is to some extent supported by this one, that doctors often are less interested in caring for geriatric patients than for those who are younger. A DRN commented that in her experience she found that "doctors frequently avoid care of the aged terminally ill and leave it all up to the nurse. Frequently there is too little rather than too much direction in this type of patient care." And the observation is again made that in some nursing homes when a patient expires, the physician does not go to the home to certify a person's death, though the doctor's signature is required on the death certificate.

It seems to be recognized by most of the respondents, whether they take an indecisive or a firm stand on the issue, that the question touches upon the currently exciting and controversial matter of independent versus dependent decision-making prerogatives of qualified professional nurses and, also, upon the potential degree of satisfaction which nurses may derive from their geriatric patient care. The issue is of sufficient importance on both counts to justify detailed examination of the DRN comments and the qualifications that they make to either negative or positive stands that they take on the question.

Negative Position

The response of this group,* summarily and bluntly stated, is:

> No. Nurses, even professional nurses, do not need more freedom than they now have; and the effects upon themselves and the patients and their relatives are not likely to be good.

However, very few of their comments are quite as bluntly expressed and with the issue closed by a period. Several of them say "no" on the premise that it would be dangerous to extend the nurse's prerogatives and would constitute intrusions into other fields such as medicine, social work, religion, and the like. Most of the negative responses are buttressed by the claim either that nurses already have sufficient freedom as well as the physician's permission and backing to exercise their potential knowledge and skills, or that it is not a question of granting more freedom to the nurse but of cultivating her intraprofessional concern and cooperation and in the development of good relations with other disciplines. This is briefly summed up by one DRN:

> If the nurse uses all the latitude she has today with the opportunity to make judgments, thinking out ways that are creative and beneficial for the welfare of the patient, I think this is enough. If she just waits until the doctor tells her what to do—if this is her policy—then I think greater freedom and exercise of independent action is indicated. In most cases the physician will be delighted if we exercise some independent judgments (with tact) and have some useful ideas to propose. (Sr. Agnes Miriam)

* 35.9 percent. See Appendix B, Table 16, Items 1 to 3.

The theme of the negative response group is that registered nurses have always had greater freedom than they have elected to accept. Freedom carries with it responsibility for the result of one's actions, and this is often frightening to the nurse. Nurses have been known to secure orders from physicians to cover a course of action they deemed best and then failed to take responsibility for any effects from such measures, saying "the doctor ordered it."

The nurse routinely exercises responsibility for keeping the physician informed on the condition and needs of a patient, for summoning him when she considers that the condition of the patients warrants such action, and for suggesting the services of other professionals when the patient indicates to her any need for their services. While nurses in recent years have been carrying out more and more procedures formerly considered solely the prerogative of the doctor, there seems to be little likelihood for any formal turning over of decision-making functions from medicine to nursing, at least not in the foreseeable future. The key functional concepts are communication, understanding, and cooperation in the care of the patient.

The nurse, however professional, still occupies a position in which she needs the physician's orders for therapy around which to plan comprehensive care, even for the dying patient; and she would seem to have already a sufficiently large professional realm within which to function effectively—without expanding her jurisdiction into other fields such as medicine, social work, religion, and the like.

Thus, according to this group, the freedom for independent action to make the last months, days, or moments of the geriatric patient more comfortable is available to the nurse if and when she determines to use it. Physicians are usually most cooperative about letting a nurse do what she proposes or wants to do and is competent to undertake. If she presents what she thinks should be done for her terminally ill aged patient to his physician, he may be glad enough to have an interested nurse share more of his responsibility for the dying person. More and more doctor's orders will conform to what the nurse thinks appropriate if her competence is established and she is able to tell the doctor details of the patient's problems and observations of how he responds to treatment. And one DRN contends that if the nurse uses a bit of womanly diplomacy, she can get many of her requests filled by the physician. "This may not be regarded as a professional approach, but it is an effective feminine approach to the dominant male."

Some of the DRN's wondered about the exact meaning of "greater freedom." They queried whether it means greater freedom than is currently practiced by nurses, greater than legally and conventionally tolerated by the public and physicians, greater than the nurse exercises with younger patients with better prospects of recovery, or more than she may have now simply by tactfully and considerately taking it? Some indicated, also, that usually there is little competition for the care of aged dying patients, particularly if they are in a nursing home or similar long-term facility. "Often no one in the health team cares for them except the nurse, and sometimes she doesn't to any noteworthy degree."

Other adherents to the negative position hold that few good effects are likely to result from the formal granting of greater freedom for independent action to the professional nurse in her care of aged terminally ill patients. They argue or imply that further withdrawal from and neglect of those patients by the medical profession would have additional adverse effects upon geriatric care, since the nurses take their cues from physicians and, hence, might become increasingly neglectful of their aged, hopelessly ill patients.

Still others indicated that there is no proof that the care of the elderly would be enhanced if medical participation were less. They emphasize that both medicine and nursing are needed in the care of the aged: "Neither without the other can be as good as both together at their very best." (Macquin, Patrick, Proctor, Puddy, Kerrigan, Vacca, Wald, White.)

Affirmative Position

More than half of the degree registered nurses took an affirmative position on this issue, but with certain qualifications.* Usually their answers, whether expressed or implied to be "yes," are followed by an interpretation on the meaning or implication of greater freedom or on grounds upon which the decision was reached. Two major provisos are repeatedly emphasized in the responses. Some would advocate greater freedom of independent action for professional nurses *if* certain limits are set and certain safeguards established, legal and otherwise; others would grant such freedom only to those nurses who by education, experience, and personal characteristics are well qualified to exercise such freedom and ready to assume responsibility for their actions and decisions.

Some of these DRN's indicated that it would be all right for the nurse to have more freedom if the physician would give routine standing orders to cover some of the more usual needs, such as medication for pain or sleep inducement, enema or laxative for sluggish bowels—remedies which are designed to alleviate mild indispositions. They held that in these areas the professional nurse should be able to exercise good judgment, know her limitations, and recognize when she should call the physician for the patient's needs beyond the regular visits, the presumption being that the doctor would continue to make regular visits.

---

* 54.0 percent. See Appendix B, Table 16, Items 4 to 6.

Some DRN's took note only of legal formalized limitations. A few would recommend greater freedom for the nurse if legal safeguards were set up to protect her or him. Others pointed to possible social as well as legal implications if the nurse were given responsibilities that are now considered to be the exclusive prerogative of the medical doctor. It was noted that at present in an emergency situation when no qualified member of the medical profession is available the registered nurse may be obliged to perform certain functions that ordinarily are considered medical, and that in most places in the United States the nurse is protected by law for this. To extend this to nonemergency situations—to make this a regular practice—would require not only a change in the laws that govern medical and nursing practice, but also a change in societal values as well. The issue extends to whether organized medicine is ready to relinquish and organized nursing ready to assume the responsibility, and also, whether the public being served is ready to accept such changes.

The largest number of DRN respondents favoring greater freedom for the professional nurse in their care of aged terminally ill patients made such freedom provisional to the qualifications of the individual nurse, recognizing that many RN's do not qualify and should not assume such responsibility.* The proposed criteria included sound nursing education and experience with special clinical training in psychology, psychiatry, and theories of human development and decline. In addition, the nurse was expected to have developed a sustaining personal philosophy of life and death and to manifest sincere interest in, and willingness to learn about, aged patients and their families. Such a nurse should be able and prepared to talk naturally and freely about death with patients and families if and when either are concerned and appear ready. She should also show firm tendencies to confer and cooperate freely with teammates and the physician about nursing plans for critically ill patients, remaining flexible and adaptive to the individuality and dignity of each patient. It was deemed essential, also, that she be prepared and willing to forthrightly accept responsibility for her independent nursing actions. Finally, it was regarded as no less important that she possess rare ability to renew and replenish her spent reserves after any very trying situation.

Some of these nurses expressed the belief that a well-prepared nurse with an adequate staff could do a better job in providing care for aged dying patients than is being accomplished at present in our care-giving institutions. Commented one DRN:

> An atmosphere of composure and security, described so well by Dr. Cicely Saunders, could be developed in such a setting. If the staff could be trained by such a well-prepared nurse and given frequent

---

* 32.6 percent. See Appendix B, Table 16, Item 5.

opportunities to plan nursing care on an individual patient basis, the level of care would almost certainly rise. Instead of abandonment and isolation, we would see closeness and security for both the patient and the family, and possibly also for the nurse. When well-prepared nurses are given greater freedom and responsibility in this care, there is very likely to appear the type of caring demonstrated by Dr. Saunders— where "the faithful hand of the living does not desert the hand of the dying." (Shumway)

Another DRN contends:

Perhaps the least, if not the best, that a nurse can do for an aged terminally ill person is to make dying as painless as possible without hastening the end. If ever an individual's personal rights and privileges are to be honored, the time comes at the ending of a long life. (Donaldson)

A very few DRN's envisioned organizational and situational changes which would promote wider liberties in which the professional nurse might exercise greater independent action. One of such changes would be the establishment of medical-nursing boards which would be charged with setting up standard procedures and delineating areas of practice. Another would involve the establishment of designated wards or "nursing beds" in the general hospital to which patients would be transferred on a referral basis by the physician:

If the practice of assigning leadership to the professional nurse for the care of aged terminally ill patients were in effect in the general hospital, I think many "heroic measures" at the time of death of elderly persons without potentials for recovery would be avoided. I see the possibility of the turning over of such patients to the nursing leadership well before the event of death to be at least as reasonable as the turning over of normal hospital deliveries to the trained nurse-midwife. The major provisos are that the nurses have special preparation for the care of the dying patient and knowingly accept responsibility for his care and that physicians be available for consultation whenever their special skills are needed. . . .

When it is clear that further medical intervention is not in the interest of the dying patient, patients might be transferred to the hospital's satellite nursing home; but they ought still to have fine medical consultation available to them for both its physical and psychological value. When a doctor is *needed,* no nurse replaces him. When a nurse is *needed,* as she is when the dying patient's requirement is for excellent nursing care, the patient will benefit by being in a special nursing unit, staffed, equipped, and placed to provide a dignified end to life . . .

Desertion of the patient by the doctor leaves a vacuum which no nurse can fill. And desertion always occurs—at least symbolically, if a doctor "pulls out" and a nurse "takes over" without planning with a

conscious patient or his family. When family and patient understand
the purpose, I have seen this transfer of responsibility work very well
indeed. (Schwartz)

Some DRN's emphasize that other positive effects would almost
naturally ensue. Improvement in the care provided for aged dying patients under the leadership of well-qualified professional nurses would
doubtless lead to improvement in the overall standards of geriatric care
—to the point where geriatrics would be considered a very prestigious
nursing specialty. From this it would almost naturally follow that promising and well qualified nurses would be attracted to this field. A DRN
briefly elaborates:

> Yes, I would recommend greater freedom for the professional nurse to
> exercise independent decision making and practice in the care of aged
> terminally ill patients and others as well. But the nurse would have to
> be prepared to accept greater responsibility and to pay the penalty
> for making bigger mistakes when she does. Some nurses, indeed many,
> are not prepared to take this kind of risk—it may have been for this
> reason that they chose nursing rather than medicine. On the other
> hand, if nurses had responsibility for independent action, in time
> women prepared to function at this level would be attracted into the
> nursing profession. It is likely that increased responsibility for inde-
> pendent action will come soonest in certain areas such as care of the
> aged because of less resistance to it there. Physicians may be glad to
> let competent nurses take over the continuing care of the aged with
> themselves performing as medical consultants. Perhaps this is what
> geriatric nursing has to offer; for it needs something special to attract
> able and promising young nurses into the field. (Conn)

Another DRN provides personal testimony supporting greater freedom and responsibility to professional nurses in their care of aged dying
patients:

> The potential effects could enhance both the care and comfort of the
> aged patient and his family. My own personal experience with the
> independent decisions and actions of nurses under the conditions of
> my father's imminent death bears this out.
>   The fact that the physician-surgeon, both the private physician
> and the hospital officer, were unable to, or disinclined to cope
> with the realities of the impending death as related either to my father
> or to me, left the nursing staff to exercise independent judgment and
> action in such an excellent manner that I feel my father received
> every detail of consideration and care that either he or I could wish
> for.
>   It started with consideration of the staff for my wishes that ex-
> traordinary lifesaving measures not be instituted and that my father's
> comfort provide the sense of direction that nursing care would follow.
> In succession came detailed judgments on what my father could and

should eat and how much to encourage him to take food or fluids and when to leave it to his expressed wishes; decisions on how to cope with his incontinence in the light of his needs for comfort and peace of mind; perception of his low tolerance for pain and his need to have natural measures applied; their way of keeping me informed on changes in his condition that signified approaching death; and, then, their calm and empathetic sharing of my grief as well as their immediate response when I impulsively turned on the call light when he expired and their staying with me until I regained control of my emotions—all these attentive considerations were immeasurable sources of support.

Their seemingly intuitive recognition of need and sense of timing and their respect for my privacy as they reminded me and made available to me the means of notifying the rest of the family and then their thoroughness in providing accommodations and privacy for me and for others as we waited for the physician were all, to us in our grief, indicative of their recognition and understanding of our needs. Incidently, such treatment leads me to feel that the nurse would generally be better equipped than the physician to obtain permission for autopsy.

It is also my feeling that medical education is sadly lacking in its foresight to prepare the physician to meet the needs of the patient of the family during the recognized period of terminal illness or actual death. The typical physician is all too obvious in his bewilderment and ineptitude or lack of interest in coping with either situation. (Quinlan)

16 Care of the Dying

The relief and comfort of aged patients should be our aim.
WORCESTER

Death has many faces and individuals meet and cope with it in very different ways. Death comes to one person suddenly and with little or no warning; to another, after repeated alarms or a prolonged illness. One is wracked with pain; another seemingly dies without pain. One appears totally unprepared; another seems ready and waiting—even praying for death. One is conscious and aware of what is happening; another unconscious and unknowing. One dies with mental poise and peace; another is fearful and greatly disturbed. One craves for, and clings to, human contacts right up to the end; another appears to want to depart entirely alone. One may have a chance to plan his passing; another may be denied such opportunity or any choice, being subject to the necessity of circumstances or the dictates of designated or responsible attendants who are "in charge." In the eyes of associates, and even attendants, one death is viewed as a lamentable defeat for all concerned; another as a commendable victory. But usually it is between these extremes that most aged persons take their places and make their exits.

Differences in the ways aged persons die, or might wish to die if and when able to exercise a choice, cover so wide a range that special caution is called for on the part of anyone who would attempt to generalize about senescent death or to identify and define patterns of uniformity in dying.*

In the present exposition, certain of the most common axioms about dying are challenged by nurses who care for dying patients. For example, the broad statement that every human being is afraid of dying does not meet with nursing consensus. Many geriatric nurses from their own ex-

* Simmons, Leo W. *Role of the Aged in Primitive Society.* New Haven, Yale University Press, 1945, Chap. 8. (It is being republished in 1970.)

periences with dying patients related instances of aged patients expressing a readiness to die, even pleading to be allowed to die. Some dying patients were said to have taken "affairs into their own hands" by refusing food offered to them or pulling out nasal tubes and needles inserted into their flesh or veins for providing their bodies with nourishment or fluids. "And these are people who know what they are doing," commented an RN who had been caring for geriatric patients for a number of years. Among the DRN's, also, this widely held view about fear of death is challenged. One of them comments as follows:

> A concern that I have had for some time is that I keep hearing professional people, especially in the psychiatric field, state quite positively that "everyone is afraid of dying."
> My own experience with many persons afflicted with long-term, chronic illness, as well as with the aged, is that I do not find this totally substantiated. For some patients, yes, of course; but I find many individuals who are not afraid of death, but are rather afraid of living, especially in the 45 to 50 age group. In the older groups, many people have said to me, "It is a relief to be able to say to a nurse, "I want to die," or "I am not afraid; I have had my life," and so forth. Some of these individuals tell me without my asking, "If I said this to So-and-so, I would be thought of as depressed. . . ."
> I cannot but wonder if we do not make it very hard for the person who isn't afraid but wants to talk over his feelings and thoughts with an understanding person who will listen and believe what he says—and whom he respects. (Taylor)

It is not difficult to find contrasting or qualifying statements on the same or similar subject. The following are a few selected anchor ideas from nurses who are concerned with caring for aged dying patients. They are drawn from the data collected for this document and represent counterpoised points of view:

1. Although death is admitted to be as inevitable as birth is natural, avoidance patterns in our contemporary culture discourage free and frank discussion of it, even with the very aged; and this has special relevance to nursing care.

2. In spite of the fact that death is viewed as the opposite of life, the progress of dying (however brief or prolonged) is generally regarded as part of living and, perhaps, a climax of it. The idea that a person's long-established "style of life" sets a pattern for the way he dies can carry important implications for his nursing care.

3. As a final expression of life on earth, dying generally takes on for human beings a special significance, both for the departing and for the

involved survivors. Certain aspects of preparedness, propriety, dignity, honor, valor, courage, self-control, endurance, peace of mind, and reverent awe are, as a rule, commendably associated with the act of dying well. Any and all of these tend to make for an appropriate fulfillment and closure to life; and the nurse is coming to hold a more and more important place in the achievement of such a closure.

4. Granting the possibility of an aware, deliberative, and participating role for the patient at one end of a continuum and an unconscious, nondeliberative and passive role at the other end, it is clarifying to recognize two practical stages in dying: the psychological death of a self-aware and responding personality and the biological death of the vital processes of the organs and the organism—and any separation in time of these two types of dying carry import for nursing care.

5. In contrast to death in childhood or youth, death in late age is generally regarded in our culture as more timely, natural, and conducive to a sense of fulfillment. However, it can and often does become a deprivating and deplorable experience—a situation that calls for correction and permits opportunities for improvements in nursing care.

6. One very promising approach to improvements in nursing care lies in a more thorough identification and understanding of the basic needs of ill and elderly persons. Once we have found what it is (it takes) to give the dying aged person most comfort and strength in the fulfillment of *his* needs, we are on the way to accomplishing as much as our earthly powers may offer.

7. Optimum nursing care of the aged dying patient stands the best chance of achievement by nurses who, in addition to their professional knowledges and skills, have come to terms with the prospect of death for themselves and are prepared and willing to go through the process of dying with each of their patients as fully as his needs require and in a manner that fits the style of his life. This calls, of course, for professional giving of the self and may also mean that while "many are called, few are chosen" for that quality of nursing.

That nurses also react in very different ways to death is, no doubt, a truism, but one that bears repeating in a discourse on care of the dying. The care that nurses provide for their aged fatally ill patients is bound to reflect, in part, their own interpretations of, and attitudes toward, death, tempered to some degree, of course, by the nursing skills and knowledge that they have acquired, plus some experience with dying patients.

Of the nursing practitioners interviewed, some regarded death as a new start in existence, the beginning of a more glorious life; others considered it to be a form of punishment or the end of everything. Commented one, "Death is man's punishment for being born." Others referred to the familiar old saying that every man owes God a death; and still others would resolve the matter simply by attributing it to the "will of God" and were seemingly unable or unwilling to elaborate on that.

Several of the registered nurses contended that the nurse aides are often reluctant to give care to a patient believed to be near death and that they may even refuse to touch or do anything for someone who has just died. A few of the nurse aides corroborated this by recalling their fears when attending a dying person or when assigned to give postmortem care. Whether fear in the presence of death is related to personal interpretation of its meaning and attitudes held toward it, or to a lack of preparation for the work they are doing, or to the fact that they become familiar with the dying person by spending a great deal of time with him (much more than the registered nurse) appears to be an open question. But it does raise the question of whether there are occasions in geriatric institutions when certain staff fears of death outdo some patients' fear of dying.

Nurses in attendance within the selected geriatric institutions seldom alluded to any special qualifications, or lack of them, for the care of aged dying persons. A few of them did voice feelings of inadequacy for the task. They were rarely specific, however, in the kinds of knowledge, skill, and experience required in helping ill and spent agers to die—much less in helping them *to die well*. This apparent minimal perception of, and concern for, becoming better prepared may be related, somewhat, to the physical, psychological, and social climate within which their assignments are made; a climate in which the subject of death is considered taboo and the signs of impending death are generally denied or ignored, especially in nursing relationships with patients. It turned out, indeed, that the nurse practitioners' responses about desirable qualifications and better preparation of personnel for the care of dying patients proved to be too scanty for any useful classification, coding, and computing.

In contrast to the nurse practitioners, the degree registered nurses made a strong plea for greater preparation of nurses for geriatric care and with special emphasis on the need for knowledge and skill in the care of dying patients. They called for extensive training both in scope and in depth to be included in basic nursing curricula, in graduate nursing programs and in in-service education. They intimated the urgent need for intensive geriatric training by calling attention to the fact that greatly increasing proportions of the population over 65 years of age are now (under Medicare) assured of more constant and improved access to organized medical and health services.

Their thinking ran as follows: in view of the mounting needs and demands for more and better qualified nurses to care for geriatric patients, the nursing profession can ill afford to neglect or postpone extensive education in gerontology and geriatrics or to continue to leave it to any form of haphazard training. Research in geriatric nursing is also greatly needed for improvement of curriculum content. Current nursing concepts and attitudes related to the care of the aged ill call for critical examination and reappraisal. Verified and useful knowledge of the processes of dying under varying conditions is and will remain in great demand. Without special training and supervised experience in the care of dying patients, nurses will continue to find it difficult to sort out their own needs and anxieties from those of their critically ill patients—a fact which so often affects present-day practices adversely. If and when nurses can develop a more objective and matter-of-fact viewpoint toward death, it may become easier and more natural for them to discuss the subject realistically with those who are involved and want to talk about it as it relates to themselves. Improved preparedness of nurses may make it possible for death to be a more manageable and constructive experience for those most intimately concerned—and the help that nurses extend to their dying patients may become far more effective in the future than it has been in the past. (V. Brown, Palmer, Camp, Duxbury, Prock)

Conceivably, there is the possibility that an open and realistic approach to the problem of senescent death may come to be regarded as indication of a general psychological and social change. Indeed, it may be considered a sign of greater cultural maturity when people are able and willing to face death and its problems in a realistic manner, without evading it on the one hand or glorifying it out of proportion on the other hand.*

According to the DRN's, the tendency to ignore or evade the realistic aspects of dying is so ingrained in our contemporary culture that not even those who teach nursing know how to relate naturally to dying persons or to cope frankly and effectively with their problems. And it is said that for a young—or even often a mature—nurse for whom death has never been a subject to be faced realistically, the dying of a particular and familiar person presents threatening aspects that may disrupt helpful relationships with the patient. DRN's emphasize that bringing about desirable changes in this area will require special education and guided experiences. (Baziak, Dithridge, Santorum, Wolanin)

It is often said, by nurses as well as others, that old age provides its own anodyne for late-in-life stresses: a certain dulling of sensations to, or

* While similar ideas were voiced by several DRN's, this particular formulation was contributed by Chaplain Victor J. Drapella, Grand Forks, North Dakota, November, 1967.

increased tolerance for pain; a lowering of the threshold for zestful living; a more temperate desire for goals difficult to obtain; an increase in or adoption of religious faith, or a personal philosophy of adaptation to, and tolerance for, conditions and circumstances in life that defy change and must be lived with. And there are, also, among the aged some individuals who seemingly come to adjusted terms with death and indicate a genuine desire to die when their "time comes." Most elders, over the years, evidently build up their own protective adaptations—each in his own individual way. In the words of one DRN:

> It would seem that many people acquire with age a growing philosophy that helps them in some ways to prepare for their last developmental task, namely, to die well. (Knowles)

SKILLS AND KNOWLEDGE

Concerning the kinds of knowledge required by nurses for the care of aged ill and dying patients, the degree registered nurses identified three major areas of interest and significance: 1) the nurse's knowledge of her patient, 2) knowledge of herself, and 3) knowledge of the processes of dying. More than a third of the DRN's stressed the importance of the geriatric nurse knowing her patient as fully as possible: his background, religio-philosophical orientation, his previous critical experiences along the life course, and the ways in which he learned to cope with them. A similar proportion of them strongly emphasized the importance of the nurse coming to know and understand herself; her own background, beliefs, personal values; and the extent to which she has come to terms with the realities of death as part of life. The third proposal, supported by about one sixth of the DRN group, recommended that the geriatric nurse acquire expert and specific knowledge on the processes of dying, encompassing the physiological, psychological and sociological spheres—especially as these relate to aged persons.

Knowledge of the Patient

A great many of the DRN's contended that the better a nurse comes to know and understand her elderly patient, the greater her chance of being of real help to him.* However this may be, a principal approach suggested by them for helping aged persons to die well is adaptation of

---

* 40.7 percent. See Appendix B, Table 17, Item 1.

nursing care to the patient's individual needs and recognizing that for coping with the crisis of his impending death a patient needs to rely upon his long-established, tried and tested ways in which he has met other crises along his life course. The time is late for unlearning old ways or for learning new ways for making the best of a stressful situation:

> A sensitive and skilled nurse in interpersonal relations will gain direction on what to do and say from accumulated interactions with, and knowledge about, her patient. Some patients will derive a sense of relief just from being able to talk; some will by preference avoid the subject entirely; and some will allude to the prospects of dying and then wait for the nurse to pursue the topic. (O'Koren)

The axiom that as a person has lived, so he will tend to die when the need arises and opportunities permit would appear to contain more than a grain of truth. To the degree that this approach is valid, geriatric nurses may come to recognize and anticipate the more constant threat of death to a person who is aged and ill in contrast to one who is younger and ailing. As a consequence, they may become more alert and sensitive in learning about the individual elder's life patterns and potential for dealing effectively with what may become his terminal illness—and by what means, as well as at what points, nursing help can be most supportive to the particular person.

Even when a threatened death does not occur, its "spectre hovers over" many aged patient-nurse encounters, especially when a person's dying is prolonged or his ailment or condition defies any meaningful prognosis, perhaps with the patient suffering several near-death crises or setbacks before death occurs.

Moreover, there are some elderly persons who are wholly unprepared or unable to meet personal death on their own basis and in a positive manner; and there is evidence, from nursing responses as well as the literature pertinent to the subject, that a great many nurses are at a loss when planning for care and support of such patients.

There is also the possibility that some nurses find the sudden and unexpected deaths of their patients the more difficult to face while others find it harder to plan for and give care in situations where death is long and drawn-out. Nevertheless, opportunities are great for the concerned and perceptive nurse to learn the individualized potentials of particular patients for coping—with help and support—with their final developmental task: dying.

Because of the influence of culture on individuals, it is considered important, also, that the geriatric nurse become familiar with the typical beliefs and attitudes about death and dying as expressed in the different cultures or subcultures from which her patients come, so that she may gain insight for cooperating constructively within the patient's own life context. For example, one person's stoicism and silent forbearance in the face of death may be as much culturally induced as are the tearful laments of another in a similar situation.

Even as culture in some ways molds the individual, so religion has an important part in the lives of many persons. Furthermore, as one grows older, one is more apt to turn to one's faith than during one's younger days —although there are notable exceptions. The nurse who has some familiarity with the different major faiths with understanding of, and respect for, the religious rituals and their symbolic meaning may be in a position of bringing special comfort to a dying patient who depends largely upon his religion to sustain him.

It has been implied and stated in the foregoing discussion that a mark of maturity in a culture or society is open and natural discussion of personal death. And a time may come before long when, even as the expectant mother (usually) makes plans and prepares for the impending birth of her child, plans will be made in advance of a person's anticipated death. Concerning senescent death, a specialist in geriatrics writes:

> Death is really retirement in its fullest sense and retirement occurs gradually. It is usually said that dying occurs in the reverse order of birth and human development or living. The older person dies sociologically, psychologically, and physiologically, in that order. (Knowles)

It is recognized that many elderly persons may have experienced something like a "sociological death" through alienation and severance of identity with their groups prior to entering a geriatric institution. Corresponding signs of "psychological death" may also have occurred, or appear bit by bit, soon after their admission, while physiological death may be greatly postponed. On the other hand, all three phases of dying may occur close together. The implications here for geriatric nursing would seem to be many and very pertinent.

If this be granted, then it certainly should be in order for the nurse to discuss with the attending physician, and perhaps with the patient's family, a nursing plan somewhat in advance of its need—ideally, long before there is need for it. To be sure, a nurse may find that a physician or family or both jointly prefer that the patient not be informed of his critical condition and that there be no discussion on the subject of death. Yet, if the patient overtly or covertly exhibits some indications that he is in need of sharing his thoughts and feelings on the matter, both the nurse and her patient stand to gain from such opportunities. Some of the DRN's propose that in situations such as this the nurse present to the physician, and to the family under his approval, her observations, appraisal, and proposal for a detailed nursing plan for meeting the patient's needs and wants—with the goal of assuring for the patient a minimum of physical and mental stress and, if possible, freedom from any sense of despair or defeat. (Declan, Gorrow, Schwartz, Shumway, Straight, Taylor, Wenrich, Wolanin)

A comprehensive listing of the kinds of information about aged persons that might be useful to a perceptive and skillful nurse in helping a patient through the terminal phase of his life would require many pages and perhaps be impractical as well. However, a brief sampling of exploratory ideas proposed by the responding DRN's may serve an important purpose:

1. It is useful for the nurse to learn, bit by bit, how aware her patient may already be of his nearness to death, how much more he would like to know, and how much in agreement his physician and his family may be in his sharing of knowledge about his terminal diagnosis.

2. It is pertinent for the nurse to know how much illness with suffering the patient has already undergone, how he takes suffering, how much he relies on drugs, and how much more discomfort he is likely to undergo.

3. Further information valuable to the nurse concerns the patient's philosophy and how firmly he adheres to it, and his religious beliefs and practices and how committed he is to them.

4. Equally relevant is knowledge of what his major goals have been, and how completed or abandoned he considers them to be and to what extent his life goals and his present concerns with dying are self-centered or directed toward others whom he considers dependent upon him.

5. On the whole, do the patient's reactions and communications imply a preference on his part to meet death in either a negative and submissive or in a rebellious and protesting way; or, on the other hand, are there indications of a reconciled, positive, and achieving or fulfilling approach? In short, were he still able to prescribe for himself and to carry out a pattern of closure conforming to his established style of life, what would it be like and to what degrees will the nurse be able to help him accomplish it "in his own way."

Nurse's Self-Knowledge

According to DRN testimony, self-knowledge on the part of the nurse is a close second to her knowledge of the patient in any prerequisites for the provision of good geriatric care.* A nurse's personal philosophy of life and death and her adaptations to the realities of illness and dying are regarded as fundamental to her capability to provide skillful and supportive care to her critically ill patients. Time after time it was affirmed that when a nurse finds herself upset and fearful of a pending death, it becomes exceedingly difficult for her to sustain a relationship with her patient within which he can sense assurance, freedom, and reinforcements for seeking some relief from, or resignation to, his loneliness or his stressful thoughts and emotions.

If, on the other hand, the nurse has been able to work through her own disturbances about recurrent death of patients and has achieved a stable and constructive stance toward the fact of mortality for everyone, she is said to possess reserves in both concrete and intangible resources for helping her patient. Probably only then will she be prepared to listen with assurance to whatever her patient would convey to her and be able to respond naturally and with genuine interest, warmth, and readiness to understand and share his experience with him. It is then, and perhaps even without knowing, that she may be able to make a significant contribution to the patient or his intimate survivors or both.

Indeed, the indications are that a nurse's remissness in attempting to clarify and resolve for herself these life-and-death matters in advance of the need to apply herself within the context of terminal crises is viewed by many nursing professionals as a major handicap for giving effective care to dying patients. Such personal life-and-death conflicts are probably intensified for both nurse and physician by their tendency to regard each death as an indication of failure on their part in most, if not all, their patient care commitments. This very tendency can interfere, sometimes drastically, with the care of a patient who cannot recover and who craves to die well, with comfort and dignity. Numerous DRN responses clearly indicate that by education, experience, and guided practice, a nurse can fortify and prepare herself and, in most cases, contribute remarkably well to the terminal needs of aged patients. (Cole, Damon, Declan, Harvey, Hughey, Smith, Wolanin)

However, attention is called to the fact that a nurse's help to a patient in coping with death is not always a "one-way exchange"; it may be reciprocal in the sense that when the nurse finds herself more upset than

---

* 38.4 percent. See Appendix B, Table 17, Item 2.

is her patient, it may be the patient who somehow is able to give the nurse more help than he receives from her. (Knowles, Steffen)

For many nurses, basic religious convictions that have been established early and that are nourished throughout life can afford strong supports for coping constructively with the events of death. The nurse is cautioned, however, that when she finds that her religious beliefs, philosophy, and attitudes toward life and death are at variance with those of her patient, she be sure to resist any attempts at controversy or proselytizing or imposing, no matter how gently or graciously, her own convictions on the patient. She can still be concerned, understanding, and supportive, however. And by her general attitude and attentive silences, she can become a constructive witness within her own faith. As one nurse expressed it, "Heaven can still be portrayed as free from suffering and sorrow and, hopefully, something more." (Baziak, Lanigan, Shaffer)

A DRN summarized the situation in part as follows:

> It deserves repeating that the nurse needs to understand her own attitude toward death and dying and the extent to which the patient threatens her own competence as a helping person. If the elderly patient is continuing to believe in his own survival, yet death is imminent, the patient's defenses should not be too hastily interfered with before he is ready to give them up on his own.
>
> It is the responsibility of the nurse to construct or maintain a milieu that will best serve the patient. Respect for the cultural, religious, and social conventions of the dying patient and his family needs to be observed. The family and the minister depend upon the nurse to tell them when the patient wants to see them, and it is her responsibility to report interests and attitudes of the patient and any changes which indicate that death is close. In our culture the dying patient may be most alone when he most needs a close continuing relationship with another human being who cares. In the hospital or nursing home, it is the nurse who by her continuing presence, actions, and words can show that she cares and can attempt to enter into and to share the experience with the patient. (Prock)

Knowledge of the Ways of Dying

The foregoing pages have dealt primarily with the *persons* involved in the crisis situation—the patient who is dying and the nurse who provides care for him—and with the knowledge, understanding, and judgment the nurse must have if she would provide comfort-care for her patient. For any degree of proficiency in the care of the dying, however, the nurse must also possess knowledge about the *process* of dying—about the experience through which a person must pass before life ends.

Many of the DRN's indicated that although the inevitability of death is a fact, accumulated knowledge about the event can and often does help the nurse to help the patient and his family in facing the event with greater composure and comfort.* Such knowledge would include the changes that can be expected during the terminal phase, the common elements as well as the possible variations on what may happen during the last hours or days preceding death. Firsthand experience and accuracy of information on what tends to occur within the crisis situation in the social and psychological as well as in the physical areas are emphasized by the DRN's. Any dependable information concerning these phases and processes in senescent dying can be of great value to geriatric nurses—when used judiciously—in helping their patients through this ultimate passage in life. Moreover, if a more matter-of-fact and realistic point of view toward death could be cultivated, the event might become easier to cope with for everyone concerned.

Some of the DRN's point out that it is as realistic to be prepared for death as for any other crisis in the life cycle and that geriatric nurses *ought* to be especially prepared to accept responsibility for helping patients and their families through such trials. Several of them envisioned a future in nursing when no nurse would care for a dying person who does not feel that she can describe the process with a high degree of reliability —if and when the patient desires to learn about it.

In present-day America, however, evading the actual facing of the fact of death has become so ingrained in contemporary attitudes that it may be folly to suggest that dying be regarded as a realistic part of life; and that it would be helpful to think of aging and dying as having begun at the moment of birth and as reaching a natural fulfillment of the cycle of life at the time of death.

A primary reason for openly facing the facts of dying and the processes involved is to allay fears and to dispel traditionally established, but often misleading, myths about dying, such as, that death is nearly always filled with pain and suffering.

The fears of patients can often be dispelled, some of them by simple items of accurate information. A person who expresses dread of pain and suffering during the final period of life might derive comfort from knowing that existing evidence points to the fact that dying usually is surprisingly peaceful.

Even if illness has been accompanied by much pain, such suffering often diminishes and may vanish altogether as death comes closer. The last hours, or even days, generally tend to be free of stress and pain, and any suffering which lingers on can be brought substantially under control by way of medication. Anxiety-producing misconceptions about how the body is treated after death can also be cleared up by simple state-

* 15.1 percent. See Appendix B, Table 17, Item 3.

ments of fact. As reported earlier, old age would seem to provide its own sedation, particularly for the very old who often are overcome by a kind of quiet lethargy days, or even weeks, before they enter their final sleep. "Dying at best is a lonely business," states one DRN. If we knew more about the physical processes involved in dying and more about their interaction with perception, we might more effectively lessen the increasing sense of isolation of the dying. (Hagen, Jayne, Duxbury)

While it is often difficult to ascertain what is on another person's mind, it may well be that all a dying person asks for is that the truth about his condition be shared with him and that he be able to voice his concerns about dying and be assured of a compassionate and attentive listener. He may find comfort and solace in the realization that he is not alone, and that he can count upon those who are about him for support. This, of course, implies a close working relationship between physician and nurse. It implies, further, close collaboration and ongoing communication among all who in one way or another care for, and about, the patient.

It is recognized that not every patient wants to know, or should know, that he is dying; but it is as important not to give false assurances as it is not to leave the patient without any hope—hope relating to possible recovery or pointing to another more ultimate hope.

A specialist in the field, Dr. Cicely Saunders (who is a nurse, a physician, and an almoner), writes that those who have established a close and continuing relationship with the patient will best be able to determine to what extent, if any, the patient wants or needs to be enlightened. But she cautions that it is rarely right for others to take the initiative in this and that even when the patient asks for the truth, it is not easy "either to decide or to carry out our decision nor that we will not have regrets."

Dr. Saunders concludes her discourse on the care of the dying with these words:

> The care of the dying should not be an individual work but one that is shared. Shared with all relations, with all the various members of the staff, spiritual, medical, and lay; and, as far as we can, with the patient himself. Where this is so we are left with a sense of fulfillment which makes this such a rewarding branch of medical and nursing care.*

* Saunders, Cicely. *Care of the Dying.* London, The MacMillan Company, 1959, page 19.

A NOTEWORTHY EXAMPLE OF COPING WITH TERMINAL ILLNESS

A recurring idea throughout these chapters is that there are some time-tested major supports which promote or make possible late life fulfillments and a commendable death in old age. These are: 1) a well-grounded and practiced religious or philosophical faith; 2) a close-knit and sustaining family unit; 3) suitable provisions for terminal illness and its care within the confines of the home with its facilities and under competent medical supervision (one which considers the individual as a person as well as a patient); and 4) some further interests to be pursued and tasks to be completed—something with which to be occupied or perhaps to complete a compelling commitment. All these four conditions appear to have been met in this noteworthy example of terminal illness.

Mr. H. was 82 when he died in the Spring of 1956. For two years before his death, he was confined to his room, partially bedfast as a result of a cardiac condition and two major operations for carcinoma.

Though more than a decade has passed since Mr. H. died, his memory lingers on, and his friends and neighbors continue to speak of him with deference. They knew him as an active, forthright, responsible, and community-minded person. He is remembered as deacon of the local Congregational Church, an exceptionally effective Bible class teacher, friend of the young people in the parish, and an especially devoted family man.

The celebration of his golden wedding anniversary at the church had been a memorable event. His eightieth birthday was observed by a large portion of the community, and he was presented on this occasion with a book of personal testimonies of appreciation signed by more than 150 persons. These dealt mainly with the constancy of his friendships, some of more than 50 years' standing; the warm understanding and the comfort he had given to individuals and families in times of stress; and the inspiring "quotes" and encouraging visits received from him. Many of the testimonials dealt with the inspiration he had been to others by his example as a devout and neighborly man: "What a wonderful thing to live 80 years, serving your God and your fellowman," or, as another family put it, "a sincere soul, a man of deep and devout faith, an example of the grace of God, and the dearest of friends."

But Mr. H. was to be honored most of all, perhaps, for the manner in which he bore his last illness, the use he made of the passing time, the way he coped with death, and the detailed planning of his own funeral, which caused relatives and friends frequently to recall and cherish the day.

By ancestry Mr. H. was a Scot. He was born in New York City, the seventh child and the second son of a Methodist minister. The father became noted for his beautiful tenor voice and his inspired singing of Christian hymns, but most of all for his faithful pastoral work in the various churches that he served over a period of 50 years. The children, including Mr. H., were deeply influenced by their father's life and faith and became devout and active Christians.

As a youth Mr. H. attended a well-known parochial school, but an accident, and later an illness, prevented him from obtaining a high school diploma, a fact that he was long to regret. He was married in 1899 to a gentle woman. An accident in her youth had left her a semi-invalid. Two children were born: a daughter who suffered an illness at an early age that left her partially permanently crippled and a son who suffered a birth injury and was subject to convulsions and emotional upsets throughout his short life and who died at the age of 21.

A continuing strong, affectionate, and mutually supportive relationship grew between father and daughter, and the daughter became a major source of strength and help to her father throughout his terminal illness. An older sister of Mr. H. also became to him a trusted and treasured ally. These two persons, mainly, made it possible for Mr. H. to live out his life at home and in the manner to be described. Though crippled, ill, and becoming very enfeebled, his wife remained a significant member of the small family unit. She survived her husband for two years.

Mr. H. never regarded himself as financially prosperous, but he was a diligent worker, lived frugally, and provided comfortably for his family. He had spent about 10 years as store manager for a paint company and more than 40 years as construction foreman for a public utility company. He treasured his economic independence and contributed substantially to the church.

He was an energetic outgoing person who spoke frankly but in a cheerful and friendly manner, showing genuine interest in those around him. With intimates, he expressed rare gifts in friendly banter without causing offense. However, he was considered to have a sharp tongue for persons whose conduct he could not condone. His quick temper was no secret to his family and to some of his friends; for his sarcasm could be biting, but it tended to quickly pass. Relatives were more aware than his friends of his moods, which in his early manhood occasionally cast melancholy over many hours at a time when he would lie in his bed, brood, and remain noncommunicative. Gradually, he learned to control these moods quite well. Frankly and purposefully a religious man with firm commitments to the Protestant faith, his religious expressions were simple, direct, and applied to daily living.

During his terminal illness he was fully aware that he would not be well again. For nearly three years he was definitely planning the closure of his life and how to spend the intervening time. His relationship with his physician was frank and trustful, and he knew that he could expect an honest answer to any question about his illness; yet Mr. H. never inquired directly whether he had cancer. Some members of his family suspected, however, that he "knew," though the subject was never discussed. His attention remained focused primarily on his ailing heart. For nearly two years oxygen was kept near his bedside to be used as needed for ease in breathing. He had medication to control pain and to induce sleep, but he used it gingerly, wishing to keep his mind clear. Near the end his doctor told him that he would probably expire in discomfort. They discussed this and a decision was reached on how to handle the situation. He seemed especially concerned about how an anguished death might distress his family. He preferred to die a natural death without any artificial or "heroic" measures to prolong life. No strong feelings were expressed for or against an autopsy; but he abhorred any thoughts of cremation. He freely discussed life and death topics in a natural, matter-of-fact manner with his physician, his family, and some of his friends. He retained the office of deacon in the church and, when he felt able, some of the small official meetings were held at his home and around his bedside.

On April 23, 1956, four days before Mr. H. died, he sent for a friend of long standing, asking him to come very soon. The friend went and afterwards prepared this memorandum:

I reached Mr. H.'s home about seven o'clock in the evening and found him lying on his bed with his little pet dog at the foot of the bed and his pet bird at his side. Ann, his daughter, remained in the room with us and was as cheerful and attentive to her father as ever. He greeted me warmly, as he always had, but appeared weary. He said he wanted to talk with me about his approaching death and that he hoped it would not disturb me, since it no longer disturbed him. His doctor had informed him that he probably would live no more than three or four days longer, that he was likely to undergo some severe choking sensations, and that he might become unconscious before the end came. He had been assured by his doctor that he would not suffer any great agony such as would greatly upset his family. The doctor also had given assurances that he would come immediately when called and be prepared to administer sufficient medication to control any intense pain and permit a natural and easy death.

Then he said he had a special favor to ask of me. With the help of Ann, he had prepared his funeral service in every important detail. He wished me to perform such functions as conducting certain parts of the service, announcing the especially chosen hymns, reading the selected Scripture passages, and offering the prayers just as they had been written out by him. He expressed a special wish that the prevailing spirit of the service be one of Christian hope and trust and that it be free of any overtones of sadness and mourning. No personal sentimentalities were expressed. At parting, we shook hands warmly—he with the greater composure, but I with an inspirational experience to be long remembered.

Mr. H. died quietly at about the time anticipated, having become unconscious about 48 hours before the end. The service was carried out exactly as he had planned. Afterwards, several persons of the large group attending said to the daughter that they had never witnessed another service so simple, bright, and hopeful in outlook and so entirely free of sadness and mourning.

Two months before his death, Mr. H. sent a letter to the above mentioned friend expressing gratitude for a small favor. Mr. H. en-

closed with the letter a quotation from James Russell Lowell, imply-
ing that the verse expressed his own philosophy of life:

> *True love is but a humble, lowborn thing, and hath its food
> served up in earthenware; it is a thing to walk with, hand in hand,
> through the every-dayness of this work-day world, a simple fireside
> thing, whose quiet smile can warm earth's poorest hovel to a home.*

The following are excerpts from some twenty-odd letters written
by Mr. H. to his beloved sister during the last years of his life.

Ann and I had a long, loving, and tender talk the other evening
regarding my "going home" which seems not far away. We want no
show at all. The minister will be apt to eulogize too much if not held
down. Ann will hand him a prepared and written-out service, even
to the Bible readings, and say to him, "This is what Dad wanted you
to use." There is nothing sad, dear, about all this preparation, nor
should there be about my going; for I am very *tired* and I will be
glad to go.

I am stronger than yesterday, for then I felt that I could not
live out another day; nor did I want to. The nights are the hardest
times, as while asleep I slip down in some position that puts pressure
on the heart, and I wake up with it sounding like a hammer, and it
takes time to get it quiet again.

Oxenham's lovely "Nightfall" describes to *perfection* how I feel
about "going home."
Fold up the tent!
Above the mountain crest,
I hear a clear voice calling, calling clear—
"To rest To rest!"
And I am ready to go,
For the sweet oil is low,
And rest is best!

Yes, Dr. Sockman's radio sermon on the "Quality of Mercy" was
a great help to me. It took care of that word "fear" which I *never*
liked. Awe also means reverence and a *kind* of fear as we sometimes
realize God's power and glory. That word "awe" just fits.

I am glad that you seem to approve of our desire about the
service of my "going home." Thank you for your prayers while you
could not sleep on Monday night. I think they must have helped for
last Tuesday night I had the best undisturbed night for at least three
weeks. Most of my nights are pretty bad, but last night was *heaven*.

My good friend, H.J., about 50 years old, had a heart attack
Monday morning about one o'clock. Result of his recent war experience, we all think. When I heard about it, I wrote to him and to
M., his wife. Then I went all to pieces—sobbed and cried. Ann had
a hard time to quiet me.

I had a heart attack at two o'clock this morning, but it was not a bad one. I have seldom, during my life, been so filled with quiet peace "that passeth understanding" as I have been the last few days. It is blessed and wonderful. I am too tired to write more now.

Today, on Radio Chapel, a heavenly voiced male quartet sang "O Love that Will Not Let me Go." I was melted to tears. Dr. McCracken followed with a talk about prayer. No words can describe the spiritual beauty and help of that sermon. Then Dr. Sockman came on with his "The Source of New Strength." Surely my soul has been fed this day. "There is a peace in my soul that the world cannot give."

After quoting some hymns today I can still hear our father's bell-like tenor voice singing the lovely soul-lifting hymn, "Come ye that love the Lord." Yes, dear, God has flooded my soul these latter days.

Time seldom hangs heavy on my hands for I am able to write. There is always someone who needs a note of comfort and sympathy, or there is a quote or two to send a friend. I can most always read, but if too weak or tired to do either, I can sleep, pray, and commune with God's spirit.

I had such a fine night's sleep last night. The night before was long and bad, so yesterday I started taking demerol tablets, every four hours, as the doctor has one do when the going gets too hard—and that kept everything quiet, inducing restful sleep. Of course it leaves me in a sort of light fog, but not having to fight for breath all the time.

My boys and girls (of the church) were home from college this past week. They were in to see me, and it did my soul good to hear them talk. A part of my task, at least, has been done well, I am glad to say.

Had callers and callers yesterday. Too many and had to take sedation in order to get to sleep and all—and now I am just stupid and in a fog. I can't think clearly at all this morning.

Yes, God's promises, handed down to us through the ages, are just as poignant as ever. We *have* to say those promises *over* and *over* in order to realize how much they can and do mean to us.

I am enclosing the lovely poem, "So be my Passing." It appeals to me lately for I am so tired, and I feel that my task is accomplished, not as well as it should be, but to a certain extent. It has been a *long, long day,* and there was a song in my heart—and I am sure that the Sundown in the Great West will be beautiful and serene. I will be glad to "go home" when the call comes.

part **III**

EPILOGUE

17 Impacts of Culture and Society on Aging

The theme was propounded earlier in this document that major gains in aging are the joint products of individual endeavor and societal develop-ment. That man does not reach a great and gratifying age solely on his own is as true as the proverb that man does not live by bread alone. Venerable age, if and when it comes to anyone, is a consequence of the adaptations of the individual *and* his society—each *to* the other rather than by any separation or withdrawal of either *from* the other. It was indicated, further, that in our so-called civilized times the youthful, up to and through their prime in life, may be able to manage well enough among themselves without reliance on old people, and that any widen-ing of the generation gap is very likely to be at the expense of the elderly, especially in their advanced aging. Moreover, there is no guarantee that any gains attained by and for the aged within a given time may not be lost again later. Indeed, the possibility looms large that in any human grouping the reciprocally supportive relationships between youth and age rest upon shifting and very tenuous equilibriums—and that senescent security, no matter how hard come by, may easily be lost.

In broad social perspective, no basic substitute has been found for reliance of the very aged upon younger persons who, through induce-ments or socially sanctioned enforcements, are willing or compelled to stand by and sustain the elderly in their helpless states. It has been as-sumed, moreover, that the youthful and their elders have found their richest opportunities in working out mutually supportive bonds within the family setting. From various aspects it has been suggested in the foregoing chap-ters that certain similarities exist between youth-age accommodations within families and within geriatric care-giving institutions such as nurs-ing homes. These similarities exist in spite of the sharp contrasts that are frequently drawn between living out life within the midst of the family and living out life within the walls of an institution.

The analogy between a family base and a geriatric care-giving fa-cility is noteworthy. Like the family base, the institution is generally re-ferred to as a "home," and the primary relationship, although generation-ally reversed, is called "nursing" and could be called "nurturing." Even

269

the childlike roles and the tendency to treat and be treated "like children" appear in both settings, but again reversed. Diapering, or its equivalents, and countless other supportive and sustaining interactions, such as "bargaining at the bedside," go on in both the family and the geriatric homes. Indeed, the possibility exists that the patterns and degrees of reciprocal reinforcements, however reversed, become potentially as complex and variable as in family settings, and their adequacy or inadequacy may span as wide a range in quality of supports provided. Some comparative analyses seem indicated, to match the contrasts that are often drawn, some of which have been referred to earlier in these pages. Indeed, such analyses might be useful in restructuring the facilities society provides for the care of the aged ill.

However that may be, it is within the larger social context than family or geriatric home that we wish now to consider the impacts of the broader cultural and societal factors on the destiny of aging persons.

THE INDIVIDUAL AND HIS ENVIRONMENT

When in conferences health professionals deliberate on patient problems, frequent reference is made to the "individual and his environment." The usage of this phrase directs attention to the vital linkages between the particular patient and his milieu. As has so often been observed throughout the present discourse, these linkages can be more delicate and their effects more significant for the individual in his tenuous old age than in his vigorous youth.

But in providing care for aged patients, the individual-environment idea, however basic and pertinent, generally appears too broad and all-encompassing to afford clarifying and useful insights into the crucial factors impinging upon the patient. The authors contend that the problems of the aged patient would have a better chance of being perceived and coped with when identified and considered in a three-fold individual-environment context.

Physical Environment

First and foremost, a patient is to be perceived and studied as a body or organism adjusting to his physical milieu. It is, of course, within this area that physicians, nurses, and other health professionals are most familiar and perceptive with respect to the patient's problem. This being so, it would seem to serve no useful purpose to elaborate upon this linkage.

Culture

In the second place, the aged patient can be viewed to considerable advantage as a person or personality within his culture. The individual begins as a *creature* of the culture and becomes bred to the culture. As an adult he becomes a recognized *bearer* of the culture, eating the prescribed food, wearing the proper clothes, using the conventional language, employing the approved techniques, subscribing to the major tenets, and trying to live up to the existing standards and the typical image of a man or woman of worth within that culture. He may also have come to play some small part as a *creator* of his culture by producing some useful inventions or innovations that are copied and perpetuated by his contemporaries or descendants. Moreover, he may have become something of a *selector* and *synthesizer* of particular elements of his culture and, perhaps, of certain other cultures, integrating and highlighting them in his patterns of personal behavior and his life-style. These elements have become "internalized," as parts of himself that are reflected in his thoughts, acts, and attitudes. Perhaps most important for our purpose, he has necessarily become a practiced *manipulator* of his culture (its folkways, norms, rules, ethical codes, practices, etc.) to some possible advantage to his own survival and welfare. If fortunate and reasonably ingenious and gamey, he may have acquired a certain capacity to marshal the cultural norms, values, and mandates in effective ways for inspiring or impelling the aid and support of certain of his associates toward fulfillment of his needs and interests far along into his enfeebled old age. Our special concern here, of course, is to discern and comprehend the manifold and subtle impacts—the assets and the limitations in opportunity— that a culture provides for a given individual to carry him through a ripe and rewarding old age.

Culture has been defined in very simple and very direct terms as learned, shared, and transmitted patterns of behavior that are usually directed toward the solving of some problem or problems experienced by human beings. A still simpler description is "the ways of life of this or that people." Like all short, crystallized definitions of general phenomena, these leave much to be said, as do similar synoptic formulations about biology, health, disease, and the like. A common characteristic recognized in all treatises on culture is *change:* a capacity to shift, accumulate, or lose components which makes culture far more flexible and variable in time and place than are the somatically determined behaviors. Without culture, man cannot live a *human* life and certainly cannot attain anything like a "good" old age.

Everyone is humanized from birth onward. One is little aware of the power of culture to mold and shape one's growth into adulthood and, later on, to determine one's decline into senescence. Perhaps a major way for an individual to begin to realize the compelling effect of culture on his personality and his life would be to grow up into prime adulthood in one culture and then to try to achieve a ripe old age in an entirely different culture, such as that of the polar Eskimo. Or it might be more tolerable and instructive to watch this as an experiment in the life of some other individual. In these times of our own rapidly paced culture, this happens to many of us in some degree, and not without accompanying problems.

The far-reaching impacts of a culture on a person's life can scarcely be exaggerated. The functions of his intelligence, for example, are multiplied a thousand-fold or more by the components of his culture—think of the modern computer for instance. Language, which opens up vast avenues for communication, accumulation, and preservation of knowledge, is the product of a man's culture. Indeed, almost all of man's advances in coping with the physical environment and his relationships with his fellows stem mainly from cultural developments. This applies also to the ways in which he copes with aging and dying. In fact, an individual's image of himself along his life course, his life goals, and his successes and failures in them are defined by, striven for, and assessed under the norms and dictates of his culture. Indeed, culture makes human for man much that would otherwise remain little more than animal; and it also fills with success or failure for him many life situations that would otherwise remain neutral or go unnoticed. While man through the centuries has created his culture and continues to modify it, the culture, in turn, *makes* the man and mirrors his life conditions for him, identifying his goals, cueing his life situations, teeing off his reaction patterns, and tallying up the score. The process continues for as long as he lives and in his declining years perhaps goes on even more impellingly and fatally than during his younger days.

Society

The third area of major import in attempting to understand what happens to an ailing and aged person, and what may be done for him, is the social milieu—the organized groups of other individuals of which he is a member and within whose society he lives out his life.

While the concept of culture may appear at first somewhat obscure and not clearly understood, elements or phenomena of one's society or social structure can become as concrete as the physical environment. Anyone who has any doubt of the realities of society around him, be he young or old, needs only to withdraw awhile from group life or to have his associates withdraw from him to discover how many of his needs, goals, activities, and reinforcements are affected. Or if he permits himself to deviate significantly from his responsibilities and thereby disrupts the affairs of his fellows, he is quick to experience the impact of their separate or combined pressures to get him back "in line." If he neglects his fellows' nudges for conforming to expectations held for him, he is soon to suffer pointed penalties for his failure to "fit in" and perform acceptably. Indeed, nonconventional behavior even in the "sick role" of an aged patient in a geriatric institution may arouse in the nursing staff and other attendants certain critical, nonsanctioning reactions.

In short, man is uniquely a societal, as well as a cultural, creature who through long periods of development has become dependent for his very existence upon system-determined aids and reinforcements of fellow members of his "in-group." He lives so much within these structured, repetitive, and interdependent relationships and in concern about fellow expectations for him that one of the greatest threats of all may be his doubt about his continued ability to live the life of an adult human being. He is threatened by the very forces in society upon which he has been dependent for nourishment, motivation, and life. He must remain a part of the system; yet he is driven to fulfill his own proclivities, even under the limitations of age; and because of his sensitive equipment, he is often pulled different ways at one time. These threats and conflicts are omnipresent and constitute for him a large portion of the stresses and strains to which he is exposed.

Man's culture sets the stage for his life, ascribes the parts to be played, and defines the terms under which the drama is to be enacted. It is, however, the other members of an individual's society—his associates in the sanctioning positions, his so-called "pressure personnel"—who check on his performance, add teeth to the cultural codes, and put the bite of discipline on individual members.

With this perspective it seems possible, and, indeed, profitable for the care and welfare of an aged patient, to study him as a continually vulnerable, but still somewhat resourceful and adaptive, human being caught within the vortex of his milieu. Though aging, it is likely that he is still endowed with certain inborn capacities for development and with sensitivity to certain goals for what remains of his life. Now in his decline he is no less a creature of his three-fold environment, undergoing stress from its three separate but related areas and suffering wear and tear along the course of his relatively long life. While making efforts to hold onto his life, he is daily confronted with the triad of environmental forces—physical, cultural, and social—that maintain him in some ways and menace him in others.

As an organism, man is borne along by his physical environment, but threatened, buffeted about, and scarred by its elements. As a person or personality, he is a product of his culture and, also, a potential victim of its norms and codes. As a social agent, or member of his society, he is still sustained and reinforced by some of his fellows if he is fortunate, and hindered and frustrated or ignored by others. Indeed, in some instances, he is subject to downright exploitation.

Such a person may be carried along more-or-less comfortably in his triple milieu for a long while, only to be torn down miserably after a time as the various environmental forces converge upon him, leaving him distraught and stranded. During stretches of time, helpful and harmful factors may have blended and balanced, permitting a safe and tolerable equilibrium amid minor fluctuations. Within the context of a geriatric facility, it is important for those responsible for the patient's welfare to be alert to the ever-present and increasing possibility that the scales may be tipped critically at any time by a clustering of stresses from any one area or from a combination of the triad of forces.

It may be that, in the study of these fairly complex components, the physical, psychocultural and social problems of the aged individual within his family and other close-knit establishments of his community (such as nursing homes) can best be discerned and coped with, and perhaps controlled. And it would appear that qualified health professionals, especially geriatric nurses, occupy strategic positions to explore these complex and compelling phenomena which are linked with the interests and welfare of their aged patients. They can observe in the same individual the biophysical and the psychosocial factors that wrack the body, or tear down the personality, or both. They are in a position to explore all three environmental areas and thereby achieve more integrative perspectives on particular patients, or perhaps categories of patients, who are caught up in physical disabilities or psychosocial predicaments or who manage to achieve a temporary recovery and rehabilitation by means of the supports available to them.

CONCEPT OF STRUCTURE

Implied in the foregoing discourse is a fundamental principle of the behavioral sciences: that peoples' behavior and relationships are subject to systematic study and possible explanations and predictions in the light of sufficient knowledge of antecedent factors. On a scientific basis we are no more free to assume caprice or accident in man's reactions on the psychosocial than on the biophysical plane; but it is not easy, even for health professionals, to hold conscientiously to this postulate in dealing with their geriatric patients.

If we are to try systematically to analyze and interpret even the stereotyped and highly repetitive behavioral patterns in institutional settings such as community, family, hospital, or nursing home, what constants can be formulated? Among the most fundamental formulations in the behavioral sciences, especially in anthropology and sociology, are *structures* of relationships and *forms* of behavior or interactions. Perhaps better known terms are *organizational systems* and *cultural patterns.*

Forms of behavior have been touched upon in the above section on the impact of culture and of society upon the geriatric patient. For our task at hand it appears relevant that structure of relationships be briefly analyzed as well.

The structured repetitive relationships of group members of the same species are apparently much older and more biologically fixed than is the phenomenon of culture. There exist forms of life subject to highly complex structural systems whose behavior appears instinctively locked into place and relatively unvariable except at the price of individual survival. Much of the insect world is characterized by this kind of "structurization" of behavior and can by no stretch of the imagination be said to possess a culture in the sense that culture is defined as learned behavior. There are apparently degrees of organically structured and determined relationships and behaviors in all forms of life that are dependent upon group orientations for survival. The greatest modifiability is open to human beings; but even in man, biologically determined components set limitations on what a specific culture may prescribe. The penalty is failure of the membership to survive as a structured group, even perhaps as individuals. Any threatened group that constitutes a structured unit is prone to sacrifice individual members at the price of survival. In complex forms of life, in fact, it is highly improbable that any social structure survives for long without some sacrifice of individual members. This is an aspect of society that has to be taken into account in all ameliorative endeavors.

Identifiable variables in apparently all structured systems, and especially among higher forms of life, include these basic elements:

1. Individual differences in capacity that are either innate or acquired.
2. Some specialization in function as a possible outgrowth of these differences.
3. Lines of domination or potential "pecking orders" also consequent to individual differences.
4. Forms of cooperative activities that may be innately established,

      as in the joint activities of ants and bees, or enforced or voluntary, as in the activities of human beings.

    5. Stations or positions held by individual members of the structured group as a consequence of the four above-mentioned components.

    6. Performance of behavior corresponding more or less to the stations occupied.

At the least, these six elements are identifiable in social structures that reach all the way from anthills and beehives to the organized systems of men, including geriatric institutions.

    The following chart may help to reflect the relationship of these basic components:

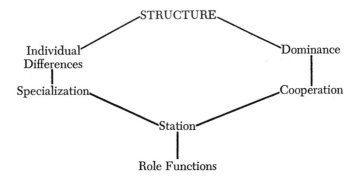

It was pointed out above that the components of society or of social structure, above all, are concrete. The reality factors in human relations are such that even an attempt by the individual just to "go about his own business" may reveal how pressing can become the demands upon him to "play his part" in the joint interests and activities of varied group memberships—and not infrequently at the expense of his own health and well-being.

CONCEPT OF INSTITUTION

    In some respects the concept of institution clarifies the related formulations of culture, society, and structure and integrates them into a more easily identifiable functional unit for analytic purposes. The idea of institution is used in both a generalized and specific sense. It may be related to a broad phase of social activity, such as economic, religious, or political phenomena, or to a specific social unit, such as family, church, hospital or nursing home, as the identifiable unit under consideration.

    The analysis of institutions provided by the anthropologist Bronislaw Malinowski is perhaps as helpful as any for a start (1944). He attempted to identify the common denominators or independent variables that appear always to be present in institutions that are structured sufficiently that they may be easily identifiable. They are:

1. The charter or set of purposes or goals for which the individuals are organized and that explain or justify to them their cooperative activities.

2. The personnel or participating membership with its structured system of relationships.

3. The rules and techniques for performance of activities believed to aid in achievement of the goals (cultural norms and rules that are prescribed).

4. The material apparatus devised and utilized in the operations of the personnel (the usable elements in the physical environment often modified into equipment and tools).

5. The recordable activities of the different participants in their several stations and in accordance with their role expectations.

6. The functional effects of the joint endeavors (results) as compared with the charter expectations.

7. The observable consequences of the performance upon the individual participants. (This special concern is not included by Malinowski.)

The essential components are portrayed in the following chart:

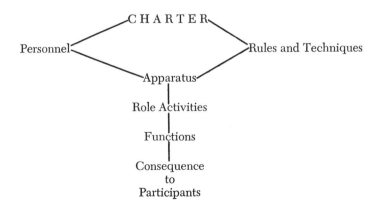

It may be possible that such a formulation of social structure and cultural pattern into the concept of institutionalized behavior will prove helpful in the analysis of interpersonal relationships that bear upon vexing questions associated with geriatric patient problems and possible therapy. The term "institutionalized behavior" is applicable, of course, to both paired and multiple relationships between persons of the same or different statuses within the structured system. Examples of such key relationships of a paired type and of different statuses would be those between clergyman and parishioner in a church, a teacher and student in a school, a parent and child in a family, a physician or nurse and a patient in a hospital or nursing home. Multiples of these relationships are easy to imagine. It is, of course, the degree to which they are structured, patterned, repetitive, and predictive that makes them useful for study, along with the *effects that they produce upon the participants.*

Within such a biosocial perspective of man in his total environment it is possible to view the individual as a vulnerable, resourceful, adaptive, and also perishable human being endowed with certain inborn capacities for development and highly sensitized goals in the adjustment of his life to surrounding circumstances. To reiterate, we see the individual as a creature of his environment who undergoes stress from various sources and suffers wear and tear in the process.

These concepts of the individual in his environment have meaning not only in relation to the aged ill and infirm patient within the institutional context, but also for the institutions organized to provide care for the aged ill as well as for the nurses entrusted with the care of geriatric patients.

18 Paradoxes Concerning Terminal Illness and Death

We are to a culture born and bred,
and within a culture we die.
ANONYMOUS

Death is a universal experience, but the awareness of the realities of death seem to be shared by human beings above any other known creatures. Humans certainly have the acquired capacity, above other forms of life, to forecast the possible approach of death for an individual member, especially under conditions of disease or other disabilities associated with old age. Within their cultural and societal developments, humans have also acquired increasing ability in planning for, and coping with, the necessities of individual deaths. In most, if not all, organized human groupings there exist conventionally prescribed devices and procedures for both the incumbent and his responsible associates in dealing with and concluding the event with relatively minimal social disruptions—permitting life to go on at a fairly even keel.

A very impressive achievement of man in modern Western civilization has been the great accumulation of a store of knowledge, facilities, and skills for coping effectively with the threats of death. Some of these potentials are manifested, for instance, in medical science, economic and social insurance, and the creation of complex and profound religious and philosophical formulations as guides for both living and dying well.

A surprising paradox appears, however, in the realization that there exist in this very complex and advanced environmental milieu strong conventional prohibitions against facing the issue of death frankly and openly and with purposive planning of means for "making the best" of the end of one's life. Recent research reflects what is already well known: that a strong tendency prevails among contemporary Americans to treat the subject of death as a "tabooed" topic and to be reluctant, evasive, and often misleading in responses made to it, especially to persons diagnosed as terminally ill, and even when they are very advanced in age and re-

279

quest to know. (Feifel, 1959) Indeed, one finds such questions raised as: "Who cares anything today for a finely finished death?" (Rilke in Sudnow, 1967) It would almost appear that death is to be viewed as something apart from life, having little or no significant relationship to it.

This paradox points up much of the ambivalence, conflict, and confusion prevalent in our contemporary attitudes and behaviors related to dying. These negative patterns are most pronounced, as has been observed, in the facing of death within intimate personal relations, such as exist between close friends or within familial and therapeutic contexts.

The paradox seemingly has taken root deeply within our culture. Since death can be such a crucial event in the lives of individuals and often in the destinies of groups and even nations, the culturally patterned reactions to dying become embedded and reflected in society's structure, its institutions, and its laws. They also bear upon the life cycle of individuals in their different stages and, not least, upon the position and destiny of elderly persons who, according to the laws of nature, are closer to the event than are younger persons. Their last days or even years can become profoundly affected by the ways in which their contemporaries and associates view, relate to, and deal with death. (Back and Baade, 1966)

Another aspect of the death paradox is apparent in the tendency which, while avoiding, isolating, or even denying death within intimate personal situations, shows much concern and preoccupation with the prevailing threats of violent, and sometimes wholesale, deaths through accidents, catastrophies, riots, warfare, and even the prospects of total annihilation.

Patterns in Facing Death

Just as it may be said that death has many faces, so in turn it is faced in very different ways by those to whom it comes. In broad human background approaches in facing death can first be divided on a dual basis: psychological denial of death as a personal, natural, and individual occurrence *or* the frank acknowledgment of its certainty and perhaps imminence. These mental stances take various forms, and the forms are subject to different coping patterns. It may be of interest to note certain of the forms that denial of death take and the types of patterns that different societies, because of their culture, permit and support for those individuals who acknowledge the certainty and imminence of their deaths.

Death Denials

Under primitive conditions, especially as reflected by the simpler cultures, death has commonly struck down children, youths, and individuals still in their prime of life more frequently than the old, for few reached old age. Consequently, death became more commonly associated with the young than with the old; and, even with the elderly, life was more often snuffed out suddenly than left to flicker and fade away by degrees.

Owing in part to its early, sudden, and unexpected impact, primitive peoples have been slow in recognizing death as natural or inevitable. Even when it was recognized as happening eventually to everyone, the tendency was to attribute the actual occurrence to a blunder or oversight of someone and most generally explaining it as caused by magic or sorcery. Countless instances are easily gathered. To illustrate:

> The Abipone in South America denied that death ever resulted from age alone; and even in cases of extreme senility, they insisted that it must be caused by accident or witchcraft. Among the Araucanians on the same continent it was claimed that though a person might die peacefully at the age of 100, even then it would be considered to be the result of sorcery. The Aurunta of Australia denied the possibility of a natural death. "However old or decrepit a man or woman may be when this takes place, it is at once supposed that it has been brought about by the magic influence of some enemy." The Bushmen of Africa denied that there could be such a thing as natural death, even for the oldest. And Malinowski wrote of the Trobianders in the South Pacific, "Natural death caused by old age is admittedly possible, but when I asked in several concrete cases, in which age was obviously the cause, why such a man died, I was always told that a sorcerer was at the back of it." He also reported, "When I asked about M'tabaly, a very old and decrepit man, whether he was going to die soon, I was told that if no evil spell were thrown on him there was no reason why he should not go on living." (Simmons, 1945, page 218)

In legend and myth we find many accounts of how death first occurred as an accident, or as an evil foisted upon man. It would seem that the fact of the naturalness of death, even for the aged, has not been generally accepted by mankind. In one study of 47 tribes in which information could be obtained, 17 of them did not regard death as natural; 26 of them only partially admitted the possibility; and only 4 appeared to frankly recognize death as a natural occurrence. Furthermore, the conviction has been perhaps even more widespread and persistent that remedies were known, or could be devised, for checking the unwelcomed onset of old age and for prolonging life, if not actually rejuvenating it.

The conviction has been equally strong and widespread, and even more persistent through almost all stages of cultural development, that although death may destroy the body, no serious damage is done to the spirit or ghost. Indeed, death might even render a service, since the spirit—the real essence of life—would be freed thereby from the bondage of the flesh. (Simmons, 1945, Chapter VIII)

Moreover, it has been quite commonly held that under favorable conditions the life of the spirit can be more noble and desirable than any earthly existence which has already become burdensome at best, and that both self-interest and personal dignity might favor the exchange of an enfeebled dotage for a life hereafter that promised richer rewards.

In the vast majority of recorded societies that have reached any complex stages of development—be they primitive or more advanced, historical or contemporary—the traditional religious beliefs and dogmas, as well as their accompanying rituals, tend to perpetuate a form of denial. They do this primarily by placing emphasis upon the survival of the ghost, soul, or spirit, and often by highlighting the possibilities to be gained in a future life.

While denial of death has its roots in most recorded human backgrounds, it may take the form either of denial of the necessity of death as a natural and inevitable occurrence in the course of every individual life, or it may lay claim to and emphasize a survival over physical death by the "essence of life" that may exist in a future and, possibly, superior state of being.

In Western civilizations, and especially here in the United States, the denial of death is more likely to take the form of a psychological and social stance. In interpersonal associations, physical death is played down by silence, by suppression, and by various forms of camouflage. The behaviors can reach certain remarkable, and perhaps, ridiculous degrees. For example, the employment of euphemisms such as "departing," "passing on," "going home," and the like. Then the common practice of making the corpse appear as lifelike as possible, to be viewed as resting peacefully for a time in a "parlor" or "slumber room" and then enclosed in a long-lasting receptacle and placed within quiet and attractive surroundings. All this, and more, testifies to deep human beliefs that, for true life, death cannot be the end.

Within the context of terminal illness, contemporary practice of this denial is likely to take the primary form of keeping the knowledge of impending death from the patient; and particular patients' preference may well be that of remaining unaware of the prognosis—but this is certainly not always so.

Two recent researchers on problems of terminal illness and death in hospitals make this summary statement. "The most standard mode—recognized by physicians and nurses themselves—is a tendency to avoid contact with those patients who, as yet unaware of impending death, are inclined to question staff members, with those who have not 'accepted' their approaching deaths, and with those whose terminality is accompanied by great pain. As our book will testify, staff members' efforts to cope with terminality often have undesirable effects on both the social and the psychological aspects of patient care and their own comfort. Personnel in contact with terminal patients are always somewhat disturbed by their own ineptness in handling the dying." (Glaser and Strauss, 1965, p. 5)

Death Recognition

Dominant categories of personal responses to recognition and acknowledgment of impending death for an individual can be typed as death defiance and death acceptance.

Death defiance on the part of anyone threatened with imminent death may take several forms or various combinations of them. The individual identifies a target which he views as the cause or the source of his plight (circumstances, an institution, other individuals, fate, God, or whatever) and vents his hostility and aggression on this target. His defiant expressions may be either vocal or other behavioral, or may be the suppression of any overt response—in the manner of passive resistance. Within a therapeutic context, the act of incontinence is not infrequently interpreted as such defiant behavior. Another type of death-defiant behavior may be the attempt of the individual to "outdo" the causal agent or factor by a suicidal act, or he may try to "head off" the adversary somewhat by living up as much of life as possible *now*, before the "bell tolls."

These few death-defiant types of response are merely illustrative. A cataloging and classification of them are not known to the authors.

Death acceptance on the part of an individual who faces imminent death is commonly characterized by at least two fairly typical stances: *passive* and *active*.

The *passive stance* may or may not be a *reconciled passive acceptance;* and the *active stance* may or may not be a *constructive active acceptance*. To be sure, a passive position toward approaching death can spring from deep undercurrents of defiance, as has been noted, and an active acceptance can be moved along by similar undercurrents of defiance. It is, perhaps, in the reconciled passive acceptance and in the constructive active acceptance that the distinction between defiant and accepting coping patterns of dying stand out clearest.

It may be that the soundest way for drawing distinctions between the two stances, passive and active, within the framework of defiance and acceptance is on a multiple and, at least, triangular basis. It is, first, to view and appraise the particular coping patterns on the basis of the manifest intent of the individual who faces death; second, to analyze them within the specific situational context where the coping patterns are carried out; and, third, to appraise them under the norms and codes of the culture within which the individual's life style has been set and his life course unfolded.

Such assessments of creditable deaths under the dictates of specific cultures are based largely on group-shared norms and ideals. These include religious beliefs and imperatives, ethical and philosophical concepts of values and morals on what is right and wrong, political ideals and goals, personal actions taken "in the line of duty," and dying for a popular cause or making noteworthy sacrifice for the "common good." Even an average individual may enhance his postmortem status by closing his life circumspectly or by conforming consistently to the end in his characteristic style of life that has become something of a trademark for him. He is often acclaimed, regardless of culture, time, and place, simply by fulfilling the special goals set for himself—even, or sometimes especially, when these are accomplished very late in life and at the price of some travail.

MODES OF DYING

It may be useful to review briefly and from a broad cultural background the modes of dying for the aged within a sampling of primitive peoples. From available records it can be observed how many different modes and means of dying have worked commendably well at some time and place in the judgment of the elders themselves as well as in the judgment of their contemporaries.

As stated in the beginning chapter, among most, and perhaps all, peoples a point is reached in aging—if death is greatly postponed—when the advantages and values of a still longer life begin to be balanced off or cancelled out, by its disadvantages and futility for both the aging individual and his associates. Then, regardless of the people, the time, and the place, the life prospects become progressively discouraging and even dismal. Soon thereafter, death appears to be, truly, the concluding solution to aging. Somewhere around this time in the life cycle, it seems pertinent, and perhaps appropriate, to wonder: How much worse off all concerned parties would be if death should really take a "holiday?"

A noteworthy contrast between cultures of primitive-historical peoples and that of contemporary western civilizations is the fact that the helpless phase of life has shifted greatly in social problems of significance. Under earlier conditions, relatively few individuals reached a great age and still fewer lasted long into its extremities of helpless dependence. Moreover, many primitive peoples found it necessary to act more forthrightly towards pronounced debilities of age; and when they did not, nature under harsh and hard circumstances took over and resolved the issue. It was also considered right and proper in many primitive societies to sanction, or even prescribe as appropriate, what is likely to be regarded in civilized times as cruel and inconsiderate measures for facilitating, or at least not delaying, a necessary and apparently timely death. These measures were nearly always sponsored and supported by the prevailing culture and often so firmly that some of the incumbents encouraged their kin to take the appropriate steps, or in some instances, requested or demanded death by the hands of a favorite kinsman as a privilege or a right.

Rather common expedients resorted to in case of the very aged or severely handicapped consisted of conventionalized neglect, abandonment, and crude or even violent forms of terminating life which were usually interpreted as dutiful responsibilities. They were frequently appraised by the groups as special acts of mercy and grace which conferred on the dying outstanding distinctions in the afterlife. Furthermore, it was not unusual for such practices to survive long after the time when physical conditions and the cultural developments had originated and justified them.

In our contemporary society with its developing lifesaving techniques and facilities, the problems involved in extending the helpless stage in senescence are taking on vastly increasing significance. With a constantly expanding proportion of the elder population reaching further extremities in decrepitation and with growing numbers of the aged likely to live out their final days or even years in institutions of perhaps questionable quality, the query may well be raised: How realistic are opportunities going to be for aged persons to achieve anything resembling a timely, appropriate, or creditable death?

Some of the very developments in our society that make it possible for multitudes of Americans to reach and be sustained in very advanced old age are tending to be something short of an unmixed blessing. Can it be that for many of the very aged and infirm, an extended life with nothing else is likely to become *nothing else*—dull prospects of day-after-day with nothing in them, a boredom not unlike despair, or out of touch with reality. If and when we face up to the position that a timely, creditable, and fulfilling closure to a life is of necessity the optimum solution for aging in the kind of world we know, can we then go on to test the premise that whether life can be "good to the last drop" or not depends primarily on how *good* the last of life can be made?

What can be learned about senescent death from the broad backgrounds of primitive and historical peoples? Their tried and tested adaptations were outgrowths of their circumstances and necessities even as ours must grow out of, and be tailored to, our times. It may be that in their solutions can be found clues and useful insights into our own exigent needs for readjusting to the Great Reaper.

It certainly is nothing new to learn that some aged individuals in relatively underdeveloped or "backward" cultures have found in their deaths opportunities for special merit and fulfillment to their lives. There is also evidence that frequently in different times and places, persons do achieve for their seniority a sense of mission or destiny and help create the situations and motivate the behaviors that culminate in a victorious and very fitting death. Thus, in important respects, the occasion, the manner, and the meaning conferred upon their deaths surpass in social significance the biological fact of the closing event.

In the transcultural study referred to above (Simmons, 1945), the following criteria were generally found to be conditioning or supportive and indicating factors for the potentialities of such deaths, though all the criteria need not be present in each instance.

1. Hard physical and environmental circumstances should require and justify the death at the time it occurs as, in the eyes of contemporaries, a very sensible choice between the available alternatives.

2. The cultural values and beliefs of the people with respect to their goals in life, the meaning of death, the nature of the Gods, and the prospects for a desirable hereafter should, together, inspire and support the step and cushion the blow.

3. Established precedents and rituals should prescribe the manner of dying and designate the "right" persons to execute and supervise the event.

4. When the anticipatory rituals are concluded, the act of dispatch should be soon over, not too long lingering with suffering.

5. A sanctioning audience (witnesses) and a possible ceremony with celebration should attend and conclude the rites.

6. If heroic or violent acts are condoned and anticipated, it is preferable that the subject, or a responsible kinsman, request, arrange for, or execute the act, and possibly as part of the ritual.

7. The individual should possess sufficient readiness or resignation along with manifest courage and character suitable to meeting the challenge and facing up to the event with commendable fortitude.

Perhaps the most important idea underlying this phenomenon and its criteria of appropriateness is the fact that while old age and death are both basically biological, the achievement of a noteworthy old age and an appropriate death are both extremely sensitive to, and dependent upon, the sociocultural milieu—and that these joint achievements challenge the organized ingenuity and the adaptability of human beings. They don't just happen. They are made possible by nature, but they are not guaranteed fruits of nature. They have to be gained and can be lost—and they are only gained by human beings *striving cooperatively*. Such evidence supports the position that it is possible for human beings working together to make of old age something worthwhile to live for and of death something more than a defeat.*

The question presents itself: Are such gains in the face of death obtainable by and for elderly persons within our contemporary culture? That they cannot be obtained in the same manner in which they occurred in former times and among other peoples and cultures seems clear. But whether any more fitting and fulfilling closure to life can be made possible for elderly patients in institutionalized settings and under modern conditions, and by what means, is a matter that calls for concerted attention and careful, as well as cautious, exploration.

In our contemporary society, as we have seen, this subject is a delicate and largely tabooed topic for frank discussion within face-to-face situations involving the death of anyone known personally—even though it be within a situational context of physician, nurse, and patient. Indeed, designated health personnel, reflecting the conventional restraints, appear to exercise more inhibitions about the subject than do many of their aged patients.

Possibly this factor explains, in part, why half the nursing personnel within the selected geriatric institutions disclaim that awareness of a terminal diagnosis has any effect on the care they provide for their aged patients. It probably also helps to explain many of the other outstanding divergences in nursing opinion concerning their geriatric patient care.

It is heartening, nevertheless, that present trends tend toward frank affirmation of differences that such care *can* and *should* make. Perhaps therein lies a promise for the aged ill of better things to come in the future of nursing.

Even under major medical advances and reasonably optimum programs of patient care, the volume of senescent deaths—now about 2,000

* Certain of these issues were discussed in great detail in Chapter 1.

per day in the United States—is almost certain to increase, and with growing proportions of elder Americans likely to die in hospitals, nursing homes, or similar institutions. Such prospects would make it appear to be of primary importance that the physician, the nurse, and other allied professionals be ever mindful and fully aware of their special opportunity and responsibility to the seriously ill aged person and his family if any. It would be well for them to remember, moreover, the admonition of the great personal physician, Oliver Wendell Holmes, that: when they cannot cure, they can ameliorate; when they can no longer ameliorate, they can comfort and ease the patient through the travail of dying.

It seems timely, indeed, that the science and the art of healing and of saving lives be matched, as a counterpart, with the science and art of helping the very aged, when their time comes, *to die well* and, if possible, with *fulfilled* and *finely finished* lives.

APPENDICES

Selected Annotated Readings

The list of books and articles given below requires a word of explanation. It is not a bibliography in the sense of being comprised of the works cited in the text or consulted in its preparation. Only a few of such works are included here. Instead, we have sought to document the central topics by pointing to materials which our readers may turn to in the pursuit of their particular aims or for elucidation of concepts explored.

The materials are classified by chapter or clusters of chapters, according to the particular topics discussed. In none of its parts, however, is the list to be considered complete. By the authors' judgment, a few of the outstanding and very relevant works have been indicated by asterisks. All are briefly annotated.

CLASSIFICATION GUIDE

ANNOTATED READINGS†

I. Society, the Aged, and Institutions‡

‡ Chapters 1 and 2.

A. ANTHROPOLOGICAL READINGS

Book References

Rosen, G. Cross-cultural and historical approaches. *In* Hoch, P. H., and Zubin, J., eds. Psychopathology of Aging. New York, Grune & Stratton, Inc., 1961, pp. 1-20.

> *An introductory overview on problems of aging in human societies. Many references.*

Simmons, L. W. Aging in primitive societies. *In* Tibbits, C., ed. Handbook of Social Gerontology: Societal Aspects of Aging. Chicago, University of Chicago Press, 1960, pp. 62-91.

> *A comparative account and appraisal of aging in primitive and contemporary societies.*

† See Name Index for alphabetical listing of authors.

——— The relation between the decline of anxiety-inducing and anxiety-resolving factors in a deteriorating culture and its relevance to bodily disease. *In* Association for Research in Mental and Nervous Diseases: Life Stress and Bodily Diseases. Baltimore, The Williams & Wilkins Co., 1950, Vol. 29, pp. 127-136.

> *A discussion of the relevance of cultural stress to psychosomatic illnesses.*

Journal References

Cowgill, D. O. The social life of the aging in Thailand. Gerontologist, 8:159-163, 1968.

> *A concise and summary statement of the status, role, and treatment of the aged in a rural and village setting.*

Simmons, L. W. Attitudes towards aging and the aged: primitive societies. J. Geront. 1:72-95, 1946.

> *A summary review of an extensive study of the position, role, and treatment of the aged in primitive societies.*

Slater, P. E. Cultural attitudes toward the aged. Geriatrics, 18:308-314, 1963.

> *Comparison of the Greek view that aging is an unmitigated misfortune with the Middle Eastern view that old age is the summit for life. Discussion of cultural paradoxes in which individuals find themselves.*

Streib, G. F. Old age in Ireland: demographic and sociological aspects. Gerontologist, 8:227-236, 1968.

> *Another good example of reporting on the social aspects of aging in different societies.*

B. SOCIOLOGICAL READINGS

Book References

Birren, J. E. The social and cultural determinants of aging. *In* Birren, J. E., ed. The Psychology of Aging. Englewood Cliffs, Prentice-Hall, Inc., 1964, pp. 25-49.

> *An analysis of how large-scale variables of social class, ethnicity, and income influence how individuals live, the patterns of their lives, and how these patterns determine their later years.*

Kuhlen, R. C. Motivational changes during the adult years. *In* Kuhlen, R. G., ed. Psychological Backgrounds of Adult Education. Chicago, Center for the Study of Liberal Education for Adults, 1963, pp. 77-113.

> *An excellent discussion of the effects of chronic frustration on motivational changes in aging. Sources of frustration are described such as age-related relationships in society, status systems that idolize youth, time and money pressures,*

physiological changes that usurp attention, technological changes that outdate the skills of the elderly, circumstantial locking-in of oldsters that makes them prisoners of stressful situations.

Moore, W. E. Aging and the social system. *In* McKinney, J. C. and de Vyver, F. T., eds. Aging and Social Policy. New York, Appleton-Century-Crofts, 1966, pp. 23-41.

A stimulating and pertinent discussion of the relationship of mortal man in his life cycle with the "immortal," yet changing, social systems and with the consequent intergenerational patterns. "This is probably the best and the worst time in history to be old—or to be young."

*Riley, M. W., and Foner, A. Aging and Society, Volume One: An Inventory of Research Findings. New York, Russell Sage Foundation, 1968.

Summarization of recent social science research findings on middle-aged and older people, and interpretations of this knowledge in terms of social theory and professional practice. Part One describes significant aspects of the societal context of today, in the recent past when today's oldsters were reared, and in the projected future when today's younger generations will have grown old. There are excellent charts on pertinent data.

*Simpson, I. H., and McKinney, J. C., eds. Social Aspects of Aging. Durham, N.C., Duke University Press, 1966.

This book deals primarily with retirement, family relations, and continued social participation in human affairs, with some consideration being given to concepts of perpetual life space. A central theme is that personal problems and the life style in old age are consistent with, and emerge out of, previous life experiences to substantial degrees.

Journal References

Burnstein, S. R. Papers on the historical background of gerontology. Geriatrics, 10:189-193, 328-332, 536-540, 1955.

Stimulating portrayal of the medical and social backgrounds in the development of gerontology and geriatrics.

Mead, M. Understanding cultural patterns. Nurs. Outlook, 4:260-262, 1956.

Another meaningful and relevant article by a renowned anthropologist. "Understanding differences among patterns of behavior in peoples of different cultural backgrounds has obvious relevance to nursing."

Palk, I. I. Aging and the elderly. Nurs. Times, 58:1235-6, 1962.

Short article stressing the need to understand the cultural and social backgrounds of the aged in order to avoid stereo-

*typing or generalizing beyond the realities of their lives. It is
claimed that the overall goal of the geriatric nurse should be
to help the elderly person to live out his life in a way that is
satisfying to him.*

Parson, T. Aging in American society. Law and Contemporary Problems, 27:22-35, 1962.

*A stimulating paper on the relationships of social changes
in American society, including shifts in value systems, and
their effects on the processes and experience of aging, especially living under the shadow of death and oriented to the
prospects of termination.*

Rienow, R., and Rienow, L. T. The desperate world of the senior citizen. Sat. Rev., January 28, 1961, pp. 11 ff.

*A brief overview of the difficulties confronting contem-
porary aged Americans.*

Simmons, L. W. Social participation of the aged in different cultures. Ann. Amer. Acad. Polit. Soc. Sci., 279:43-51, 1952.

*Description of social opportunities that different societies
and cultures provide for aging persons to continue participation and to gain further prerogatives, prestige, and rights, or
to hold on to what they have.*

C. PSYCHOLOGICAL READINGS

Book References

Birren, J. E. Behavioral theories of aging. *In* Shock, N., ed. Aging: Some Social and Biological Aspects. Washington, American Assn. for the Advancement of Science, 1960, pp. 305-332.

*Discussion of social science theories of aging: counter-
part theory, development theory, personality theories, etc.*

———— Personality of aging. *In* Birren, J. E., ed. The Psychology of Aging. Englewood Cliffs, N.J., Prentice-Hall, Inc., 1964, pp. 223-251.

*Discussion of definitions and types of personalities; per-
sonality changes occurring with age; and change in interests,
attitudes, and capacities such as social, sexual, and mental.*

———— ed. The Psychology of Aging. Englewood Cliffs, Prentice-Hall, Inc., 1964.

*A stimulating and informative book on the psychological
components in aging. An authoritative source.*

Chown, S. M., and Heron, A. Psychological aspects of aging in man. *In* Farnsworth, P. K., ed. Annual Review of Psychology. 16:417-450, 1965.

*An excellent review of contemporary attitudes toward
aging and the aged.*

Kastenbaum, R., ed. Contributions to the Psychology of Aging. New York, Springer Publishing Co., Inc., 1965.

> This book contains a selection of nine papers constituting a symposium held in 1964 by the Division of Maturity and Old Age of the American Psychological Association. There are chapters with theoretical formulations on the psychosocial aspects of aging; engrossment and time perspective in aging; engagement-disengagement theory as related to personality types; and adaptive techniques used by oldsters in situations of threatening self-esteem.

———— New Thoughts on Old Age. New York, Springer Publishing Co., Inc., 1964.

> A collection of papers on recent theories related to aging. Emphasis is placed largely upon developmental theory—that senescence and death are natural processes concluding the life cycle.

Tibbitts, C., ed. Handbook of Social Gerontology: Societal Aspects of Aging. Chicago, University of Chicago Press, 1960.

> Nineteen papers on the social science aspects of aging by leading scholars in their specialties.

Journal References

Birren, J. E. A brief history on the psychology of aging. Gerontologist, 1:127-234, 1961.

> Very useful outline of developments in gerontology to 1960.

Kastenbaum, R. Theories of human aging: the search for a conceptual framework. J. Soc. Issues, 21:13-36, 1965.

> A summary of contemporary theories of human aging, simply and attractively described.

D. THE AGED AND THEIR HEALTH PROBLEMS

Book References

Brody, E. M. Aging as a family crisis: implication for research and planning. Proceedings of the 7th International Congress of Gerontology, June 26 to July 2, 1966, pp. 49-52.

> Stresses the relevance of the family as a significant factor in the older person's functioning as health declines—the problems of the aged cannot be isolated from the family.

Busse, E. W. Social forces influencing the care and health of the elderly. *In* McKinney, J. C., and de Vyver, F. T., eds. Aging and Social Policy. New York, Appleton-Century-Crofts, 1966, Chapter 9.

> A valuable review of contemporary social factors and their effects upon the aged, especially with respect to their health.

Clark, M., and Anderson, B. G. Culture and Aging: An Anthropological Study of Older Americans. Springfield, Ill., Charles C Thomas, Publisher, 1967.

> *A carefully planned study of aged persons who were treated in a mental hospital compared with aged persons who did not reach a mental hospital. An arresting finding is the damaging effects of the hospital upon the persons who were later returned to the community.*

Knowles, L. N., ed. Maintaining High Level Wellness in Older Years. Gainesville, Fla., University of Florida Press, 1965.

> *A symposium directed to the goal of a high level of wellness in old age that is based on "integrated functioning" directed toward maximizing the potentials of which the individual is capable. Four major contributors.*

*Shanas, E. The Health of Older People: A Social Survey. Cambridge, Mass., Harvard University Press, 1962.

> *Summary of the findings of a 1957 survey on the health needs of older people based on a nationwide sample of persons 65 years or over.*

Journal References

*Ellison, D. L. Work, retirement, and the sick role. Gerontologist, 8:189-192, 1968.

> *An insightful analysis and comparison of retirement and the sick role and their reciprocal effects upon each other, especially for the aging.*

Kastenbaum, R. The reluctant therapist. Geriatrics, 18:296-301, 1963.

> *It is suggested by the author that the reluctance of psychotherapists to work with the aged ill is due to attitudes and values uncritically absorbed from popular opinion. Such stereotypes lead to unwillingness to enter a low status relationship, avoidance of unpleasant interactions, and calculated risks that the aged ill will not live long enough to "pay back" the therapist's "investment" in him.*

McLeod, K. Well Oldsters health conferences. Nurs. Outlook, 6:207-208, 1958.

> *A physician proposes "Well Oldsters Clinics" to protect the health of the elderly, somewhat like "Well Baby Clinics" safeguard the health of infants and children.*

Parsons, T. Toward a healthy maturity. J. Health Hum. Behav., 1:163-182, 1960.

> *Analysis of the effects of a society oriented toward the achievement of goals and how these factors shape or influence opportunities for aging successfully.*

Phillips, H. T., and Lambert, C., Jr. Survey of health needs of older citizens and their potentials in home health work. Public Health Rep., 79:571-576, 1964.

> *This survey explores the health needs of older citizens and their potential for meeting each other's needs.*

Simmons, L. W. Impact of social factors upon human adjustment within a community. Amer. J. Psychiat. 122:990-998, 1966.

> *This discourse deals primarily with social agencies and processes in caring for the mentally ill.*

*Townsend, G. Care of the aged in the community. Nurs. Times, 57:257, 1961.

> *A British physician critically examines some commonly accepted cliches about old people that underlie both the definition of their problems and attempts that are made to solve them.*

Zeman, F. D., et al. Everyday problems in the care of the aged. Bull. N. Y. Acad. Med., 32:577-602, 1956.

> *Transcription of an interdisciplinary panel meeting. Other participants were Norton S. Brown, Robert McGraw, Marian Randall, and Ollie A. Randall. Many useful suggestions are presented.*

E. PERSONAL TESTIMONIALS AND NOTEWORTHY QUOTATIONS ON AGING

Book References

*Brigham, J. The Youth of Old Age. Boston, Marshal Jones Company, 1934.

> *A librarian who lived to be an octogenarian and who chose early as his avocation the collection of noteworthy statements on aging. The book provides a rich sample from 283 authors and notable persons, both ancient and modern, to which the author has added his own observations, delightfully enlivened by his wit and dry humor.*

*Scott-Maxwell, F. The Measure of My Days. New York, Alfred A. Knopf, Inc., 1968.

> *A fresh and delightful book for broadening insights on the personal experience of growing old in contemporary society. The author is a retired psychiatrist who was born in America but spent much of her life in England. Should be of special interest to geriatric nurses.*

*Tibbitts, C. Aging in the Modern World: A Book of Readings. Ann Arbor, The University of Michigan Press, 1957.

> *An excellent selection of readings, drawn from ancient and modern times, which are valuable both for instruction and for reading pleasure.*

Vischer, A. L. Old Age: Its Compensations and Rewards. New York, The Macmillan Company, 1947.

> *This physician, who worked for 20 years with old people in Basle, brings to the subject a freshness, a uniqueness of insights and a ripe wisdom. His simple and precise descriptions of the problems and his seasoned judgments on how to cope with them helps the reader to capture a genuine feeling for the positive and compensatory side of aging.*

F. INSTITUTIONS

Book References

Garvin, R. M., and Burger, R. E. Where They Go To Die: The Tragedy of America's Aged. New York, Delacorte Press, 1968.

> *This is a caustic, sensational, and somewhat disturbing book. It obviously lacks an objective and balanced treatment of the subject. It does arouse, however, some justified concern for what goes on in many institutions established for the care of the aged.*

Goldfarb, A. I. Current trends in the management of the psychiatrically ill aged. *In* Hoch, P. H., and Zubin, J., eds. Psychopathology of Aging. New York, Grune & Stratton, Inc., 1961, pp. 248-265.

> *A review of trends in old age homes, state hospitals, and nursing homes in New York State. The findings are that in spite of constant improvements over many years, the conditions remain far from admirable or even adequate.*

Gurel, L. A Survey of the Self-Care Dependent in Selected V.A. Hospitals. Washington, V.A. Hospitals, 1963.

> *This is a study of self-care dependency by a sample of 12,836 patients in 11 V.A. Hospitals. More than a third of the geriatric patients were self-care dependent as compared with slightly more than a tenth of the total patient group. Contains much pertinent information on prolonged care of long-term chronically ill patients.*

Henry, J. Culture Against Man. New York, Random House, Inc., 1963.

> *Chapter 10 provides an anthropologically oriented comparison of three institutions for the care of the aged ill: a public institution, an inexpensive private nursing home, and an expensive one.*

—— Personality and aging. *In* McKinney, J. C., and de Vyver, F. T., eds. Aging and Social Policy. New York, Appleton-Century-Crofts, 1966, pp. 281-301.

> *A provocative and disturbing analysis of the depersonalization of many public institutions and cheap nursing homes upon aged patients they serve.*

Mauksch, H. O. The organizational context of nursing practice. *In* Davis, F., ed. The Nursing Profession. New York, John Wiley & Sons, Inc., 1966, pp. 109-137.

> *A description of the institutional structure and system within which the profession operates.*

Pearson, L., ed. Death and Dying: Current Issues in the Treatment of the Dying Person. Cleveland, The Press of Case Western Reserve University, 1969.

> *Five social scientists and clinicians examine the sociological, psychological, and physical phenomena of dying. Interest is directed to the interactions between the dying person and significant figures associated with the closure of his life.*

Riley, M. W., and Foner, A. Aging and Society, Volume One: An Inventory of Research Findings. New York, Russell Sage Foundation, 1968, Chapter 25.

> *This chapter, "Roles in Institutions," provides a good summary of research findings on the attitudes and reactions of old people, their families, and the public toward services provided in institutions for the aged and the aged ill. The assessments are, on the whole, cautionary and critical.*

Simmons, L. W., and Wolff, H. G. Social Science in Medicine. New York, Russell Sage Foundation, 1954.

> *Observations and interpretations of "Hospital Practice in Social Science Perspective," not especially related to the aged, but focused on interpersonal relationships.*

Sklar, J., and O'Neill, F. T. Experiment with intensive treatment in a geriatric ward. *In* Hoch, P. H., and Zubin, J., eds. Psychopathology of Aging. New York, Grune & Stratton, Inc., 1961, pp. 266-273.

> *On a special ward where teamwork and personal attention were given to patients, surprising improvements were achieved and significant results reported.*

Solon, J. A. Nursing home and medical care. *In* DeGroot, L. J., ed. Medical Care: Social and Organizational Aspects. Springfield, Ill., Charles C Thomas, Publisher, 1966, p. 198.

> *Pertinent cross-sectional and comparative data. For example, in 1961 virtually no proprietary nursing home had a full-time physician; only 44 percent had a full-time registered nurse and 14 percent had no trained nurses.*

*Sudnow, D. Passing On: The Social Organization of Dying. Englewood Cliffs, N.J., Prentice-Hall, Inc., 1967.

> *This book contains striking contrasts in the treatment that the dying receive in two hospitals under different controls and financing systems. While neither hospital is limited to the care of the aged, many aged patients were found in both of them. A very impressive documentation.*

*U.S. Department of Health, Education, and Welfare. Nursing Home Utilization and Costs in Selected States, Health Series No. 8, February 1968.

> *Excellent source of recent information on some 2,600 nursing homes from 5 selected states, plus summary data drawn from relevant reports of homes in the other states from 1960 to 1965. Very useful document.*

Journal References

Bell, T. The relationship between social involvement and feeling old among residents in homes for the aged. J. Geront., 22:17-22, 1967.

> *Calls attention to this phenomenon as a major defect in many geriatric institutions.*

Brody, E. M., and Spark, G. M. Institutionalization of the aged: a family crisis. Family Process, 5:76-90, 1966.

> *First rate article on family crises involving an aged member in which the institution becomes a "dumping place for spent and ailing individuals who have worn out their welcome."*

―――― The impaired aged: a follow-up study of applicants rejected by a voluntary home. J. Amer. Geriat. Soc., 14:414-420, 1966.

> *The findings indicate that within one and one half years, two thirds of the rejected patients had either died in a proprietary home or were still living in such facilities.*

Editorial. St. Christopher's Hospice, Lawrie Park Road, London. Nurs. Times, July 28, 1967.

> *Description of the opening of a modern hospice that has been planned, built, and staffed under the guidance of Dr. Cicely Saunders to enable patients who are in the last stages of their illness to have a peaceful and, above all, a tranquil closure to life and to be supportive to the patients' relatives and friends in their bereavement. "Contrary to common belief, patients in the proper atmosphere, and helped by modern medicine and nursing, can be maintained in an alert and peaceful frame of mind to the last . . . ."*

Morris, E. Choosing a nursing home. Amer. J. Nurs., 61:58-61, 1961.

> *Guide on how a nurse may assist an aged person and his family in choosing a nursing home. Sources of information are indicated.*

Randall, O. A. The situation with nursing homes. Amer. J. Nurs., 65:92-97, 1965.

> *A noted social worker and gerontologist reports that despite some improvements in nursing home care, the "problems overshadow the gains." She finds that "nursing homes are too widely considered a business first and a service second, and while they offer nursing as their main commodity,*

*the nursing care provided is usually far below minimal stand-
ards." The author challenges nurses to become involved and
not remain silent concerning these problems.*

Savitz, H. A. Humanizing institutional care for the aged. J. Amer. Geriat.
Soc., 15:203-210, 1967.

> *A physician-in-chief, emeritus, of a rehabilitation center
> presents a challenge for reform.*

Taubenhaus, L., Walker, J., and McCormick, J. A public health approach
to nursing home care. Amer. J. Public Health, 54:53-59, 1964.

> *A discussion of the isolation of the proprietary nursing
> home from the mainstream of medical resources. This is re-
> garded as a major obstacle to quality care for the aged ill and
> dying patients.*

Wald, F. S. "To everything there is a reason and a time for every purpose."
The New Physician, 18:278-285, April 1969.

> *The author comments perceptively on certain critical and
> unresolved problems linked with death and bereavement in
> contemporary society. She then describes how many of these
> problems are dealt with and often resolved at St. Christo-
> pher's Hospice in London, England, where she, as a nurse,
> spent some time in participant observation.*

II. The Project, Problems, and Methodology

Chapter 3.

A. RESEARCH IN NURSING

Book References

Fox, D. J. Fundamentals of Research in Nursing. New York, Appleton-
Century-Crofts, 1966.

> *This book is addressed to the potential researcher. It
> will stimulate her interest and clarify concepts and procedures
> in research that she may undertake. Especially commendable
> is the directness and simplicity with which research methods
> are presented and illustrated.*

———— and Kelly, R. L. The Research Process in Nursing. New York,
Appleton-Century-Crofts, 1967.

> *"A general book of readings of the kind presented here
> is a special kind of reference in that it selects from among
> the many reports and articles available those readings which
> the authors believe best exemplify important areas of content
> in nursing research and which will serve to best introduce
> the student of research to an overview in the field." (page vi)
> Each section and each reading has an introduction by the
> authors.*

Simmons, L. W., and Henderson, V. Nursing Research: A Survey and Assessment. New York, Appleton-Century-Crofts, 1964.

> *Records are reviewed on the beginnings of nursing research, the directions that the research has taken, and the forces that have impeded or promoted its development. Existing research studies are analyzed and appraised, indicating areas in which progress has been made.*

Wooldridge, P. J., Skipper, J. K., Jr., and Leonard, R. C. Behavioral Science, Social Practice, and the Nursing Profession. Cleveland, The Press of Case Western Reserve University, 1968.

> *The book clarifies the manner in which behavioral science theories and methods can be adapted to nursing research and utilized in the improvement of nursing practice. The author's concern is with the challenging task of designing and carrying out research in nursing which leads to findings related to both practice theory and behavioral science.*

B. STATISTICAL METHODS

Book References

Blalock, H. M. Social Statistics. New York, McGraw-Hill Book Company, 1960.

> *An excellent book on the subject.*

III. The Aged Ill and Their Care

Chapters 4 to 9.

A. CONCEPTS, PROBLEMS, ATTITUDES, AND REACTIONS RELATED TO THE AGED ILL

Book References

Black, K. W., and Gergen, K. J. Individual orientation and morale of the aged. *In* Simpson, I. H., and McKinney, J. C., eds. Social Aspects of Aging. Durham, N.C., Duke University Press, 1966, Chapter 19.

> *A survey indicating that not every older person wishes for a very long life. Only about half of the respondents wanted to live 150 years, with older persons less interested in doing so than younger people.*

Coser, R. L. Life in the Ward. East Lansing, Michigan State University Press, 1962, pp. 84-95.

> *Contains an interesting discussion of "Laughter in the Ward." There is presented a dynamic account and analysis of the role and function of humor and jocularity as a means of coping with stress.*

Exton-Smith, A. N., Norton, D., and McLaren, R. An Investigation of Geriatric Nursing Problems in Hospital. London, The National Corporation for the Care of Old People, 1962.

An intensive study was made in a British hospital on such physical nursing needs as feeding requirements and techniques, the care of the incontinent patient, the provision of suitable clothing, effective ward furniture and equipment, and general nursing practice suited to geriatric patient care. Emphasis is placed on classifying patients according to their needs and on individualized nursing care.

Flugel, J. C. Humor and laughter. *In* Gardner, L., ed. Handbook of Social Psychology, Volume 2. Cambridge, Addison-Wesley Press, 1954, pp. 709-734.

A psychoanalytic and social interpretation of the use of humor that is easily applicable to aged persons.

Freud, S. Humor. *In* Collected Papers. London, Hogarth Press, 1950, pp. 215-221.

An extremely perceptive treatment on a psychoanalytic basis.

Masters, W. H., and Johnson, V. E. Human Sexual Response, Boston, Little, Brown and Company, 1966.

Chapters 15 and 16 deal with geriatric sexual responses and may be useful to the nurse in understanding some of the unconventional behavior of the aged ill.

Simmons, L. W. Prestige. *In* The Role of the Aged in Primitive Society. New Haven, Yale University Press, 1945, pp. 50-81.

There is documented here the considerable respect and prestige achieved and accorded to aged men and women, but especially men, within a wide variety of primitive societies.

Stotsky, B. The Elderly Patient. New York, Grune & Stratton, Inc., 1966.

An up-to-date treatment by a physician who reviews and discusses selected findings in the behavioral sciences, clinical practice, and programs of service, institutional as well as other, concerning varied geriatric patient care problems, including death and bereavement.

U.S. Public Health Service, National Institutes of Health. Mental Disorders of the Aged. Washington, U.S. Government Printing Office, 1965.

In this valuable document it is suggested that the cause of childish behavior in the aged, whether it is physical or emotional, needs exploration to determine whether or not it is due solely to the absence of love and personal attention.

Journal References

Age Center of New England. Seven sins of society against older people. Practical Nurs., 8:8, 1958.

> *Seven "sins" are indicated and it is proposed that the nurse avoid these to insure a better relationship with aged patients.*

Butler, R. M. The life review: interpretation of reminiscence in the aged. Psychiatry, 26:65-67, 1963.

> *Postulates and discusses a "universal occurrence of an inner experience or mental process of reviewing one's life in older people" as part of preparing for death. A summary review of the literature.*

Coser, R. L. Some social functions of laughter: a study of humor in a hospital setting. J. of Human Relations, 12:171-182, 1950.

> *An interesting and suggestive article on the utilization of humor by stressful or frustrated patients as a means of release, defense, and social integration of the patient group. The functions of humor are well analyzed, many valuable references are provided on the subject, and its relevance to aged patients is easy to see. Strongly recommended.*

Freeman, J. T. Sexual capacity in the aging male. Geriatrics, 16:37-43, 1961.

> *Describes the wide range in potential sexual drive and behaviors. Has pertinence for understanding unconventional patient behavior which the geriatric nurse may encounter.*

Hulicka, I. M. Fostering self-respect in aged patients. Amer. J. Nurs., 64:84-88, 1964.

> *Discourse by a psychologist on the behavior, and bases for the behavior, of elderly hospitalized patients. Contains very useful suggestions for making the lives of these patients a little happier and their behavior more acceptable to the staff.*

Kastenbaum, R. Wine and fellowship in aging: an exploratory action program. J. of Human Relations, 13:266-276, 1965.

> *A demonstration is described on the use of wine and a social hour to refresh the spirits of aged patients and to stimulate and smoothe their interpersonal relationships.*

Neylan, M. P. Anxiety, Amer. J. Nurs., 62:110-111, 1962.

> *For patients to exhibit anxiety in unfamiliar or stressful situations is normal and to be expected. This behavior must be understood and causes ascertained by the nurse in order to be helpful to the patient.*

Wolanin, M. O. They called the patient repulsive. Amer. J. Nurs., 64:73-75, 1964.

>*An excellent description of the reactions of a nursing staff to a patient's incontinence, sloppy self-feeding, and obscene language and of how to deal with it.*

Wolk, R. L., Rustin, S. L., and Scotti, J. The geriatric delinquent. J. Amer. Geriat. Soc., 11:53f, 1963.

>*Discussions concerning aged persons who act out their conflicts in unconventional ways.*

B. READINGS ON GERIATRIC CARE

Book References

ANA Regional Clinical Conferences. Exploring Progress in Geriatric Care. New York, American Nurses Association, 1966.

>*A series of six papers on various aspects of geriatric nursing presented at the 1965 ANA regional clinical conferences.*

Blumberg, J. E., and Drummond, E. Nursing Care of the Long-term Patient. New York, Springer Publishing Co. Inc., 1963.

>*The authors propose concepts and guidelines for the care of the long-term patient.*

Gubersky, B. Geriatric nursing. *In* Cowdry, E. V., ed. The Care of the Geriatric Patient. St. Louis, The C. V. Mosby Co., 1958, pp. 214-238.

>*A nursing service director in a large and well-known home and hospital for the aged discusses some psychological as well as physical aspects of care. She makes the point that it is the knowledge that each nurse has of the patient that makes for the varying degrees of quality nursing and satisfactory accomplishments in geriatric nursing.*

Hodkinson, M. Nursing the Elderly. Oxford, Pergamon Press, Inc., 1966.

>*This small book from England is reviewed by one American nurse as a "real find to add to the somewhat limited literature on geriatric nursing."*

*Newton, K., and Anderson, H. C. Geriatric Nursing. St. Louis, The C. V. Mosby Co., 1966.

>*This is a standard text in its fourth edition. Surprisingly little space or attention is devoted to the care of the dying patient or to coping with problems of dying and bereavement.*

Rudd, T. N. The Nursing of the Elderly Sick. Philadelphia, J. B. Lippincott Co., 1964.

>*A British physician stresses such care components as respect for the individual, coordinated health team endeavors, programs of rehabilitation, and keeping the patient at home as long or as much as possible. He also stresses changes in the philosophical and cultural values in society toward greater support of opportunities and provisions for the aged to con-*

tinue finding "fulfillments" for their lives in their postretirement period.

Schwartz, D., Henley, B., and Seitz, L. The Elderly Ambulatory Patient. New York, The Macmillan Company, 1904.

> A very useful book based on extensive research and experience. Comprehensive care of out-patients 60 years or older and having two or more chronic illnesses is attempted and appraised.

Stevens, M. K. Geriatric Nursing for the Practical Nurse. Philadelphia, W. B. Saunders Company, 1965.

> A reasonably comprehensive and well balanced treatment that is recommended for the practical nurse.

U.S. Department of Health, Education, and Welfare, Public Health Service. Nursing Care of the Aged: An Annotated Bibliography for Nurses. Washington, D.C., U.S. Printing Office, 1967. The authors of the bibliography are Myrtle I. Brown, Priscilla H. Basson, and Dorothy E. Burchett.

> A rather comprehensive bibliography of sources published between the years 1954 to 1965. A valuable source of reference.

Worcester, A. The Care of the Aged, the Dying, and the Dead. Fourth Edition. Springfield, Ill., Charles C Thomas, Publisher, 1961.

> A medical classic unique in its eloquent simplicity, wisdom, skill, and warmth of interpersonal relationships in the care of the aged. No comparable counterpart has appeared in the nursing literature.

Journal References

Brooks, H. L. The golden rule for the unconscious patient. Nurs. Forum, 3:12-18, 1965.

> Interestingly presented portrayal of the needs and rights of unconscious patients.

Brown, J. New concepts in geriatric nursing. Canad. Nurse, 53:289-93, 1957.

> Discourse on some of the special needs of elderly patients, and nursing measures for meeting such needs.

de Lourdes, Mother M. B. Trends in nursing in a residential facility for the elderly. Practical Nurs., 14:2-21, 1964.

> The team approach in nursing homes is stressed, and suggestions are made concerning desirable qualities for nursing personnel.

Feltz, P. My most unforgettable patient. RN, 27:76-79, 1964.

> This nurse relates how she aided an aged patient to regain an interest in living.

Gerletti, J., Crawford, C. C., and Perkins, D. Rx for your geriatric patient. RN, 25:88f, 1962.

Useful suggestions to nurses for safeguarding the dignity of elderly patients.

Martin, J. Caring for the geriatric patient with stroke. Nurs. Mirror, 116:7-11, 1963.

A registered nurse calls attention to the problems of care for the conscious and the unconscious patient following a stroke. An arresting case history is presented.

Michelle, Sister M. Personalized care for the aged and chronically ill. Health News (New York State), 42:5-11, 1965.

New nursing objectives and methodology developed at Sanatorium Gabriels (now Uihlein Mercy Center, Lake Placid, N.Y.) to provide personalized care for the institutionalized aged and chronically ill.

Novick, L. J. Understanding makes the difference. Canad. Nurse, 61:728-730, 1965.

Insightful article on the nurse's need for understanding of the aged patient.

Randall, O. A. Nursing care of the aged. Nurs. World, 130:10-12, 1956.

Noted social worker and gerontologist suggests five ways a nurse can strengthen an aged patient's "wish to live" and, thus, his "will to live."

Rudd, T. N. Geriatric long-stay wards as therapeutic communities. Nurs. Times, 57:1156-61, 1961.

In this discourse on therapeutic communities for the care of aged patients, the author points out that among the requisites for effective geriatric nursing are sensitivity, human warmth and understanding, and sociological knowledge.

C. PSYCHIATRICALLY ORIENTED READINGS

Book References

Berezin, M. A., and Cath, S. H., eds. Geriatric Psychiatry: Grief, Loss, and Emotional Disorders in the Aging Process. New York, International Universities Press, 1965.

A good treatment by a number of authors.

Busse, E. W. Psychoneurotic reactions and defense mechanisms in the aged. *In* Hoch, P. E., and Zubin, J., eds. Psychopathology of Aging. New York, Grune & Stratton, Inc., 1961, pp. 274-284.

Study and report on a community sample of aged persons and the prevalence of neuroses among them, defense patterns for these abnormalities, and the problem of treating them.

Group for the Advancement of Psychiatry. Psychiatry and the Aged: An Introductory Approach. New York, GAP, 1965.

> *A summary analysis, formulated by the committee on aging under the chairmanship of Alvin I. Goldfarb, of basic data and definitions, dimensions of the problem, classification of the mental and emotional disorders of the aged, and a formulation of goals and expectations in treatment. An informative overall introduction, with references and suggested readings.*

*Post, F. The Clinical Psychiatry of Late Life. London, Pergamon Press, 1965.

> *An excellent brief treatise, useful and easily understood.*

Zinberg, N., and Kaufman, I. Normal Psychology of the Aging Process. New York, International Universities Press, 1963.

> *The physiological, psychological, and social aspects of the progress of aging are linked together in the area of gerontological psychiatry in an effort to formulate theories about the problem and treatment of personality disorders in the aged.*

Journal References

Gibson, J. Mental diseases of old age. Canad. Nurse, 56:604f, 1960.

> *Brief discourse by a British psychiatrist on some of the more common mental disorders, their symptoms, and causes.*

Kramer, J. R. and Kramer, C. H. Helping staff understand our philosophy of patient care. Geriat. Nurs., 3:20-26, 1967.

> *This administrator and medical director, respectively, of a proprietary nursing home, having found that "the most puzzling and difficult problems which geriatric patients present are mental and emotional behavioral disturbances," instituted an ongoing in-service program to help staff become more aware and understanding of factors involved in patient behavior. They describe the program and report that it has resulted in improved staff performance.*

Simon, A. The geriatric mentally ill. Gerontologist, 8:7-17, 1968.

> *A brief, but good overview of the aged mentally ill and their care in America.*

IV. The Critically Ill and Dying Patient

Chapters 10 to 12.

A. CONCEPTS, PROBLEMS, ATTITUDES, AND REACTIONS TO DEATH AND DYING

Book References

Back, K. W., and Baade, H. W. The social meaning of death and the law. *In* McKinney, J. C., and de Vyver, F. T., eds. Aging and Social Policy. New York, Appleton-Century-Crofts, 1966, pp. 302-329.

> *A penetrating analysis of the implications of dominant attitudes held toward death in American society and some of the alternative attempts at coming to grips with the inherent problems.*

Borkenau, F., The concept of death. *In* Fulton, R., ed. Death and Identity. New York, John Wiley & Sons, Inc., 1965, pp. 42-56.

> *There are traced some of the conflicting attitudes toward death in different cultures and historical epochs: death denial; death defiance; death embracing. "In regard to our special problem we may assume that the denial of death is the most deeply rooted of the archetypes, since it is structurally, and in all probability chronologically, tied to the awareness of human mortality."*

*Choron, J. Death and Western Thought. New York, Collier-Macmillan, 1963.

> *This book provides a rich survey of the philosophers' "answers" to the problem of death and dying. The author's professed intent was to "fill the gap" in the philosophical literature on the subject and to throw some light on the possible impact of the fact of death and the attitudes toward it on philosophical thinking.*

*——— Modern Man and Mortality. New York, The Macmillan Company, 1964.

> *The author presents a penetrating and provocative discussion of supports for and against belief in life after death. Varieties of death fears, especially by older persons, and some evidence is presented for the claim that fear in the face of death is not an inevitable experience. Ways of alleviating the fear of death are recorded and discussed in some detail.*

Diggory, J. C., and Rothman, D. Z. Values destroyed by death. *In* Fulton, R., ed. Death and Identity. New York, John Wiley & Sons, Inc., 1965, pp. 152-160.

> *The findings indicate that the concomitants, or consequences, of a person's death which he fears most are influenced largely by the role he has or expects to have and, thus, by the goals to which he is committed.*

Feifel, H. Attitudes of mentally ill patients toward death. *In* Fulton, R., ed. Death and Identity. New York, John Wiley & Sons, Inc., 1965, pp. 131-142.

> *The author reports that the study showed that the degree of mental disturbance in patients has little seeming effect on their overall attitudes toward death.*

*——— Attitudes toward death in some normal and mentally ill populations. *In* Feifel, H., ed. The Meaning of Death. New York, McGraw-Hill Book Company, 1959, pp. 114-130.

This chapter stresses the idea that man's birth is an un-controlled event in life but that he often can have something to do with the manner of his departure from life and that his philosophy of life and death may carry profound psychosocial connotations, especially for his manner of dying.

———— Death. *In* Farberow, N. L., ed. Taboo Topics. New York, Atherton Press, 1963, pp. 8-21.

An impressive and clarifying article on contemporary American tendencies to deny and defy the facts of death, especially in personal reference.

Fulton, R., and Geis, G. Death and social values. *In* Fulton, R., ed. Death and Identity. New York, John Wiley & Sons, Inc., 1965, pp. 67-75.

The idea is presented that death in America has ceased to be merely a religious and philosophical concern and has become a subject of scientific investigation. It is also emphasized that in personal context death has become a taboo subject to be avoided and disguised.

Nagy, M. H. The child's view of death.† In Feifel, H. ed. The Meaning of Death. New York, McGraw-Hill Book Company, 1959, pp. 79-98.

Describes three major stages of development in children of their ideas about the nature of death. Between three and five, children tend to highlight the denial of death as an inevitable and final process. Between five and nine or ten, death seems to be personified. Between nine and ten, it is recognized as a process that takes place in everyone with the dissolution of the physical life.

Simmons, L. W. Reactions to death. *In* The Role of the Aged in Primitive Society, New Haven, Yale University Press, 1945, pp. 217-243.

A summary cross-cultural survey of reactions to death by certain primitive and historical peoples.

Solnit, A. J., and Green, M. The pediatric management of the dying child. Part II: The child's reaction to the fear of dying. *In* Modern Trends in Child Development. New York, Indiana University Press, 1963.

This is an excellent follow-up on Part I: Psychological Considerations in the Management of Death on Pediatric Hospital Services listed under Journal References.

Wahl, C. W. The fear of death. *In* Fulton, R. ed. Death and Identity. New York, John Wiley & Sons, Inc., 1965, pp. 56-66.

A review of man's fear of death and some of the paradoxes involved in his irrational copings with this fear. It is suggested that children's reactions to death may provide some useful clues for the understanding of adult behavior.

† The references on the reactions of children to death are included here because of their usefulness for the contrast that appears in the reactions of adults and aged persons.

Journal References

Kastenbaum, R. The realm of death: an emerging area in psychological research. J. Human Relations, 13:538-552, 1965.

> *Short summary on concepts and attitudes about death and their implications.*

Parsons, T. Death in American society. Amer. Behav. Scientists, 6:61-65, 1963.

> *A good brief analysis of denial of death in American life.*

Solnit, A. J., and Green, M. Psychologic considerations in the management of death on pediatric hospital services. Part I. The doctor and the child's family. Pediatrics, 24:106-112, 1959.

> *Useful for purposes of comparing patterns of coping with death of the young and the old.*

B. ATTITUDES AND REACTIONS OF THE AGED TO DEATH AND DYING

Book References

Kastenbaum, R. The Mental Life of the Dying Geriatric Patient. Proceedings of the International Congress of Gerontology. Vienna, June 26 to July 7, 1966. No. 842, pp. 153-159.

> *There is discussion on preparing the way for more effective research in this important subject. The approach here is limited to three variables: the mental status of the patients, their explicit references to death, and the degree to which these patients become well-known to the hospital staff. Tentative findings fail to support the popular assumption that most aged patients are in poor mental contact when they reach the stage of dying.*

Munnichs, J. A. M. Old Age and Finitude: A Contribution to Psychogerontology. Basle, Switzerland, S. Karger, 1966.

> *"Finitude" is used here to mean "knowing and realizing that one's life will come to an end." The major questions discussed are: how central is the experience of finitude in old age; are old people more sensitive and fearful or acceptive of the end; and is such acceptance, when it occurs, related to identifiable degrees of maturity in the individual? It is a thoughtful, carefully organized, and very suggestive book based on interview studies in the town of Nijmegen, Netherlands.*

Swenson, W. M. Attitudes toward death among the aged. *In* Fulton, R., ed. Death and Identity. New York, John Wiley & Sons, Inc., 1965, pp. 105-111.

> *Attempts were made to obtain objective measures of the death attitudes of a cross-section of aged persons who appeared to the author to be aging successfully. It is reported*

that conscious fear of dying was found to be rare among this sample of aged persons.

Wolff, K. Personality Type and Reaction toward Aging and Death. Presented at the Gerontological Association Convention in Los Angeles, California, St. Louis, the Gerontological Society, November, 1965.

> *A psychiatrist, through depth interviews, studied the emotional reactions toward death by aged patients. He noted that the strongest predictive factor is the person's previous pattern of lifelong defenses.*

Journal References

Feifel, H. Older persons look at death. Geriatrics, 2:127-130, 1956.

> *A summary report of attitudes and views of the aged on death.*

Lipman, A., and Marden, P. W. Preparation for death in old age. J. Geront., 21:426-431, 1966.

> *A statistical study by interview of 119 aged persons who lived alone and were "poor"—with a median annual income of $840.00. The two statistically significant variables shown to be related to responsibility in preparation for dying were race and educational background—whites and higher education correlated with higher responsibility assumed by the respondents.*

C. RECORDS AND TESTIMONIALS ON PERSONAL EXPERIENCE WITH IMPENDING DEATH

Book References

Choron, J. The problem of easy dying. *In* Modern Man and Mortality. New York, The Macmillan Company, 1964, pp. 91-103.

> *Presents the thesis that the way to mitigate fear of death depends on the kind of fear and its intensity. The coping patterns of famous persons are cited. Perhaps the most striking example is that of the English philosopher David Hume who appears very successfully to have come to terms with death. "On April 16, 1776, I was struck with a disorder in my bowels, which at first gave me no alarm, but has since, as I apprehend it, become mortal and incurable. I now reckon upon a speedy dissolution." Hume lived several months with this knowledge of approaching death and tried heroically to come to constructive terms with it. His friends and physicians were unanimous in their admiration of his serenity.*

de Beauvoir, S. A Very Easy Death. New York, G. P. Putnam's Sons, 1965.

> *This well-known French writer gives a detailed account of her 78-year-old mother's terminal illness and death in a nursing home in Paris. The mother sustained injuries during a fall in the apartment house where she lived. While a patient in "one of the best" nursing homes in Paris, a diagnosis of*

cancer was made and surgery performed. The book contains a day by day account of what was happening, including attitudes and behavior of doctors and nurses who cared for the patient. Her two daughters kept the diagnosis from their mother, but the reader gets the impression that the mother was aware of her condition. She had told her one daughter that she would never return to her flat and had said to the other that "death itself does not frighten me, it is the jump I am afraid of." There are flashbacks, which reveal life patterns of the mother. This is a powerful and moving, and sometimes shocking, document, beautifully written.

Goldsmith, N. Multiple sclerosis. *In* Pinner, M., and Miller, B. F., eds. When Doctors are Patients. New York, W. W. Norton & Company, Inc., 1952, pp. 157-168.

When this report was published, Dr. Goldsmith was practicing dermatology in Lancaster, Pa. For many years he had suffered from multiple sclerosis in its slow and insidious development. "At best now I walk with great difficulty, rarely leave my home, and I am just this side of a wheelchair. I used to improve irregularly, but for more than two years now I have failed to enjoy anything except the slightest transitory remissions, and am slowly but relentlessly deteriorating." He describes with skill and valuable insight the symptoms of his illness, the effects they have upon him as a person, and his ingenious and successful coping adaptations. The effect is very inspiring.

Meyerson, A. Vascular disease. *In* Pinner, M., and Miller, B. F., eds. When Doctors are Patients. New York, W. W. Norton & Company, Inc., 1952, pp. 183-200.

Dr. Meyerson spent many years in research, practice, and teaching of psychiatry in Boston. He gives a remarkably detailed account of the development of his heart disease over a period of eleven years, up to a few months of his death, and provides with amazing objectivity an intimate account of his mental, emotional, and interpersonal problems and how he coped with them in the face of impending death. A very impressive and illuminating document.

*Moran, Lord. The following account is taken from the Diaries of Lord Moran, The Struggle for Survival 1940-1965. Boston, Houghton Mifflin Company, 1966.

An amazingly detailed picture of the British statesman Sir Winston Churchill's attitude toward death and how he coped with the problems as they appeared to him can be abstracted from Lord Moran's diary notes.

Pinner, M. Chronic heart disease. *In* Pinner, M., and Miller, B. F., eds. eds. When Doctors are Patients. New York, W. W. Norton & Company, Inc., 1952, pp. 18-30.

Dr. Pinner, Chief of Division of Pulmonary Diseases at Montefiore Hospital, New York City, describes his instantaneous recognition of angina in himself and the slow but continuous development of a fatal heart disease. He illustrates the unfortunate failure of fellow physicians to be frank with him about his condition and his personal mistake of trying to keep secret his awareness of impending death. A remarkable document.

Sigerist, H. E. Living under the shadow. *In* Pinner, M., and Miller, B. F., eds. When Doctors are Patients. New York, W. W. Norton & Company, Inc., 1952, pp. 3-17.

Dr. Sigerist, a physician and eminent medical historian, describes with skill and intimate personal detail how he lived and continued to labor with reasonable mental poise under the shadow of a critical heart ailment, "my third incurable disease which is a serious one, a killer."

*Tolstoy, L. The Death of Ivan Ilych and Other Stories. New York, The New American Library of World Literature, 1960, pp. 95-156.

Here is a famous literary classic first published in Russia in 1886. It is a very dramatic short story from the pen of the famous author. The story is about a Russian official of good conventional character and average ability. It tells of his promotion to a judgeship, his marriage, entanglement with family functions and their frictions and routine and, also, of his affliction with an incurable illness. There is developed a striking dual account of a deteriorating body and a soul or mind that awakens first to the horrors of dying but finally appears to transcend death into a calm peace and "light."

*Troyat, H. Tolstoy. Translated from the French by Nancy Amphoux. Garden City, Doubleday & Company, Inc., 1967.

From original sources, family diaries mainly, a detailed and extensive account is recorded about the great and continuous fear of death that Leo Tolstoy suffered in his old age and how he attempted, perhaps not too successfully, to cope with it within what was for him a harrowing family situation.

Wertenbaker, L. T. Death of a Man. New York, Random House, Inc., 1957.

Charles Christian Wertenbaker was a professional writer who was living in Paris, France, at the time of his voluntary death, following a diagnosis of cancer. He consented to exploratory surgery, but before doing so he stipulated that no drastic surgery be done. The surgeon complied with the patient's wishes. As related in this book by his wife, Charles Wertenbaker loved life, but preferred death rather than to go on living dependent upon others. He wanted to die a whole man, and with his faculties intact, which he feared he would not be able to do if he permitted the doctors to cut him up and he became bedridden. So he took matters into his own hands. Sometime before he died, he worked on an outline for a book to be called "Sixty Days in a Lifetime," expressing his feelings about his situation. Death of a Man is a striking, detailed, and at times shocking, account of his terminal illness and voluntary death by his wife and of the actively supportive role she played.

Journal References

Lewis, W. R. A time to die. Nurs. Forum 4:6-27, 1965.

Author relates two case studies and draws some interesting conclusions.

MacDonald, A. Death psychology of historical personages. Amer. J. Psychol., 32:552-556, 1921.

A useful discussion of the age, manner of death, and need of final communication manifested by historically prominent persons.

Peterson, R. The advantages of growing old. Nurs. Outlook, 11:26-27, 1964.

This article contains a discussion of Cicero's views on old age and death. Cicero, in his DE SENECTUTE, points out that old age has its compensations, and loss of physical vigor and withdrawal from activity can be considered invitations to further one's intellectual potential; for he believes that age does not necessarily weaken the mind and points to a number of aged individuals who occupied prestigious positions. Another interesting observation of Cicero's is that man experiences death in a number of ways during his life time: the death of infancy; the death of adolescence; the death of middle age, and he suggests that man is prepared to face the inevitable.

Saunders, C. A patient. Nurs. Times, March 31, 1961.

A remarkable and inspiring account of a young wife and mother who suffered long in dying and gave as much or more than she got from very faithful supporters—suggests the possibility that some individuals who suffer most have most to give.

D. SHOULD THE PATIENT BE TOLD THE TRUTH ABOUT A TERMINAL PROGNOSIS

Book References

Benet, S. V. No visitors. *In* Selected Works. New York, Henry Holt and Company, 1940.

A notable literary plea is made for the patient to be told the truth about his diagnosis if he seems able to take it and wants it.

Fox, R. Experiment Perilous. New York, The Free Press, 1959.

> *A poignant description of a hospital system where pronounced open awareness prevails with respect to terminal diagnosis and with pertinent effects upon the social structure and the interpersonal relations.*

Glaser, B. G., and Strauss, A. Awareness of Dying. Chicago, Aldine Publishing Company, 1965.

> *An analysis of types of awareness context and degrees of awareness of impending death on the part of patients and those who attend them. Chapters 8 to 10 carry useful interpretations of the dynamics involved in the varying critical situations and the pros and cons of communicating what to whom and in what manner. No special attention is directed to aged dying patients.*

*Goldfarb, A. I. (Moderator). Death and Dying: Attitudes of Patient and Doctor. New York, Group for the Advancement of Psychiatry, 1965.

> *This symposium, sponsored by the Group for the Advancement of Psychiatry, presents some fresh and provocative ideas on attitudes of patients toward death and how physicians may cope with problems related to them.*

*Verwoerdt, A. Communication with the Fatally Ill. Springfield, Ill. Charles C Thomas, Publisher, 1966.

> *This book presents reflections of medical views of caution in communicating terminal diagnoses to patients. The author, who is a psychiatrist, addresses his discourse primarily to physicians.*

Wolff, I. S. The magnificence of understanding. *In* Standard, S., and Nathan, H., eds. Should the Patient Know the Truth. New York, Springer Publishing Co., Inc., 1955.

> *An exceptionally fine and sensitive statement by a nurse.*

Journal References

Brauer, P. H. Should the patient be told the truth. Nurs. Outlook, 8:672-676, 1960.

> *Emphasizes the query, "Pray, which patient, and what truth?" Interesting and provocative comments out of observations and clinical experience of a physician. There are also some useful clarifications on the varied meanings of "terminal." Observation is made that it is the time element involved in terminal that is most tricky.*

Cappon, D. How the living look at dying. RN, 28:45-48 and 110-113, 1965.

> *An interesting and pertinent summary of a physician's study which sought answers from 254 persons—varying in age and ranging from healthy to dying. Explored were such ques-*

tions as: the extent of information desired on their pending death; their preferred way of dying; any preferences for euthanasia; fear of dying; and the relation of their value systems to their attitudes toward death.

Christ, A. E. Attitude toward death among a group of acute geriatric psychiatric patients. J. Geront., 16:56-59, 1961.

Report of a study on how a group of 100 aged psychiatric patients felt about the topic of death. A large majority reportedly manifested fears about death; but 87 percent of those responding stated that they had never talked about death or dying to any staff member before this interview for the study.

Kalish, R. A. A social psychological view (on death and responsibility). Psychiat. Opinion, 3:14-19, 1966.

A constructive discussion on who is responsible, when, and how, for telling a patient about his impending death.

Kramer, C. H., and Dunlap, H. E. The dying patient. Geriat. Nurs., 2:15-20, 1966.

Discusses the challenge of resisting and fighting death in old age and the problem of whether to tell the patient about his fatal illness.

Oken, D. What to tell cancer patients. JAMA, 175:1120-28, 1961.

The claim is made and partially demonstrated that the major reason of physicians to justify not telling their patients when their diagnosis is terminal has not been really tested from their "clinical experience." According to Dr. Oken, physicians often claim that the patient is apt to go to pieces when informed that he is fatally ill, and in actual fact, such a generalization is not well-grounded on objective data.

Quint, J. C. Obstacles to helping the dying. Amer. J. Nurs., 66:1568-1571, 1966.

Discussion of how nurses are hindered in their care when patients have not been told they are fatally ill and when the patients' terminal behavior is counter to the nurse's expectations.

Saunders, C. A medical director's view (on death and responsibility). Psychiat. Opinion, 3:28-34, 1966.

Some excellent ideas are shared on how to tell, or not to tell, a patient of his approaching death, helping him to die peacefully and, also, to live until he dies.

Sheff, T. J. Rules, types of error, and their consequences in medical diagnosis. Behav. Sci., 8:97-107, 1963.

An instructive analysis on why there are fewer risks for physicians in not communicating a very poor prognosis.

E. A CRITICAL ISSUE IN LIFE OR DEATH

Book References

Cabot, N. H. You Can't Count on Dying. Boston, Houghton Mifflin Company, 1961.

> *A protest against extraordinary prolongation of life.*

Dorozynski, A. The Man They Wouldn't Let Die. New York, The Macmillan Company, 1965.

> *Dramatic account of society's attempt to prolong the life of a valued scientist.*

Glaser, B. G., and Strauss, A. L. Time for Dying. Chicago, Aldine Publishing Company, 1968.

> *Descriptive data on dying patients focused on the process of dying, the variable of the time involved, and the reaction of those who attend the dying. Observations are set within the context of sociological theories. Little special attention is given to senescent deaths.*

Journal References

Blaker, C. W. Thanatopsis. The Christian Century, December 7, 1966, pp. 1503-1506.

> *Record of an 8-year medical prolongation of the life of an unconscious man and its social implications and consequences.*

Deutsch, F. Euthanasia: A clinical study. Psychoanal. Quart., 5:347-368, 1936.

> *Report on various clinical cases involving euthanasia.*

Duke, T. W. Artificial prolongation of life. Presbyterian Life, January 1, 1967, pp. 15-17.

> *A physician's simple and clear account of what is meant by artificial prolongation of life and its implications for medical and nursing care.*

Editorial. What they (nurses) say about the right to die. RN, 27:64-70, 99, 1964.

> *Nurses' reasons for and against the "right to die" for very old and ill patients. See also RN, 28:72-3, 1965.*

Fletcher, J. The patient's right to die. Harpers Magazine, October, 1960, pp. 141f.

> *Considers pros and cons of the right to die.*

Glaser, B., and Strauss, A. L. Temporal aspects of dying. Amer. J. Sociol., 71:48-59, 1965.

> *Interesting discussion of significant favorable and unfavorable aspects of the time factor in geriatric deaths.*

Kalish, R. A. A continuum of subjectively perceived death. Gerontologist, 6:73-76, 1966.

> *This article utilizes the concepts of social death, psy-chological death, physical death, and "social immortality" in exploring the speculation that "subjectively perceived death can occur at various times in various degrees as a function of the interaction between the perceiver and the perceived dying . . ."*

Kastenbaum, R. As the clock runs out. Ment. Hyg., 50:332-336, 1966.

> *An interesting presentation of a conceptual context within which time, aging, and death converge in a special personalized experience.*

Shideler, M. M. Coup de Grace. The Christian Century, December 7, 1966, pp. 1499-1506.

> *Description of a case of prolonged irreversible illness and the arguments supporting euthanasia.*

Weisman, A. Appropriate death. Int. J. Psychiat., 2:190-93, 1966.

> *Proposes criteria for an appropriate death. Among these, emphasis is placed on the kind of death a person would choose for himself in facing impending death.*

V. Bereavement†

† Chapters 13 and 14.

Book References

Agee, J. Death in the Family. New York, Avon Books, 1951.

> *Documentation and discussion of family and relatives' in-volvement with death in homes 50 years ago. Provides good basis for comparison of then and now.*

Anonymous. A way of dying. *In* Skipper, J. K., Jr., and Leonard, R. C. Social Interaction and Patient Care. Philadelphia, J. B. Lippincott Co., 1965.

> *A striking testimonial from a shocked and grieving wife who describes how her husband suffered a prolonged and agonizing death within a hospital setting.*

Birren, J. E. Reaction to loss and the process of aging: Interrelationships of environmental changes, psychological capacities, and physiological status. *In* Berezin, M. A., and Cath, S. H., eds. Geriatric Psychiatry: Grief, Loss, and Emotional Disorders in the Aging Process. New York, International Universities Press, 1965.

> *Summary of concepts about early and late life relation-ships as related to life reviews covering the age phases of ex-pansion, stability, and contraction. Reported findings signify*

*the great importance of the family to the aged and indicate
that the widowed, the single, and the divorced are less favored in late life.*

Eliot, T. D. Bereavement: Inevitable but not insurmountable. *In* Becker,
H., and Hill, R., eds. Family Marriage and Parenthood. Boston,
D. C. Heath & Company, 1955, 641-668.

*A sociological discussion of the patterns and functions of
bereavement in family and community context.*

Glaser, B. G., and Strauss, A. L. Awareness of Dying. Chicago, Aldine
Publishing Company, 1965.

*Chapter 9, "The Unaware Family" (of terminal illness
in the patient), suggests that a dying patient's family creates
a chronic problem for nurses, especially in a "closed" awareness context. The authors describe the problems that arise
and the often awkward and feeble staff patterns for coping
with them.*

*Chapter 10, "The Aware Family," describes the different
kinds of problems that arise for the staff when the family
knows about the terminal prognosis, a critical variable being
whether the patient also knows about his being fatally ill. It is
indicated that full awareness by both the family and patient
eases the communication problems for the staff, but many
other problems remain and some new ones are likely to
appear.*

Gorer, G. Death, Grief and Mourning in Contemporary Britain. London,
Cresset Press, 1965.

*This book provides an excellent basis for drawing com-
parisons between English and American practices associated
with death and funerals.*

Mitford, J. The American Way of Death. New York, Simon & Schuster,
Inc., 1963.

*A somewhat sensational, but reasonably valid, account of
funeral practices in the United States.*

Schwab, Sister M. The nurse's role in assisting families of dying geriatric
patients to manage grief and guilt. *In* ANA Clinical Sessions, American Nurses Association. New York, Appleton-Century-Crofts, 1968.

*A short, but excellent paper based on the assumption
that grief is normally a process that reaches a stage of resolution. The observation is made that guilt frequently comes into
play when the grieving process is resolved before actual death
takes place. Three instructive case histories are provided.*

Shorr, A. L. Filial Responsibility in the Modern American Family. Washington, D.C. U.S. Department of Health, Education, and Welfare.
1960.

A notable article indicating how the American family has constituted a solid core of interpersonal responsibility and a chief anchor to aging and dying. The author evaluates current practices of filial responsibility in the United States and the relationship of this to the Social Security Program.

*Townsend, P. The Family Life of Old People: An Inquiry in East London. London, Routledge and Kegan Paul, 1957.

An excellent description of social and interpersonal relationships in contemporary family life.

Volkart, E. H., and Michael, S. T. Bereavement and mental health. *In* Leighton, A. H., Clausen, J. A., and Wilson, R. N., eds. Explorations in Social Psychiatry. New York, Basic Books, Inc., Publishers, 1957.

An analysis of the processes of bereavement and the social role of funerals.

Journal References

Eliot, T. D. Of the shadow of death. Ann. Amer. Acad. Polit. Soc. Sci., 229:87-99, 1943.

A very suggestive article of potential usefulness to nursing personnel.

———. The bereaved family. Ann. Amer. Acad. Polit. Soc. Sci., 160:184-190, 1932.

A useful sociological analysis of the dynamics and processes in family grief.

Engel, G. L. Grief and grieving. Amer. J. Nurs., 64:93-98, 1964.

Discussion on how nurses may be helped to provide aid and comfort to grieving families and patients.

Simmons, L. W. Aging in primitive societies: a comparative survey of family life and relationships. Law and Contemporary Problems, 27:36-51, 1962.

Summary of family relationships and their effects upon aging in primitive societies.

VI. *The Geriatric Nurse Practitioner*

Chapters 15 and 16.

A. THE NURSE IN GERIATRICS: SATISFACTIONS, FRUSTRATIONS, NEEDS, AND RESPONSIBILITIES

Book References

Argyris, C. Interpersonal Competence and Organizational Effectiveness. Homewood, Ill., Dorsey Press, 1962.

This book contains an excellent treatise (pp. 1-37) on the social responsibility of institutions and the effects of an organization on human behavior. Questions are raised about the assumptions underlying currently accepted principles of organization.

—————— Personality and Organization. New York, Harper and Brothers, 1957.

Another very useful sourcebook by the same author. The nurse occupying a leadership position in a geriatric institution will find here much pertinent material on the interrelationship of the formal social structure and the people who work within it. There is presented an insightful treatise on the ways in which the behavior of individuals is affected depending upon the particular type of organizational structure within an institution.

Barnes, E. People in Hospital. London, Macmillan and Company, 1961.

While the author addresses herself primarily to the hospital situation, the document has pertinence for nurses in geriatric facilities as well. Chapter 4 contains a description of possible demands on nurses by patients and the satisfactions the nurse derives from being needed. In Chapter 9, the author discusses interpersonal relationship problems that may have dire effects on patient care. Some of the special problems related to institutionalization of older persons are also discussed.

Barrett, J. The Head Nurse: Her Changing Role, Second Edition. New York, Appleton-Century-Crofts, 1968.

Part I of this edition presents a new role for the head nurse. There are excellent discussions on institutional organization and the kind of relationships which must be established between the head nurse and other health personnel in order to provide effective and optimum care for patients and their families. While the author directs herself to the hospital head nurse, the document has as much pertinence for any nurse who occupies a leadership position in a geriatric institution. Contains a wealth of annotated references as well as exercises for teaching purposes.

Brown, E. L. Newer Dimensions of Patient Care, Part II: Improving Staff Motivation and Competence in the General Hospital. New York, Russell Sage Foundation, 1962.

This is the second of three volumes on NEWER DIMENSIONS OF PATIENT CARE. It contains useful suggestions for raising the staff's self-confidence and self-esteem. Volume One: THE USE OF THE PHYSICAL AND SOCIAL ENVIRONMENT OF THE GENERAL HOSPITAL FOR THERAPEUTIC PURPOSES and Volume III: PATIENTS AS PEOPLE also contain a great deal of useful information for nursing.

Strauss, G., and Sayles, L. K., The Human Problems of Management. Englewood Cliffs, N.J., Prentice Hall, 1960.

A very useful book on working with people. Has sections on the meaning of work, rewards the worker expects, and skills needed for effective supervision.

Journal References

Artwein, C. Geriatric nursing is rewarding. Practical Nurs., 12:19, 1962.

> *Discourse on how rewarding work with the aged ill can be.*

Blancher, G. C. Some satisfactions in geriatric nursing. Amer. J. Nurs., 60:1635, 1960.

> *According to this nurse, one of the satisfactions to be derived from working with the aged ill is the degree to which it is possible to get to know the patient and to learn to anticipate his needs.*

Clemente, Sister M. Existentialism: a philosophy on commitment. Amer. J. Nurs., 66:500, 1966.

> *This inspiring account on the meaning of commitment makes the point that being committed means being personally involved—the results are intangible rewards for the nurse who becomes "involved."*

Davis, B. A. Coming of age: a challenge for geriatric nursing. Jour. Amer. Geriat. Soc., 16:1100-1106, 1968.

> *A brief, but useful, historical review of geriatric nursing in this country "with a focus on the work being done in this area by the geriatric division of the American Nurses Association."*

Jones, E. M. Who supports the nurse? Nurs. Outlook, 10:476, 1962.

> *A discourse on the need of the nurse to receive support —from her peers, immediate superiors, or other co-workers—in order to give support to her patients.*

Goodland, N. L. Putting the patient in the picture. Nurs. Mirror, 121:7, 1965.

> *The point is made that patients must have their questions answered truthfully if their minds are to be at ease. It is proposed that if physicians fail to satisfy the patients' need for information, it behooves the nurse to assume this responsibility. Possible reasons for the nurse's reluctance to answer patients' questions are also discussed.*

Knowles, L. N. Nursing care of the geriatric patient. J. Nurs. Educ., 4:13, 1965.

> *According to the author of this discussion on three phases of nursing care for the aged, geriatric nursing can be rewarding even when the patient may be dying.*

Kron, T. Nurses' aides need clearer directions. Amer. J. Nurs., 63:118, 1963.

In this article the point is made that the nurse who is responsible for care given by ancillary personnel must make sure that her directions and instructions are clearly understood by them. Numerous illustrations of misunderstanding of such instructions are included.

Marie, Sister C. Nursing needs more freedom. Amer. J. Nurs., 62:53, 1962.

The proposal is made that nurses be allowed more freedom than they presently have in evaluating patients' needs and planning patient care; but the caution is expressed that nurses may not be ready to make proper use of such freedom —they should have preparation for it.

Peplau, H. E. The heart of nursing: interpersonal relationships. Canad. Nurse, 61:273, 1965.

If nurses accept the premise that interpersonal relations are the heart of nursing, it behooves them to look at and examine their relationships not only with patients but with other disciplines as well.

Raphael, W. Nurse, nurse, for better or worse. Nurs. Times, 61:1686, 1965.

A research consultant reports the findings that the comments patients made on the care they received centered around two aspects: nurse-patient relationships and skill, with relationships being mentioned much more often than skill.

Reiter, F. Choosing the better part. Amer. J. Nurs. 64:65, 1964.

This nurse educator suggests that "the long-term care setting is the place in which some of the problems of independence in nursing practice may be resolved." Implications for the geriatric nurse are easy to see.

Scriver, I. Nursing home care in geriatrics. Canad. Nurse, 65:110, 1965.

A director of nursing services at a Canadian geriatric center identifies nine personality characteristics especially needed by nurses caring for the aged ill.

Weinsaft, P., and Friedman, D. In-service program offers continuous improvement in geriatric care. Hospitals, 39:55, 1965.

The authors describe an ongoing in-service program on geriatric nursing which resulted in increased motivation and job satisfaction as well as in improved patient care.

B. ATTITUDES, KNOWLEDGES, AND SKILLS THE NURSE NEEDS FOR OPTIMUM CARE OF DYING PATIENTS

Book References

Aguilera, D. C. Crisis: Death and Dying. *In* ANA Clinical Sessions, American Nurses Association. New York, Appleton-Century-Crofts, 1968.

A revealing paper by a nurse on how nurses react to death and dying. There is also a pertinent brief coverage of the literature interspersed with useful suggestions to geriatric nurses.

Birren, J. E. Life review, reconciliation, and termination. *In* Birren, J. E., ed. The Psychology of Aging. Englewood Cliffs, N.J., Prentice-Hall, Inc., 1964, pp. 25-49.

> *The idea is presented with impressive insight and wisdom that when an aged person comes near to the end of his life, he needs more and more psychological support from fewer and fewer trusted individuals. This becomes especially crucial when the situation provokes for the patient a life review. There is thus need for a sophisticated terminal counselor to help the dying, his relatives, and friends, lest past conflicts get increasingly distorted and perpetuated.*

*Bowers, M. K., Jackson, E. N., Knight, J. A., and LeShan, L. Counseling the Dying. New York, Thomas Nelson and Sons, 1964.

> *A very suggestive and practical guide is provided on how to communicate and provide support to the dying. The authors include a psychoanalyst, a psychiatrist, a chaplain, and a clergyman.*

Eisler, K. R. The Psychiatrist and the Dying Patient. New York, International Universities Press, 1955.

> *Many excellent suggestions from a physician who is sensitive to the need of safeguarding the self-image and dignity of a terminally ill person of whatever age.*

*Hinton, J. Dying. Baltimore, Penguin Books, Inc., 1967.

> *A useful book by a British psychiatrist who combines knowledge of medicine and the social sciences in producing a splendid humane approach and interpretation of death and with helpful suggestions applicable to nursing.*

Howe, M. J. The issue of dying. *In* Exploring Progress in Geriatric Nursing Practice. New York, American Nurses' Association, 1966, pp. 24-32.

> *Drawing upon the literature as well as upon her own experience, this nurse educator challenges nurses to face the issue of death realistically.*

Loether, H. J. Problems of Aging. Belmont, Cal., Dickenson Pub. Co., Inc., 1967.

> *Chapter 8 carries a stimulating discussion of death in old age and the problems associated with it.*

O'Connor, Sister M. C. The Art of Dying Well: The Development of Ars Moriendi. New York, Columbia University Press, 1942.

> *Contains very pertinent suggestions for the geriatric nurse.*

*Quint, J. C. The Nurse and the Dying Patient. New York, The Macmillan Company, 1967.

> *This is an especially valuable book in planning courses and teaching nurses how to provide superior care to dying patients. It is not directed primarily to problems of the aged ill.*

*Saunders, C. Care of the Dying. Nursing Times Reprint. London, Macmillan and Company, 1959.

> *This booklet contains reprints of the articles by Dr. Cicely Saunders (who is a nurse, doctor, and almoner) published in the* Nursing Times *during 1959. Euthanasia, control of pain in terminal cancer, and mental distress in the dying are among the subjects discussed. Also included are useful suggestions related to nursing care. These articles clearly reveal Dr. Saunders' philosophy and practice in a terminal home which assures each patient of personalized and supportive care and permits him to die in his own way.*

Journal References

Baker, J. and Sorensen, K. C. A patient's concern with death. Amer. J. Nurs., 63:90-92, 1963.

> *Consideration is directed to the function of the nurse in talking with a dying patient. The main idea is that the nurse restrain expression of her own thoughts and feelings while she listens to and encourages the patient to express his fears or concerns and helps him formulate his own philosophy.*

Boekelheide, B. Dealing with your feelings of failure. RN, 25:50-56, 1962.

> *A nurse educator suggests that when caring for a patient afflicted with an incurable illness, comfort rather than curative nursing measures should be the first consideration.*

Folta, J. R. The perception of death. Nurs. Research, 14:232-235, 1965.

> *Here is a report on a study of perceptions of impending death by nursing personnel and their reactions to the dying of patients. It was found that most of the nurses viewed death in the abstract as a peaceful, controllable, and common phenomenon; but when death became personalized, it was likely to be perceived with great anxiety.*

Fulton, R., and Langdon, P. A. Attitudes toward death: an emerging mental health problem. Nurs. Forum, 3:104-112, 1964.

> *This is a discourse on the need by nursing and medical personnel, as well as by lay persons, for reorientation to death and dying. The authors suggest that present day practices concerning death and dying are hypocritical.*

Goetz, H. Needed: a new approach to care of the aging. RN, 25:60-62, 1962.

> *While recognizing that by the nurse recovery of the patient is viewed as "success" and his death tends to be interpreted as "failure," this writer stresses the point that termi-*

nal care can be successful. Suggestions are given for the care of the dying.

Ingles, T. Death on a ward. Nurs. Outlook, 12:28, 1964.

> *In this brief statement, striking comparisons are drawn between death on an American ward and death in a Colombian hospital. It provides a graphic description of how freedom is permitted for patients and relatives to express their grief in Colombia and how it usually is restricted in the United States.*

Kastenbaum, R., Cutler, D. R., Kalish, R. A., Weisman, A. D., and Saunders, C. Death and responsibility (symposium), Psychiat. Opinion, 3:41, 1966.

> *Views of a minister, psychologist, social psychologist, psychiatrist, and a medical director on responsibilities when a person is dying. "Our responsibility is to help them to do this as themselves. Not in desperation or distress but in quietness and fulfillment and readiness." Dr. Cicely Saunders, page 34.*

Lieberman, M. A. Observations on death and dying. Gerontologist, 6:70, 1966.

> *This is the report of a study based on data gathered from 22 older people who died from a week to a year after completing a 12- to 15-hour interview and testing. The major observation was that, "viewing the dying process as extending over a relatively long time, I think it is reasonable to say that psychological changes associated with the dying process can be identified and that these changes are specifically related to the time line defined in terms of distance from death." page 72.*

Noles, E. Nursing a geriatric patient. Amer. J. Nurs., 63:63-74, 1963.

> *Here is a suggestive example of providing something like comprehensive care for an aged ill person. Constructive responses are made to the patient's depression, anxieties, and concerns over impending death.*

Northington, J. Comfort for your dying patient. RN, 25:63-64, 1962.

> *A physician describes and evaluates the symptoms of approaching death and suggests things to do to alleviate the patient's discomfort.*

Quint, J. C. Awareness of death and the nurse's composure. Nurs. Research, 15:49-55, 1966.

> *There is a discussion of the influence a ward's social structure exerts upon nurse's composure when a patient is dying.*

Ristau, R. The loneliness of death. Amer. J. Nurs., 58:128-134, 1958.

> *A nursing student gives a vivid account of the evident comfort afforded a dying patient by the nurse's presence during the period of his travail.*

Saunders, C. Terminal illness. Excerpts from papers read before the Health Congress of the Royal Society of Health at Blackpool, 24-28 April 1961, London.

> *A valuable source for gaining insights about the personal aspects of dying as they relate to both the patient and the nurse. It brings out clearly that ". . . we will fail our dying patients if we always remain hidden behind our technical functions and avoid the true personal contact for which they are so often longing."*

———— The last stages of life. Amer. J. Nurs. 65:70-75, 1965.

> *A noted British nurse-physician demonstrates in practice the provision of opportunities for positive achievements and fulfillments in the patient's experience of dying.*

Strauss, A., Glaser, B., and Quint, J. The nonaccountability of terminal care. Hospitals, 38:73-77, 1964.

> *The authors recognize that a degree of responsibility to terminal patients, and for which the nursing staff is not accountable, is probably necessary and desirable, but they also stress the need for improvement, through training, of the nonaccountable psychological aspects of this nursing care. Room for improvement is strongly implied.*

Vanden Bergh, R. L. Let's talk about death to overcome inhibiting emotions. Amer. J. Nurs., 66:71-73, 1966.

> *A physician's plain and sensible discourse on the need for, and ways of, overcoming inhibiting emotions related to death and dying—and the important role the nurse has in the accomplishment of this. There is also a critique on existing patterns in hospitals with respect to this matter.*

Vreeland, R. and Ellis, G. L. Stresses on the nurse in an intensive care unit. JAMA, 208:332-334, 1969.

> *Two nurses describe vividly the stresses, and certain rewards, they have observed or experienced in an intensive-care ward where a patient's life and death hangs so constantly in the balance.*

Wilmhurst, M. More thoughts about dying. Nurs. Times, 55:441-442, 1959.

> *A nurse challenges the position of refusing to tell a dying patient about his fatal illness while at the same time disclosing it to his relatives. She claims that such a situation creates a barrier around the patient at a time when he sorely needs intimate understanding and support.*

Wolff, I. S. Should the patient know the truth? Amer. J. Nurs., 55:546-548, 1955.

> *A delicate and perceptive statement that notes the danger of the nurse's own needs, her approach to, and her potential for, helping the patient most effectively.*

VII. Impact of Culture and Society on Aging and Dying

Chapters 17 and 18.

Book References

Blauner, R. Death and social structure. *In* Neugarten, B. L., ed. Middle Age and Aging: A Reader in Social Psychology. Chicago, Chicago University Press, 1968, pp. 531-540.

> *Summary studies are made on the role of death within the social structure on a wide cross-cultural basis and with a valuable bibliography of anthropological and social character.*

Cumming, E. New thoughts on the theory of disengagement. *In* Kastenbaum, R., ed. New Thoughts on Old Age. New York, Springer Publishing Company, Inc., 1964, pp. 3-18.

> *Attempts are made to elaborate upon and broaden the original disengagement theory to take into account numerous psychological and social factors that affect the aging process.*

────── and Henry, W. E. Growing Old: The Process of Disengagement. New York, Basic Books, Inc., 1961.

> *The authors develop a theory of aging as the "inevitable mutual withdrawal or disengagement resulting in decreased interaction between the aging person and others in the social system to which he belongs." The book has sparked considerable controversy.*

Koller, M. R. Social Gerontology. New York, Random House, Inc., 1968.

> *For a beginning student, here is a brief introductory book on gerontology that touches upon historical backgrounds and recent developments in theories and research. It can be useful in seeking a quick preview of the field; but it may appear superficial to students schooled in either gerontology or geriatrics.*

Kroeber, T. Ishi in Two Worlds: The Biography of the Last Wild Indian in North America. Berkely, University of California Press, 1962.

> *The extinction of a California Indian tribe and the striking story of its last survivor who emerged from the stone age into the modern worlds in 1911, after having tried to live entirely alone in the wilderness.*

Kutner, B., Fanshel, D., Togo, A., and Langner, T. Five Hundred Over Sixty. New York, Russell Sage Foundation, 1956.

> *Insightful explorations are made into the problems of personal and social adjustments of the aged. Attention is directed primarily to issues related to personal morale, marriage and family relations, employment, alienation, and isolation.*

Lasagna, L. Life, Death and the Doctor. New York, Alfred A. Knopf, Inc., 1968.

In Chapter 12, the author presents a striking account of the "tyranny of senescence" as it is lived out in our contemporary culture and society—and from the viewpoint of a physician. Paradoxes that confront the aged patient and the doctor are not difficult to discover. The same can be said of Chapter 13, "Preparing for death."

——— The Doctor's Dilemmas. New York, Harper and Brothers, 1962.

Arresting account of the problems faced by the doctor in treating the dying.

*Lehman, H. C. Age and Achievement. Princeton, N.J., Princeton University Press, 1953.

Striking and inspiring examples out of history of the personal accomplishments of individuals in late age.

Lewis, O. La Vida: A Puerto Rican Family in the Culture of Poverty— San Juan and New York, 1965. New York, Random House, Inc., 1965.

Presented in first person biography is the life of a Puerto Rican mother and her grown-up children under continuing conditions of poverty in two separate and sharply contrasted cities. The implications for illness and aging are pronounced.

Linton, R. The Cultural Background of Personality. New York, D. Appleton-Century Company, Inc., 1945.

Here is a provocative description and interpretation of the dynamic interrelation of culture, society, and the individual.

Lowenthal, M. F., and Haven, C. Interaction and adaptation: Intimacy as a critical variable. In Neugarten, B. L., ed. Middle Age and Aging: A Reader in Social Psychology. Chicago, University of Chicago Press, 1968.

This excellent article explores the significance of intimate relationships as a moral builder in the lives of the aged. The authors "were struck with the fact that the happiest and the healthiest among them often seemed to be people who were or had been involved in one or more close personal relationships. It appeared that such relationships might serve as a buffer against age-linked losses and this explains some of the seeming anomalies." page 390.

*Malinowski, B. A Scientific Theory of Culture and Other Essays. Chapel Hill, University of North Carolina, 1944.

This small book contains a useful analysis and interpretation of the nature of culture and its function in human relations.

Neugarten, B. L., Moore, J. M., and Lowie, J. C. Age norms, age constraints, and adult socialization. In Neugarten, B. L., ed. Middle Age and Aging: A Reader in Social Psychology. Chicago, University of Chicago, University of Chicago Press, 1968, pp. 22-28.

> *An overall discussion of age as one of the bases for ascription of status and function in social organization and a major factor in the regulation of social interaction.*

Reichard, S., Livson, F., and Peterson, P. Aging and Personality. New York, John Wiley & Sons, Inc., 1962.

> *A valuable study of the influence of social and psychological variables, particularly those of personality, upon the status and adjustment patterns of aged and retired men in industrial society.*

Riley, M. W., and Foner, A. Aging and Society. New York, Russell Sage Foundation, 1968.

> *Parts 2 and 3 present the research findings on age-related changes in the human organism and sum up the personality and psychological characteristics associated with old age as compared with youth. Valuable information is also provided on the attitudes and reactions of the aged toward self-identity, life satisfactions, threats to health, mental disorders, including suicidal tendencies, and the anticipation of death. pp. 184-406.*
>
> *Part 4, on "Social Roles," analyzes the structure of roles and digests the research data on change in the roles which old people tend to make or have imposed upon them in work and retirement patterns, family relationships, political interests and activities, religious concerns and observances, membership in voluntary associations, leisure time pursuits, and general social participation.*

Rose, A. M. The subculture of aging: A topic for sociological research. *In* Neugarten, B. L., ed. Middle Age and Aging: A Reader in Social Psychology. Chicago, University of Chicago Press, 1968, pp. 29-34.

> *A discussion of how older persons create mutually shared values and behavioral patterns that constitute what may be called a subculture. The special relevance of this to segregation of the aged is suggested.*

Shock, N. W. Trends in Gerontology. Stanford, Calif. Stanford University Press, 1951.

> *This book presents a multidisciplinary approach to the study of aging, dividing gerontology into the biological and physical; the psychological, the pathological and disease processes; and the sociological spheres.*

Simmons, L. W., ed. Sun Chief: The Autobiography of a Hopi Indian. New Haven, Yale University Press, 1942.

> *A frank and intimate account of 50 years in the life of a Hopi Indian. It attempts to describe in considerable detail how he came to be the person that he is; how he thinks, feels,*

and behaves; and how he copes with aging and illness—being the product of two sharply contrasting cultures.

———— The Role of the Aged in Primitive Society. New Haven, Yale University Press, 1945. (This book is being republished in 1969)

An anthropological study of the status, role, and treatment of the aged in a representative sample of 71 primitive and historical societies.

———— and Wolff, H. G. Social Science in Medicine. New York, Russell Sage Foundation, 1954.

A medico-social science treatise on the interrelationships of society, culture, and the individual with respect to illness and health. Attention is called especially to Chapters 3, 4, and 5.

Sussman, M. B., and Burchinal, L. Kin family network: Unheralded structure in current conceptualization of family functions. *In* Neugarten, B. L., ed. Middle Age and Aging: A Reader in Social Psychology. Chicago University of Chicago Press, 1968, pp. 247-255.

The popular theory of prevalent nuclear family is challenged, and the proposal is made that it be replaced with concepts of a "modified and extended" family system that operates within the network of informal but independent functions. In short, there still exists an American kin family system with complex matrices of aid and service activities that link together the component units into a functional network; and within this system, members of all ages become involved.

Townsend, P. The emergence of the four-generation family in industrial society. *In* Neugarten, B. L., ed. Middle Age and Aging: A Reader in Social Psychology. Chicago, University of Chicago Press, 1968, pp. 255-257.

Attention is called to the existence in Western nations of increasing proportions of elderly persons with great grandchildren. This is regarded as a new and significant phenomenon in human societies, the implications of which may be very great.

von Mering, O., and Weniger, F. L. Social-cultural background of the aging individual. *In* Birren, J. E., ed. Handbook of Aging and the Individual. Chicago, University of Chicago Press, 1959.

An instructive account on the role of culture in the life of the aging individual.

*Williams, R. H., and Wirths, C. G. Lives Through the Years. New York, Atherton Press, 1965.

In this study the theory of disengagement is refined and extended to become an important basis for much of the theoretical work done in the area of aging. The various con-

*ditions for successful and unsuccessful aging are examined
and illustrated by many extensive personal histories.*

Journal References

Barron, M. L. Minority group characteristics of the aged in American
society. J. Geront., 8:472-482, 1958.

> *The aged in America display varied typical minority
> group characteristics. They are stereotyped by younger age
> groups, suffer from prejudices and discrimination in employ-
> ment, feel some subordination, and manifest certain amounts
> of hypersensitivity and defensiveness on their status.*

Glaser, B. A. The social loss of aged dying patients. Gerontologist, 6:77-
80, 1966.

> *How the impact of social value of the aged ill patient
> affects the kind of nursing care that he is likely to receive
> in his terminal stage is pointed out.*

Kutner, B., Socio-economic impacts of aging. J. Amer. Geriat. Soc., 14:
33-40, 1966.

> *Valuable interpretation of socio-economic factors on
> aging.*

Rosenberg, G. S., Age, poverty, and isolation from friends in the urban
working class. J. Geront., 23:533-538, 1968.

> *A systematic study is reported on how dissimilar social
> characteristics (age, income, occupation, and race) affect
> working class persons with respect to their isolation from
> friends and close associates within an urban, neighborhood
> context.*

Shock, N. W. Age with a future. Gerontologist, 8:147-152, 1968.

> *A summary review on the future prospects for aging
> long and well within modern cultures with their developed
> technologies and social systems.*

Statistical Data
Pertaining to Chapters 4 to 16

LIST OF TABLES

1. Childlike treatment of the aged ill as viewed by nurse aides, licensed practical nurses, registered nurses, and degree registered nurses. Chapter 4.

2. The use of kidding, joshing, and humor in staff-patient relationships as viewed by nurse aides, licensed practical nurses, registered nurses, and degree registered nurses. Chapter 5.

3. Coping with mistrust and aggression by aged patients as viewed by nurse aides, licensed practical nurses, registered nurses, and degree registered nurses. Chapter 6.

4. Coping with breakdowns in conventional proprieties as viewed by nurse aides, licensed practical nurses, registered nurses, and degree registered nurses. Chapter 7.

5. Coping with hallucinations and other delusory experiences as viewed by nurse aides, licensed practical nurses, registered nurses, and degree registered nurses. Chapter 8.

6. Differences in nursing care of conscious and unconscious aged patients as viewed by nurse aides, licensed practical nurses, registered nurses, and degree registered nurses. Chapter 9.

7. Differences in nursing care of aged patients based on prognosis as viewed by nurse aides, licensed practical nurses, registered nurses, and degree registered nurses. Chapter 10.

8. Use of "heroic" or "artificial" life-sustaining measures for aged dying patients as viewed by nurse aides, licensed practical nurses, registered nurses, and degree registered nurses. Chapter 11.

9. Aged patients' attitudes toward death and dying as perceived by nurse aides, licensed practical nurses, and registered nurses. Chapter 12.

333

10. Discussing death and dying with aged ill persons as viewed by nurse aides, licensed practical nurses, registered nurses, and degree registered nurses. Chapter 12.

11. Reactions of fellow patients to a death as perceived by nurse aides, licensed practical nurses, and registered nurses. Chapter 13.

12. Coping with patients' stresses when death takes one of them as viewed by nurse aides, licensed practical nurses, registered nurses, and degree registered nurses. Chapter 13.

13. Aiding and supporting bereaved relatives and friends as viewed by nurse aides, licensed practical nurses, registered nurses, and degree registered nurses. Chapter 14.

14. Best liked things or conditions in geriatrics as viewed by nurse aides, licensed practical nurses, and registered nurses. Chapter 15.

15. Least liked things or conditions in geriatrics as viewed by nurse aides, licensed practical nurses, and registered nurses. Chapter 15.

16. Granting greater freedom to the professional nurse for independent action and practice in geriatric care as viewed by degree registered nurses. Chapter 15.

17. Facts about, or attitudes toward, death that tend to help nurses and aged patients cope with this event as viewed by degree registered nurses. Chapter 16.

Statistical Tables

Table 1

CHILDLIKE TREATMENT OF THE AGED ILL
AS VIEWED BY
NURSE AIDES, LICENSED PRACTICAL NURSES, REGISTERED NURSES,
AND DEGREE REGISTERED NURSES

Coded Items	NA's (%) (N=102)	LPN's (%) (N=53)	RN's (%) (N=81)	DRN's (%) (N=95)
TOTAL	100.0	100.0	100.0	100.0
AFFIRMATIVE POSITION				
1. Yes, to make them feel wanted	0.0	1.9	1.2	1.1
2. Yes, to gain their cooperation	7.8	0.0	2.5	0.0
3. Yes, because they behave like children	13.7	7.5	2.5	1.1
SUBTOTAL	21.5	9.4	6.2	2.2
CONDITIONAL POSITION				
4. This depends upon the patient's state of mental health	32.3	11.3	21.0	6.3
5. Patient's personality and background are deciding factors	4.9	3.8	3.7	4.2
6. Personality of staff is a factor	0.0	0.0	0.0	2.1
SUBTOTAL	37.2	15.1	24.7	12.6
NEGATIVE POSITION				
7. Aged patients should never be treated like children	7.8	0.0	12.3	77.9
8. They should be treated with respect and dignity	32.4	73.6	55.6	6.3
SUBTOTAL	40.2	73.6	67.9	84.2
Ambiguous statements	1.1	1.9	1.2	1.1

Table 2

THE USE OF KIDDING, JOSHING, AND HUMOR IN
STAFF-PATIENT RELATIONSHIPS
AS VIEWED BY
NURSE AIDES, LICENSED PRACTICAL NURSES, REGISTERED NURSES,
AND DEGREE REGISTERED NURSES

Coded Items	NA's (%) (N=102)	LPN's (%) (N=53)	RN's (%) (N=82)	DRN's (%) (N=98)
TOTAL	99.9	100.1	100.0	100.0
AFFIRMATIVE POSITION				
1. Yes, as a means of making them feel wanted	18.4	20.8	25.6	5.1
2. Yes, as a means of gaining patient's cooperation	2.9	3.8	6.1	0.0
3. Yes, without amplification	18.4	11.3	3.7	2.0
SUBTOTAL	39.7	35.9	35.4	7.1
NEGATIVE POSITION				
4. Never, various qualifications or none given	3.9	1.9	6.1	26.5
5. No, accord aged patients respect and dignity	2.9	7.5	22.0	7.1
SUBTOTAL	6.8	9.4	28.1	33.6
CONDITIONAL POSITION				
6. This depends upon the patient's health, mental and physical	11.6	5.7	4.9	2.0
7. It depends upon a patient's personality and background	38.8	45.3	29.3	52.0
8. Personality of staff a factor	2.9	1.9	2.4	3.1
SUBTOTAL	53.3	52.9	36.6	57.1
Ambiguous statements	0.0	1.9	0.0	2.2

Table 3

**COPING WITH MISTRUST AND AGGRESSION BY AGED PATIENTS
AS VIEWED BY
NURSE AIDES, LICENSED PRACTICAL NURSES, REGISTERED NURSES,
AND DEGREE REGISTERED NURSES**

Coded Items	NA's (%) (N=102)	LPN's (%) (N=52)	RN's (%) (N=82)	DRN's (%) (N=84)
TOTAL	99.9	99.9	99.9	100.2
NEGATIVE ACCEPTANCE				
1. No experience with this	15.7	7.7	6.1	0.0
2. Shifting responsibility	10.8	3.8	2.4	3.6
3. Use of medications, restraints	0.0	1.9	1.2	2.4
4. Use of diversional tactics	5.9	7.7	4.9	0.0
5. Resort to reason and persuasion	7.8	11.5	2.4	1.2
SUBTOTAL	40.2	32.6	17.0	7.2
POSITIVE ACCEPTANCE				
6. Change of staff with supportive attitude	18.6	9.6	30.5	17.9
7. Acceptance with attempts to reassure	34.3	38.5	24.4	2.4
8. Support to extent of not permitting suffering	2.9	1.9	14.6	28.6
9. Acceptance and attempts to ascertain basic cause	0.0	0.0	7.3	40.5
SUBTOTAL	55.8	50.0	76.8	89.4
Ambiguous statements	3.9	17.3	6.1	3.6

APPENDIX B

Table 4

COPING WITH BREAKDOWNS IN CONVENTIONAL PROPRIETIES AS VIEWED BY NURSE AIDES, LICENSED PRACTICAL NURSES, REGISTERED NURSES, AND DEGREE REGISTERED NURSES

Coded Items	NA's (%) (N=102)	LPN's (%) (N=52)	RN's (%) (N=82)	DRN's (%) (N=82)
TOTAL	100.1	99.8	100.1	99.9
NEGATIVE ACCEPTANCE				
1. No experience with this	7.9	1.9	8.5	0.0
2. Shifting responsibility	4.0	1.9	4.9	2.4
3. Use of medication, restraints	1.0	9.6	4.9	8.5
4. Diversional tactics	17.8	11.5	11.0	3.7
5. Resort to reasoning and persuasion	14.9	19.2	3.7	6.1
SUBTOTAL	45.6	44.1	33.0	20.7
POSITIVE ACCEPTANCE				
6. Change of staff with supportive attitude	5.0	1.9	7.3	20.7
7. Acceptance with simple attempts to reassure	40.6	36.5	28.0	2.4
8. Support to extent of not permitting suffering	6.9	13.5	22.0	28.0
9. Acceptance and attempt to ascertain basic cause	1.0	1.9	9.8	22.0
SUBTOTAL	53.5	53.8	67.1	73.1
Ambiguous statements	1.0	1.9	0.0	6.1

Table 5

**COPING WITH HALLUCINATIONS AND OTHER DELUSORY EXPERIENCES
AS VIEWED BY
NURSE AIDES, LICENSED PRACTICAL NURSES, REGISTERED NURSES,
AND DEGREE REGISTERED NURSES**

Coded Items	NA's (%) (N=103)	LPN's (%) (N=52)	RN's (%) (N=82)	DRN's (%) (N=83)
TOTAL	100.2	100.0	100.0	100.0
NEGATIVE ACCEPTANCE				
1. No experience with this	10.7	0.0	3.7	0.0
2. Shifting responsibility	7.8	3.8	2.4	3.6
3. Use of medications, restraints	0.0	1.9	3.7	2.4
4. Use of diversional tactics	6.8	5.8	4.9	3.6
5. Resort to reason and persuasion	11.7	5.8	1.2	0.0
SUBTOTAL	37.0	17.3	15.9	9.6
POSITIVE ACCEPTANCE				
6. Change of staff with supportive attitude	0.0	1.9	1.2	6.0
7. Acceptance with attempts to reassure	31.1	25.0	19.5	49.4
8. Support to extent of not permitting suffering	28.2	38.5	45.1	19.3
9. Acceptance and attempt to ascertain basic cause	0.0	7.7	17.1	13.3
SUBTOTAL	59.3	73.1	82.9	88.0
Ambiguous statements	3.9	9.6	1.2	2.4

Table 6

DIFFERENCES IN NURSING CARE OF CONSCIOUS AND UNCONSCIOUS AGED PATIENTS AS VIEWED BY NURSE AIDES, LICENSED PRACTICAL NURSES, REGISTERED NURSES, AND DEGREE REGISTERED NURSES

Coded Items	NA's (%) (N=104)	LPN's (%) (N=53)	RN's (%) (N=81)	DRN's (%) (N=101)
TOTAL	100.1	100.0	100.0	100.0
NEGATIVE POSITION				
1. There are no differences in nursing care	45.2	45.3	35.8	25.7
2. Possible differences are not related to mental state	5.8	9.4	18.5	1.0
SUBTOTAL	51.0	54.7	54.3	26.7
POSITIVE POSITION				
For the conscious patient				
3. More physical care	0.0	0.0	0.0	0.0
4. More psychological care	9.6	15.1	19.8	13.8
5. More physical *and* psychological care	3.8	3.8	1.2	4.0
Total of more care for the conscious patient	13.4	18.9	21.0	17.8
For the unconscious patient				
6. More physical care	12.5	11.3	7.4	10.9
7. More psychological care	0.0	1.9	0.0	10.9
8. More physical *and* psychological care	5.8	3.8	4.9	30.7
Total of more care for the unconscious patient	18.3	17.0	12.3	52.5
9. Yes, but differences are not specified	8.7	9.4	9.9	3.0
SUBTOTAL (yes, there are differences in care)	40.4	45.3	43.2	73.3
Ambiguous statements	8.7	0.0	2.5	0.0

Table 7

DIFFERENCES IN NURSING CARE OF AGED PATIENTS
BASED ON PROGNOSIS
AS VIEWED BY
NURSE AIDES, LICENSED PRACTICAL NURSES, REGISTERED NURSES,
AND DEGREE REGISTERED NURSES

Coded Items	NA's (%) (N=104)	LPN's (%) (N=53)	RN's (%) (N=82)	DRN's (%) (N=102)
TOTAL	99.9	99.9	100.0	100.1
NEGATIVE POSITION				
1. No difference: God determines life and death	6.7	9.4	6.1	1.0
2. No difference: Nurses have moral commitment to help the living	16.3	11.3	8.5	5.9
3. No differences: general statements	24.0	9.4	22.0	0.0
4. Possible differences are not related to prognosis	4.8	18.9	14.6	22.5
SUBTOTAL	51.8	49.0	51.2	29.4
AFFIRMATIVE POSITION				
5. Yes, more physical care for the dying	11.5	0.0	4.9	3.9
6. Yes, more psychological care for the dying	8.7	22.6	7.3	15.7
7. Yes, more physical and psychological care for the dying	25.0	22.6	29.3	48.1
8. Yes, general statements, including those indicating more care for the recovering patient	1.0	3.8	6.1	2.0
SUBTOTAL	46.2	49.0	47.6	69.7
9. Ambiguous statements	1.9	1.9	1.2	1.0

Table 8

USE OF "HEROIC" OR "ARTIFICIAL" LIFE-SUSTAINING MEASURES
FOR AGED DYING PATIENTS
AS VIEWED BY
NURSE AIDES, LICENSED PRACTICAL NURSES, REGISTERED NURSES,
AND DEGREE REGISTERED NURSES

Coded Items	NA's (%) (N=88)	LPN's (%) (N=53)	RN's (%) (N=82)	DRN's (%) (N=98)
TOTAL	100.0	99.8	100.0	99.9
AVOIDING THE ISSUE				
1. Physician should make the decision	10.2	11.3	11.0	10.2
2. Determined by policy and philosophy of institution	0.0	0.0	0.0	11.2
3. It is a moral and religious issue	28.4	17.0	3.7	2.0
4. Issue resolved in nursing standards and ethics	1.1	0.0	2.4	0.0
SUBTOTAL	39.7	28.3	17.1	23.4
OPPOSING THEIR USE				
5. Let the aged terminally ill patient die in peace and comfort	13.6	17.0	39.0	10.2
SUPPORTING THEIR USE				
6. Full support: justified "unto death"	20.5	24.5	24.5	14.3
7. Conditional: decision on individual patient basis	8.0	20.8	15.8	25.5
8. Rights of patient/family should be respected	2.3	1.9	2.4	21.4
SUBTOTAL	30.8	47.2	42.7	61.2
Ambiguous statements	15.9	7.3	1.2	5.1

Table 9

**AGED PATIENTS' ATTITUDES TOWARD DEATH AND DYING
AS PERCEIVED BY
NURSE AIDES, LICENSED PRACTICAL NURSES, AND REGISTERED
NURSES** [*]

Coded Items	NA's (%) (N=89)	LPN's (%) (N=53)	RN's (%) (N=78)
TOTAL	100.0	100.0	100.0
PRESENTS NO PROBLEMS			
1. Patients are not concerned about death	30.3	26.4	29.5
2. Environment not conductive to "death talk"	0.0	1.9	2.5
SUBTOTAL	30.3	28.3	32.0
FEAR OF DEATH IS NORMAL			
3. Fear of death is part of human nature	11.2	17.0	16.7
4. Such fear is related to dying alone	4.5	5.7	3.8
SUBTOTAL	15.7	22.7	20.5
PATIENTS' ATTITUDES DEPEND ON DIVERSE FACTOR			
5. Fear of death is very individual	22.5	13.2	16.7
6. Attitude is related to state of health	23.6	13.2	9.0
7. Attitude related to religio-philosophical orientation	7.9	22.6	20.5
SUBTOTAL	54.0	49.0	46.2
8. Ambiguous statements	0.0	0.0	1.3

[*] Data not available from the degree registered nurse respondents.

Table 10

DISCUSSING DEATH AND DYING WITH AGED ILL PERSONS
AS VIEWED BY
NURSE AIDES, LICENSED PRACTICAL NURSES, REGISTERED NURSES,
AND DEGREE REGISTERED NURSES

Coded Items	NA's (%) (N=101)	LPN's (%) (N=53)	RN's (%) (N=79)	DRN's (%) (N=95)
TOTAL	100.1	100.0	100.0	100.1
NEGATIVE APPROACH: SUBJECT IS TABOO				
1. Avoid and discourage discussion of death	52.5	34.0	30.4	2.1
2. Topic not mentioned; problem does not exist	5.0	9.4	10.1	0.0
SUBTOTAL	57.5	43.4	40.5	2.1
NEUTRAL STAND: TOPIC TOLERATED				
3. Tolerate discussion, but make noncommittal remarks	36.6	43.4	17.7	7.4
4. If patient initiates topic, make guarded remarks	4.0	1.9	10.1	16.8
SUBTOTAL	40.6	45.3	27.8	24.2
POSITIVE APPROACH				
5. Discuss meaningfully if patient takes initiative	1.0	7.5	12.7	37.9
6. Discuss meaningfully whenever opportunity arises	0.0	0.0	5.1	26.3
7. Have policy to provide opportunities for discussion	0.0	1.9	2.5	3.2
8. Patient has right to know and to have discussion	1.0	1.9	3.8	3.2
SUBTOTAL	2.0	11.3	24.1	70.6
Ambiguous statements	0.0	0.0	7.6	3.2

Table 11

REACTIONS TO DEATH OF A FELLOW PATIENT
AS PERCEIVED BY
NURSE AIDES, LICENSED PRACTICAL NURSES, AND REGISTERED
NURSES *

Coded Items	NA's (%) (N=97)	LPN's (%) (N=53)	RN's (%) (N=79)
TOTAL	99.9	100.0	100.2
PRESENTS NO PROBLEM			
1. Patients show no conscious concern about death	44.3	37.7	38.0
2. Environment not conducive to "death talk"	13.4	5.7	16.5
SUBTOTAL	57.7	43.4	54.5
FEAR OF DEATH IS NORMAL HUMAN BEHAVIOR			
3. Fear of death is part of human nature	11.3	18.9	8.9
4. Such fear is related to being alone when dying	0.0	0.0	0.0
SUBTOTAL	11.3	18.9	8.9
PATIENT'S ATTITUDE DEPENDS ON DIVERSE FACTORS			
5. Grief is related to closeness of relationship and suddenness of death	14.4	7.5	7.6
6. Attitude is related to state of health	9.3	17.0	12.7
7. Attitude is related to religio-philosophical orientation	4.1	9.4	12.7
SUBTOTAL	27.8	33.9	33.0
Ambiguous statements	3.1	3.8	3.8

* Data not available from the degree registered nurse respondents.

Table 12

**COPING WITH PATIENTS' STRESSES WHEN DEATH TAKES
ONE OF THEM AS VIEWED BY
NURSE AIDES, LICENSED PRACTICAL NURSES, REGISTERED NURSES,
AND DEGREE REGISTERED NURSES**

Coded Items	NA's (%) (N=101)	LPN's (%) (N=53)	RN's (%) (N=82)	DRN's (%) (N=93)
TOTAL	100.0	100.0	100.0	100.0
NEGATIVE APPROACH: SUBJECT IS TABOO				
1. Avoid and discourage discussion of death	57.4	28.3	29.3	7.5
2. Topic not mentioned; patients not informed	1.0	13.2	4.9	0.0
SUBTOTAL	58.4	41.5	34.2	7.5
NEUTRAL STAND: TOPIC TOLERATED				
3. Tolerate discussion, but make noncommittal remarks	25.7	32.1	17.1	23.7
4. If patient initiates topic, make guarded remarks	0.0	1.9	1.2	5.4
SUBTOTAL	25.7	34.0	18.3	29.1
POSITIVE APPROACH				
5. Discuss meaningfully if patient takes initiative	0.0	1.9	1.2	11.8
6. Discuss meaningfully whenever opportunity arises	10.9	3.8	17.1	14.0
7. Have policy to provide opportunities for discussion	3.0	7.5	13.4	33.3
8. Patients have right to know and to have discussion	0.0	0.0	1.2	0.0
SUBTOTAL	13.9	13.2	32.9	59.1
Ambiguous statements	2.0	11.3	14.6	4.3

Table 13

AIDING AND SUPPORTING BEREAVED RELATIVES AND FRIENDS
AS VIEWED BY
NURSE AIDES, LICENSED PRACTICAL NURSES, REGISTERED NURSES,
AND DEGREE REGISTERED NURSES

Coded Items	NA's (%) (N=101)	LPN's (%) (N=52)	RN's (%) (N=81)	DRN's (%) (N=90)
TOTAL	100.0	100.1	99.9	100.0
NEGATIVE APPROACH: PROBLEM DOES NOT EXIST				
1. Patients don't have relatives, or they don't care	20.8	23.1	22.2	0.0
2. Aged person's death not upsetting; no grieving	1.0	5.8	16.0	0.0
SUBTOTAL	21.8	28.9	38.2	0.0
3. AIDING THE BEREAVED IS RESPONSIBILITY OF OTHERS	61.4	40.4	22.2	1.1
POSITIVE APPROACH				
4. Assist if bereaved seek help or seem to need help	9.9	15.4	13.6	46.7
5. Have planned policy to provide aid and comfort to them	1.0	5.8	17.3	52.2
SUBTOTAL	10.9	21.2	30.9	98.9
Ambiguous statements	5.9	9.6	8.6	0.0

Table 14

BEST LIKED THINGS OR CONDITIONS IN GERIATRICS
AS VIEWED BY
NURSE AIDES, LICENSED PRACTICAL NURSES, AND REGISTERED
NURSES

Coded Items	NA's (%) (N=102)	LPN's (%) (N=52)	RN's (%) (N=81)
TOTAL	100.1	100.0	100.0
PRACTICAL OR MATERIAL ITEMS			
1. Physical plant; location; equipment; etc.	4.9	1.9	4.9
2. Policies; work schedule; salaries and other benefits	4.9	5.8	11.1
3. Functions: nursing procedures, treatments, techniques	3.9	3.8	0.0
SUBTOTAL	13.7	11.5	16.0
RELATIONSHIPS; ATTITUDES			
4. Harmonious personnel relationships	8.8	5.8	6.2
5. Harmonious patient-nurse relationships	36.3	40.4	33.3
6. Attitude of patients' relatives or society at large	0.0	0.0	0.0
SUBTOTAL	45.1	46.2	39.5
OTHER POSITIVE STATEMENTS			
7. Altruistic responses, including references to religion	27.5	28.8	21.0
8. General positive statements about work with the aged	11.8	13.5	21.0
SUBTOTAL	39.3	42.3	42.0
Ambiguous, including negative statements	2.0	0.0	2.5

Table 15

**LEAST LIKED THINGS OR CONDITIONS IN GERIATRICS
AS VIEWED BY
NURSE AIDES, LICENSED PRACTICAL NURSES, AND REGISTERED
NURSES**

Coded Items	NA's (%) (N=90)	LPN's (%) (N=50)	RN's (%) (N=72)
TOTAL	100.0	100.0	99.9
PRACTICAL OR MATERIAL ITEMS			
1. Physical plant; location; equipment; etc.	4.4	4.0	9.7
2. Policies; work schedule; salaries and other benefits	33.3	20.0	22.2
3. Functions: nursing procedures, treatments, techniques	5.6	10.0	4.2
SUBTOTAL	43.3	34.0	36.1
RELATIONSHIPS; ATTITUDES			
4. Frustrating personnel relationships	6.7	16.0	22.2
5. Frustrating patient-nurse relationships	21.1	12.0	6.9
6. Negative attitude of patients' relatives or society at large	0.0	10.0	6.9
SUBTOTAL	27.8	38.0	36.0
GENERAL NEGATIVE STATEMENTS			
7. General frustrations	1.1	0.0	4.2
8. Negative responses about work with the aged	0.0	0.0	1.4
SUBTOTAL	1.1	0.0	5.6
Ambiguous, including positive statements	27.8	28.0	22.2

Table 16

GRANTING GREATER FREEDOM TO THE PROFESSIONAL NURSE FOR INDEPENDENT ACTION AND PRACTICE IN GERIATRIC CARE AS VIEWED BY DEGREE REGISTERED NURSES [*]

Coded Items	DRN's (%) (N=89)
TOTAL	100.0
NEGATIVE POSITION	
1. General negative statements	4.5
2. No. the nurse has sufficient freedom to exercise her potential	15.7
3. No. It is not a question of more freedom, but cultivating interprofessional concern and cooperation and developing good relations with other disciplines	15.7
SUBTOTAL	35.9
POSITIVE POSITION	
4. Yes, if certain limits were set up and legal safeguards established	7.9
5. Yes, for nurses with credentials supporting suitable qualifications	32.6
6. Yes, general positive statements	13.5
SUBTOTAL	54.0
Ambiguous statements	10.1

[*] Data not available from nurse practitioner groups.

Table 17

FACTS ABOUT, OR ATTITUDES TOWARD, DEATH THAT TEND TO HELP NURSES AND AGED PATIENTS COPE WITH THIS EVENT AS VIEWED BY DEGREE REGISTERED NURSES [*]

Coded Items	DRN's (%) (N=86)
TOTAL	100.0
1. Knowledge of the patient in terms of the past and the present, including his religio-philosophical orientation	40.7
2. Self-knowledge on the part of nurses	38.4
3. Knowledge of the processes of dying	15.1
4. Open positive attitude toward dealing with death	3.5
5. Ambiguous statements	2.3

[*] Data not available from nurse practitioner groups.

Statistical Profile
of Study Participants

STATISTICAL PROFILE OF STUDY PARTICIPANTS

LIST OF TABLES

351

STATISTICAL TABLES

Table C-1

**SELECTION FORMULA FOR NURSING PERSONNEL
TO BE INTERVIEWED**

Number of Full-time Nurse Aides, Licensed Practical Nurses, and Registered Nurses Employed by Institution	Number of Nurse Aides, Licensed Practical Nurses, and Registered Nurses to be Interviewed in the Institution
1 to 3	1
4 to 6	2
7 to 12	3
13 to 20	4
21 to 30	5
31 to 50	6
51 to 100	7
101 to 200	8
201 to 500	9
500 or more	10

Table C-2

**AGE OF STUDY PARTICIPANTS:
NURSE AIDES, LICENSED PRACTICAL NURSES, REGISTERED NURSES,
AND DEGREE REGISTERED NURSES**

Ages	NA's (N=104)	LPN's (N=53)	RN's (N=82)	DRN's (N=102)
Younger than 26 years	12	7	2	0
26–35	20	9	17	11
36–45	39	17	16	38
46–55	18	11	33	27
56 or older	15	9	14	19
Age not reported	0	0	0	7

Table C 3

CIVIL STATUS OF STUDY PARTICIPANTS:
NURSE AIDES, LICENSED PRACTICAL NURSES, REGISTERED NURSES,
AND DEGREE REGISTERED NURSES

Civil Status	NA's (N=104)	LPN's (N=53)	RN's (N=82)	DRN's (N=102)
Single	17	9	14	43
Married	66	28	49	32
Widowed	11	5	9	4
Separated or Divorced	10	7	4	10
Religious Sister	0	4	6	6
Not reported	0	0	0	7

Table C-4

RELIGION OF STUDY PARTICIPANTS:
NURSE AIDES, LICENSED PRACTICAL NURSES, REGISTERED NURSES,
AND DEGREE REGISTERED NURSES

Religion	NA's (N=104)	LPN's (N=53)	RN's (N=82)	DRN's (N=102)
Catholic	46	26	40	26
Protestant	55	25	32	62
Hebrew	0	1	8	2
Other or undeclared	3	1	2	5
Not reported	0	0	0	7

Table C-5

GENERAL EDUCATION OF STUDY PARTICIPANTS: NURSE AIDES, LICENSED PRACTICAL NURSES, AND REGISTERED NURSES [*]

Education	NA's (N=104)	LPN's (N=53)	RN's (N=82)
Elementary School	22	2	
Attended High School	40	10	
High School Graduate	42	41	81
Baccalaureate Degree (liberal arts)			1

[*] Degree registered nurses were asked about "highest academic degree earned." See Table C-6.

Table C-6

VOCATIONAL OR PROFESSIONAL PREPARATION OF STUDY PARTICIPANTS: NURSE AIDES, LICENSED PRACTICAL NURSES, REGISTERED NURSES, AND DEGREE REGISTERED NURSES [*]

Vocational/Professional Program	NA's (N=104)	LPN's (N=53)	RN's (N=82)	DRN's (N=102)
No formal preparation	58			
Some classroom instruction while working	46			
No formal course, licensed by waiver		6		
Vocational high school practical nurse program		9		
Hospital practical nursing program		37		
R.N. hospital diploma program			52	
Hospital diploma program plus some college credits			18	
Hospital diploma program plus B.S. degree			5	
Associate degree (2-year community college program)		1	3	
Baccalaureate nursing program			4	
B.A. or B.S.				5
M.A. or M.S.				83
Ed.D.				3
Ph.D.				5
Not reported				6

[*] Figures for degree registered nurses indicate highest academic degree earned

Table C-7

POSITIONS HELD BY STUDY PARTICIPANTS:
NURSE AIDES, LICENSED PRACTICAL NURSES, REGISTERED NURSES,
AND DEGREE REGISTERED NURSES

Position	NA's (N=104)	LPN's (N=53)	RN's (N=82)	DRN's (N=102)
General staff, providing direct patient care	104	26	13	0
In charge of a unit: A.M., P.M., or night tour of duty	0	24	33	0
Supervisor, director, administrator, or in-service educator	0	3	36	32
Instructor or assistant professor	0	0	0	25
Dean and/or professor in nursing education	0	0	0	36
Position other than above, i.e. consultant, researchers, or not reported	0	0	0	9

Table C-8

NUMBER OF YEARS WORKED IN GERIATRIC INSTITUTIONS:
NURSE AIDES, LICENSED PRACTICAL NURSES, REGISTERED NURSES,
AND DEGREE REGISTERED NURSES [*]

Work Experience	NA's (N=104)	LPN's (N=53)	RN's (N=82)	DRN's (N=102)
Less than 1 year	5	4	9	4
1 year, but less than 2 years	11	4	12	5
2 years, but less than 3 years	16	9	10	8
3 years, but less than 5 years	32	4	18	9
5 years, but less than 7 years	9	7	8	8
7 years, but less than 10 years	15	7	9	1
10 years, but less than 15 years	12	9	11	15
15 years, but less than 20 years	3	8	3	5
20 years or longer	1	1	2	3
Number of years not indicated				15
None or not reported				29

[*] Figures for degree registered nurses indicate work experience in geriatrics *or* chronic illness.

Table C-9

INSTITUTIONAL SETTING OF STUDY PARTICIPANTS: NURSE AIDES, LICENSED PRACTICAL NURSES, REGISTERED NURSES, AND DEGREE REGISTERED NURSES

Institutional Setting	NA's (N=104)	LPN's (N=53)	RN's (N=82)	DRN's (N=102)
University				61
Hospital: nursing service or education				30
Church-oriented institution for the aged: Catholic	27	8	21	
Church-oriented institution for the aged: Jewish	23	12	17	
Church-oriented institution for the aged: Protestant	24	16	20	
Proprietary nursing home	25	13	18	1
Tax-supported homes for the aged	5	4	5	
Other, or not reported				10

Table C-10

SIZE OF EMPLOYING INSTITUTIONS AND NUMBER OF NURSING PERSONNEL INTERVIEWED: NURSE AIDES, LICENSED PRACTICAL NURSES, AND REGISTERED NURSES

Bed capacity*	NA's (N=104)	LPN's (N=53)	RN's (N=82)
50 beds or less	19	15	15
51–100 beds	34	14	27
101–200 beds	45	20	34
More than 200 beds	6	4	6

* Number of beds licensed as "nursing home beds."

Table C-11

AREA OF SPECIALIZATION OF DEGREE REGISTERED NURSES

Specialization Area	DRN's (N=102)
Geriatric Nursing	5
Public Health Nursing	13
Psychiatric/Mental Health Nursing	16
General Nursing; medical/surgical; or no specialization	55
Other	7
Not reported	6

Table C-12

INSTITUTIONS, ACCORDING TO TYPE OF CONTROL, BED CAPACITY, FULL-TIME NURSING STAFF, AND NUMBER OF STAFF INTERVIEWED

Type of Control	Number of Beds*	Number of Full-time Nursing Staff				Number of Staff Interviewed			
		NA's	LPN's	RN's	Total	NA's	LPN's	RN's	Total
Church-oriented: Catholic	352	262	31	59	352	27	8	21	56
Church-oriented: Jewish	621	322	83	76	481	22	12	17	51
Church-oriented: Protestant	338	105	35	43	183	22	14	20	56
Other nonprofit institutions	302	209	48	41	298	8	6	6	20
Proprietary nursing homes	560	199	37	47	283	25	13	18	56
Total:	2,173	1,097	234	266	1,597	104	53	82	239

* In homes for the aged, the number of beds refers to "infirmary" or "nursing unit" beds.

D Degree Registered Nurse Respondents

Aiello, Hertha E.
Alderson, Mary L.
Alexander, Florence M.
Baziak, Anna T.
Bixby, Kathryn S.
Boris, Joan
Braun, Beate M.
Brown, Mrs. Everett S.
Brown, Myrtle Irene
Brown, Virginia
Browne, Louise J.
Bryce, Ruth H.
Byers, Virginia B.
Camp, Ruth P.
Carlton, W. Louise
Charbenau, Charlotte P.
Cole, Dorothy J.
Conn, Mrs. Rex
Corona, Dorothy F.
Damon, Margaret N.
Declan, Sister M.
de Tornyay, Rheba
Diller, Doris
Dithridge, Eileen H.
Dixon, Dorothy M.
Donaldson, Irene B.
Dunn, Florence
Duxbury, Vivian M.
Field, Margaret M.
Foley, Mary J.
Frenay, Sister Mary Agnes C.
Gabrielle, Sister Mary
Gorrow, Mary W.
Hadley, Betty Jo
Hagen, Sister M.P. Damien
Haglund, Elizabeth J.

Hall, Mary
Hamrick, Mabel
Harvey, Lillian H.
Horn, Barbara J.
Hughey, George Ann
Huntington, Arria S.
Jayne, Martha P.
Kerrigan, Sister M. Ruth
Ketcham, Katherine
Klein, Helen C.
Knowles, Lois N.
Kurtz, Gail
Lanigan, Barbara T.
Lindstrom, Teresa
Louise, Sister Mary
Lufkin, Sylvia R.
MacPhetridge, L. Mae
Macquin, Hazelle B.
Maliepaard, Nora
Matthews, Barbara E.
Mendel, Mabel P.
Mertz, Hilda
Miller, Helen S.
Miriam, Sister Agnes
Muir, Gladys
Nagy, Loraine M.
Nelson, Katherine R.
Ogden, Ruth P.
O'Koren, Marie L.
Olsen, Edith
Olsen, Elizabeth C.,
    and selected students
Palmer, Mary Ellen
Patrick, Maxine
Prock, Valencia
Proctor, Frances J.

Pol, Madeleine
Puddy, Marjorie G.
Quinlan, Mary E.
Reiter, Frances
Russell, Ruth C.
Santorum, Catherine D.
Santos, Maria
Schwartz, Doris
Shaffer, Mary E.
Shumway, Sandra S.
Smith, Alice E.
Smith, Helen Curtis
Somers, Majorie P.
Sperry, Ruth E.
Steffen, Anna M.
   and selected faculty members
Stern, Catherine G.
   and 3 graduate students

Straight, Ruth B.
Swarney, Jane
Swinburne, Margaret
Sylvester, Dorothy Metz
Taylor, Margaret S.
Torrens, Iva F.
Travelbee, Joyce
Vacca, Christine
Wald, Florence S.
Wenrich, Marian
Whidden, Ann
White, Anna A.T.
Wilkinson, Elizabeth
Windeler, Edith M.
Wolanin, Mary Opal

E ☐ Data-Gathering Forms

YALE UNIVERSITY SCHOOL OF NURSING

*Interview Guide used for nurse practitioner group: nurse aides,
licensed practical nurses and registered nurses*

1. What would you say are some of the differences, if any, between caring for an aged patient who is expected soon to die and one who is expected to recover?
2. In what ways, if any, does your care differ depending on whether the patient is fully conscious and mentally alert, or is semi- or unconscious or under heavy sedation. Which challenges you more? What do you think about the use of medication so that the patient is not so aware of his state?
3. What is the determining factor on whether or not you urge natural or artificial lifesaving measures or both? How far into the terminal phase of life do you think it important to urge such measures?
4. What do you do when an aged patient pleads "not to suffer" during his or her last days on earth?
5. Under what conditions, if any, do you resort to "kidding" or "joshing" with aged ill patients? Under what conditions, if any, do you treat them "like children"?
6. How do certain facts about, or attitudes toward, death influence your care of an aged ill person? Does your care differ, depending on whether the patient seems ready to die, even wishing for death, or resists or fears death? If so, how? What, if any, differences have you

360

observed between an aged patient whose terminal illness is related to a lesion or disease and one who is dying of "old age"?

7. How do you cope with the following situations:
   a) when there is a breakdown of conventional proprieties on the part of an aged ill person;
   b) when the patient shows mistrust and/or aggression toward those caring for him or her;
   c) when an aged patient hallucinates, has visions, or other illusory experiences such as hearing voices, seeing absent or deceased persons, etc.;
   d) when an aged ill person appears to take advantage of nearness of death for gaining special or forbidden favors?

8. What are some ways in which you "keep in touch" or communicate with aged dying patients?
   a) by means of the senses (sight, hearing, smell, taste, hunger, thirst);
   b) manipulation of the environment (light, sound, familiar settings);
   c) ministrations (rituals, religious symbols, keepsakes)?

9. How do you deal with the possible stresses of fellow patients when death is taking one of them?

10. How do you deal with situations such as the following:
    a) when relatives or close friends are present during a person's dying days or hours;
    b) when a doctor, lawyer, religious advisor, or social worker is present;
    c) when the presence of one or the other seems indicated?

11. What part do you have, if any, in aiding and supporting the bereaved?

12. What are two or three things or conditions:
    a) that you *like best* about your work with the aged ill;
    b) that you *like least* about your work with the aged ill?

QUESTIONNAIRE

Questionnaire: Nursing Leadership

1. How may one say that nursing care differs for an aged ill person who is expected soon to die in contrast to one who is expected to recover?

2. How may one say that nursing care differs for an aged critically ill person who is conscious and mentally alert in contrast to one who is semi- or unconscious or under *heavy* sedation?

3. How far into the terminal phase of life may a nurse justifiably urge

natural and/or artificial life-sustaining measures or promote self-care and rehabilitative procedures?

4. What may a nurse do when an aged dying patient pleads "not to suffer" through his or her last days on earth?

5. Under what conditions, if any, may a nurse resort to "kidding" or "joshing" aged ill patients or treat them "like children"?

6. How may certain facts about or attitudes toward death tend to help nurses and aged patients to cope with this event? Under what conditions should a nurse discuss, or *not* discuss, the prospects of death with an aged ill person?

7. Suggest and appraise possible ways of coping with the following situations:
    a) when there is a breakdown of conventional proprieties on the part of an aged ill person;
    b) when the patient shows mistrust and/or aggression toward those caring for him or her;
    c) when an aged ill person hallucinates, has visions, or other illusory experiences such as hearing voices, seeing absent or deceased persons, etc.;
    d) when the aged ill patient appears to take advantage of nearness of death for gaining special and/or forbidden favors?

8. Suggest and appraise possible ways of keeping in contact, or communicating, with dying aged persons:
    a) by means of the senses (sight, hearing, touch, smell, taste, hunger, thirst);
    b) manipulation of environmental factors (light, sound, familiar settings, etc.);
    c) ministrations such as religious symbols, rituals, keepsakes, etc.?

9. What are some ways in which a nurse may deal with stresses experienced by fellow patients when death is taking one of them?

10. How may a nurse make constructive use of the following situations:
    a) when relatives or close friends are present during a person's dying days or hours;
    b) when a doctor, lawyer, religious advisor, or social worker is present;
    c) *or* when the presence of one or the other of those persons seems indicated?

11. In what ways may the nurse render aid and support to the bereaved?

12. What would be the potential effects of granting greater freedom to the professional nurse for independent action and practice in the care of aged terminally ill patients? Would you recommend this, and if so, under what circumstances?

    We would welcome any other thought, on any part of this subject, that you would be willing to share with us.

NOTE: When responding to these questions, please distinguish between RN, LPN, and NA.

Index of

Names

Index of

Subjects

Abipone, view of death among, 281
Adjustment, of patient to institutional setting, 22-23
Administration
  influencing factor on patient behavior, 69
  philosophy and policy a factor in nursing practice, 129-130
Adult relationship
  importance of maintaining, 44
  nurse-patient, 43-49
Aged
  exhibiting regressive traits, 35
  individual differences of the, 36-37
  living creative lives, 35
  population, 3
  predicament in contemporary society, 3
  threats to good living, 5-6
Aged ill, trends toward institutionalization, 27
Aged patient See Patient(s)
Ager,
  a creature of his three-fold environment, 274
  cultural norms and values important in support of, 271
  definition of, 4
Aggressions, patients', a problem for nursing staff, 66
Aggressive behavior See Behavior disorders
Aging See also Old age; Retirement; Senescence
as an achievement, 4-7
characteristics associated with, 36
contrast in, primitive and contemporary cultures, 284-285
into decrepitude a social problem, 285-288
fulfilling old age a joint endeavor, 269
growing old, 3
and humor in primitive cultures, 52

Aging (*cont.*)
  in primitive societies, 4
  requisites for aging well, 4-5
  into senescence a joint accomplishment, 4, 10, 12
Araucanians, view of death among, 281
Artificial life-sustaining measures See Heroic life-sustaining measures
Attitude(s)
  importance of in nursing care, 34
  of nurses toward aged persons, 35
  of nurses toward bereaved, as viewed by relatives, 211-212
  of nurses toward bereaved relatives, 210-228
  of nurses toward unconscious patient, 114
  of physicians toward geriatrics, 229-230, 241-242
  reflecting kind of nursing care, 34
  relevant to care of the dying, 260
  toward aged an element in patient care, 151
  toward aged culturally determined, 5
  toward death, 127-133
  toward elderly related to status of geriatrics, 229
  toward youth versus aged in U.S.A., 49
Aurunta of Australia, view of death among, 281

Basic motivations See Fundamental needs
Behavior
  affected by institutional system, 69
  aggressive, a problem for nursing staff, 66
  hostile patient, as survival assets for individual, 68-69

Behavior (*cont.*)
  related to social structure of institution, 278
  subject to systematic study, 274-276
  unconventional patient, a problem for nursing staff, 66
Behavior disorders
  behavior versus person engaging in, 92
  complexities, 108
  failings as part of aging, 84
  figures on, juxtaposed, 110
  guidelines for coping with, 73-74, 102
  indications of patient's needs, 90-91
  institutional setting, effect on, 66-69
  internal and external bases, 68-69
  need for further exploration of, 111
  negative coping patterns, 70-72, 87-90, 97-99
  nurses' major position on, 81-82, 94-95, 109-111
  nurses' reactions to, 87
  positive coping patterns, 72-80, 91-93, 99-108
  possible causes of, 66-69, 85
  a problem for nursing staff, 66
  reinforcements for the nurse when coping, 79-80
  relationship of disorders to the aging process, 108-109
  view of, in institutional settings, 84, 86
Behavioral science, fundamental principle of, 274-275
Bereaved
  aiding relatives during bereavement following death of kinsman, 221-225
  aiding relatives during predeath bereavement, 219-221
  considerations when aiding relatives, 223-224
  discrepancy between perception of stress and nursing practice, 198-199
  giving aid and comfort to, 216-227
  needs of, when fellow patient dying, 206-207
  nurses coping with stresses of, 198-207
  relatives' reaction toward nursing personnel on dying kinsman's death, 211-212
  support of, in institutional death, 192-194

Bereavement
  aiding relatives before event of death, 219-221
  coping with, issue explored, 32
  following death, aiding relatives, 221-225
  nurses' views on reactions of relatives when patient dying, 211
  stages of mourning, 219-225
  universal experience, 210
Best geriatric nursing practice, definition of for present project, 29-30
"Best" nursing care *See* Guidelines, Nursing care practice
Breakdowns in conventional behavior *See* Improprieties
Bushmen of Africa, view of death among, 281

Care *See also* Care of the dying; Nursing; Nursing care; Nursing practice
  effect of conflicting policy on patient, 25
  enhancement of, if nurses more independent practitioners, 245-248
  "equal care" concept for dying and recovering patients, 133-137
  patient's responsiveness, implications for, 113-117
  positive approaches on coping with patients' stresses in event of death, 202-207
  of senile patients, 37
Care of the dying *See also* Care; Death; Dying
  care and comfort dominant goal in, 157-158
  collaboration and communication important in, 261
  concept of individualized care important, 144-146
  consideration of patient-oriented goals, 139, 140-141
  dilemma for nurses, 127-133
  discrepancy between perception of patient's view of death and nursing practice, 179
  dominant goal is care and comfort, 157-158
  expediency versus quality nursing, 154
  exploratory ideas, 257